Dysphagia Following Stroke

Third Edition

Clinical Dysphagia

Series Editors
John C. Rosenbek and Harrison N. Jones

Dysphagia Following Stroke, Second Edition
Stephanie K. Daniels and Maggie-Lee Huckabee

Dysphagia in Neuromuscular Diseases
Robert M. Miller and Deanna Britton

Dysphagia Post-Trauma
Elizabeth C. Ward and Angela T. Morgan

Dysphagia in Rare Conditions, An Encyclopedia
Harrison N. Jones and John C. Rosenbek

Dysphagia in Movement Disorders
John Rosenbek and Harrison Jones

Dysphagia Following Stroke

Third Edition

Stephanie K. Daniels, PhD
Maggie-Lee Huckabee, PhD
Kristin Gozdzikowska, PhD

PLURAL PUBLISHING INC.

PLURAL PUBLISHING
INC.

5521 Ruffin Road
San Diego, CA 92123

e-mail: information@pluralpublishing.com
Website: http://www.pluralpublishing.com

Typeset in 10.5/13 Garamond by Flanagan's Publishing Services, Inc.
Printed in the United States of America by Integrated Books International

Library of Congress Cataloging-in-Publication Data

Names: Daniels, Stephanie K., author. | Huckabee, Maggie Lee, author. | Gozdzikowska, Kristin, author.
Title: Dysphagia following stroke / Stephanie K. Daniels, Maggie-Lee Huckabee, Kristin Gozdzikowska.
Description: Third edition. | San Diego, CA : Plural Publishing, [2019] | Includes bibliographical references and index.
Identifiers: LCCN 2018054958| ISBN 9781635500301 (alk. paper) | ISBN 1635500303 (alk. paper)
Subjects: | MESH: Deglutition Disorders—etiology | Stroke—complications
Classification: LCC RC815.2 | NLM WI 258 | DDC 616.3/23—dc23
LC record available at https://lccn.loc.gov/2018054958

Contents

Foreword

When asked to write a foreword for the new edition of *Dysphagia Following Stroke* from the perspectives of patient and caregiver, it made sense. My husband, Adan, suffered a brainstem CVA during a coronary angioplasty procedure in 2012. Dysphagia has been part our family's daily life for six years. We began this journey late one Wednesday night. The stubborn man had been complaining of a chest cold for a couple of days, and he finally agreed to go to the hospital when he realized that the pain in his shoulder might be something heart related. When the ER staff told us that they suspected a blockage and might need to put in a stent, we never thought of potential complications. We would never have imagined a brainstem stroke. The next year, filled with physical therapy, occupational therapy, and speech therapy, was so busy that we did not register that swallowing was an issue until after he came home.

In terms of rehabilitation hospital statistics, Adan counted as a positive outcome. He was admitted after a brainstem stroke, NPO, and with a PEG tube inserted. At discharge, he was fully dependent on oral feeding. Modified barium swallow (videofluoroscopy) testing showed minor penetration with nectar-thick liquids, but no aspiration. His volitional cough was gone for the most part, but his reflexive cough was strong. With a modified diet, he would be safe to return home.

Adan's outpatient experience shows what can happen when that team is no longer in place. When he switched providers, a different speech pathologist—who may not have had full access to his medical records—tried having him practice effortful swallows for two or three months. The harder my husband tried to follow the directions, the less success he experienced. (A later chapter in this book hints at why this may have been the case.) I also made major mistakes with his diet. I provided Adan with prepackaged dysphagia food and drink but failed to consider that he had a hearty appetite. A year after his stroke, his cardiologist discovered that his triglycerides were sky-high and he had gained 40 pounds. As a runner and cyclist who was no longer as active, his caloric requirements were much lower than before. His appetite was not reduced, and unlike some patients with dysphagia, he had enthusiasm and energy to eat even when it was a challenge. If a team including a speech pathologist and nutritionist, informed by data of his lesion location and the results of his swallowing assessments, had been monitoring his status, he would not have had to unlearn the effortful swallows or work hard to lose weight.

In reflecting on the differences between his inpatient and outpatient experiences, I realize that the dysphagia rehabilitation system did not fail Adan. The goal was to prevent him from aspirating, and to keep him safe. In the five and a half years since the stroke, he has never had aspiration pneumonia, but he has significant dysphagia. He is grateful to have progressed beyond the PEG tube he remembers from the hospital. But with little improvement in his ability to swallow, approximately a year and a half after the stroke, treatment for Adan's dysphagia was discontinued. He was 49 years old. Adan comes from a long-lived family. He is discouraged by the notion of spending the next 30 or 40 years of life drinking nectar-thick liquids and eating pureed foods.

Managing meals and drinks has become a blur of thickener and blender. We learned tricks from the speech therapists, from books, and from more mistakes than I care to admit. Gluten is the devil for purees. Packaged gravy has a billion calories and too much salt. Rice will blend, but it works better if it is overcooked a bit. Cream of rice is better. Baby food pouches are great for travel. Over the past five and a half years, we have collected quite a list of lessons. The most important is this: *Dysphagia is relentless*. It invades every meal and infuses every drink.

A perfect illustration comes from a recent weekend trip to a fishing cottage near the coast in South Texas. Our plan was to drive the six hours to meet Adan's parents and siblings for a celebration of his father's 94th birthday. Having traveled before, I knew to pack food and drink for Adan. We brought yogurt, milk, baby food fruit and veggie squeeze pouches, baby cereal, bananas, and plenty of powdered (low-cal) sports drinks and bottles of water to keep him hydrated. I always have thickener in his backpack for travel, a small chopper to puree, and a cover up in case of spills. A normal road trip in the U.S. means grabbing a quick meal at a fast food restaurant along the road. With dysphagia, a meal means squeeze pouches in the parking lot or stares from curious customers who wonder why the adult is eating baby food.

Breakfast in South Texas brings breakfast tacos with homemade salsa. All of those things are not on my husband's diet. He can clear carefully scrambled eggs on a good day when the wind is blowing from the right direction, but eggs mixed with chorizo sausage and chopped onion is a no-go situation. Baby cereal was his option on our visit. He likes oatmeal baby cereal when traveling. It is easy, tastes good, and travels well.

The afternoon meal was a grill-centric affair. The portable chopper enabled Adan to eat some grilled chicken and rice. Nevertheless, he coughed one hard cough—the type that triggers vasovagal syncope for him. Adan's mom is becoming accustomed to the momentary dips in consciousness; she no longer prays aloud when his head slumps to the right.

For those who are relatively young and fortunate enough to return home, dysphagia after stroke joins the family like an unwanted guest. You know that things could be worse, but it is inconvenient and annoying and gets in the way of your social life. If only it would leave.

When asked to share our thoughts as patient and caregiver, I asked if I might read the book. I expected to learn more about the latest research in dysphagia and stroke. I was surprised by the number of times I found myself saying, "Yes!" to something the authors described or recommended. From the value of a team approach, to the importance of nutrition and oral hygiene, to the central role of medical history and data, and even the observation that one should not assume that patients who do not perform a task cannot perform the task (Adan hated one physician in ICU, so pretended he was asleep when that doctor rounded), this book speaks to our experience as patient and caregiver. That said, we find the final chapters about the future of the field profoundly exciting. They give us new directions to explore and new horizons to watch. It is an exciting time.

Karen French Montoya

Preface

This text is geared toward clinicians working with patients with stroke-related dysphagia in all settings: hospitals, rehabilitation centers, outpatients, and long-term care. However, it may also be useful as an entry level textbook, supplemented by other etiologic-specific readings, for students in professional training programs. It is intended as a practical sourcebook. In addition to a thorough overview of dysphagia diagnosis and management, this book focuses heavily on evaluation and management of stroke. The clinician will want to refer to other texts for coverage of specific issues or techniques related to other etiologies. We recognize that survivors of stroke can present as patients with complex needs. The full range of clinical encounters cannot be addressed; thus, we focus specifically on the effects of stroke and not the potential complicating features of the critically or chronically ill patient.

In this third edition, chapters on assessment have been expanded to include new and emerging instrumental technologies, including high resolution manometry, impedance, and ultrasound. For the chapters on management, we have included description of the newly described International Dysphagia Diet Standardization Initiative but have also included new research that emphasizes caution in diet modification. We have provided a significantly expanded framework for rehabilitation, reflecting our shift from peripherally focused rehabilitation to neuromodulation of cortical swallowing control. All chapters have been updated with the latest research and trends in clinical practice.

Acknowledgments

The third edition was more challenging than anticipated. This is a reflection of the rate at which our research and practice patterns in dysphagia diagnosis and management change. Kristin (Lamvik) Gozdzikowska moved from assistant to author in this edition and was welcomed warmly. It was great to have another perspective, particularly from someone who is part of the next generation of clinicians-researchers.

There are many, many people who have contributed to our clinical and research practice; however, there are two in particular to whom we would like to give a shout out: Jay Rosenbek and Art Miller. Both Jay and Art have inspired us through the quality of their seminal work, their generosity with their time in mentoring, and their overall kindness. They continually make us want to do more and better, and we feel privileged that they are our friends.

As clinicians at heart, we give tribute to our patients. The inherent idiosyncrasies of dysphagia following stroke make writing a book on this topic a challenging task. But it is through those who live with this condition that we all learn to be critical of what we think we know, impatient with our failures to know more, and driven to develop better clinical practices. Many thanks to Karen and Adan for contributing their thoughts to this book.

The first edition of this book followed on the footsteps of Hurricane Katrina and the levee breaches in New Orleans. The second edition followed on the footsteps of the Christchurch earthquakes. These two events affected us personally and professionally. The writing "home" for this third edition is the bruised, battered, and nonetheless resilient Kaikoura, New Zealand following the 2016 earthquake. It is no surprise that *Dysphagia Following Stroke* has an increasing emphasis on rehabilitation! We three believe strongly in the capacity for recovery and regeneration at many levels.

Abbreviations

AHA/ASA = American Heart Association/American Stroke Association

AIS = acute ischemic stroke

A-P = anterior-posterior

BA = Brodmann's area

BOT = base of tongue

CAD = coronary artery disease

CDS = Clinical Dysphagia Scale

CEA = carotid endarterectomy

CIMT = constraint-induced motor therapy

CN = cranial nerve

CNS = central nervous system

CP = cricopharyngeus

CPG = central pattern generator

CRT = cough reflex test

CSA = cross-sectional area

CSE = clinical swallowing examination

CT = computed tomography

CTAR = chin tuck against resistance

DiSP = dysphagia in stroke protocol

DOSS = Dysphagia Outcome and Severity Scale

DWI = diffusion-weighted imaging

EAT-10 = Eating Assessment Tool

ED = emergency department

E-E = expiration-expiration

E-I = expiration-inspiration

EMG = electromyography

EMST = expiratory muscle strength training

FDS = Functional Dysphagia Scale

FIM = functional independence measure

fMRI = functional magnetic resonance imaging

HLC = hyolaryngeal complex

HRM = high resolution manometry

I-E = inspiration-expiration

I-I = inspiration-inspiration

ICC = intraclass correlation coefficient

IDDSI = International Dysphagia Diet Standardization Initiative

IOPI = Iowa Oral Pressure Instrument

LES = lower esophageal sphincter

LHD = left hemisphere damage

LMN = lower motor neuron

LMS = lateral medullary syndrome

LOC = level of consciousness

MASA = Mann Assessment of Swallowing Ability

MBSImP = Modified Barium Swallow Impairment Profile

MDTP = McNeil Dysphagia Treatment Program

MEP = motor evoked potential

mL = milliliter

MRI = magnetic resonance imaging

NA = nucleus ambiguous

NGT = nasogastric tube

NIH-SSS = National Institutes of Health-Swallowing Safety Scale

NMES = neuromuscular electrical stimulation

NPO/NBM = nil per os/nothing by mouth

NPV = negative predictive value

NTS = nucleus tractus solitarius

OTT = oral transit time

P-A = penetration-aspiration

PEG = percutaneous endoscopic gastrostomy

PES = pharyngeal electrical stimulation

PPS = pulses per second

PPV = positive predictive value

PPW = posterior pharyngeal wall

PTT = pharyngeal transit time

PVWM = periventricular white matter

PWI = perfusion-weighted imaging

QoL = quality of life

RHD = right hemisphere damage

RIG = radiologically inserted gastrostomy

rTMS = repetitive transcranial magnetic stimulation

SA = swallowing apnea

SAD = swallowing apnea duration

sEMG = submental electromyography

SMA = supplementary motor area

SPM = swallows per minute

SST = swallowing screening tool

STD = stage transit duration

SWAL-QoL = Swallowing Quality of Life

SWI = swallow risk index

tDCS = transcranial direct current stimulation

TOMASS = Test of Masticating and Swallowing Solids

TTA = thermal-tactile application

TVF = true vocal fold

TWST = Timed Water Swallowing Test

UES = upper esophageal sphincter

UMN = upper motor neuron

VDS = Videofluoroscopic Dysphagia Scale

VEES = videoendoscopic evaluation of swallowing

VFSS = videofluoroscopic swallowing study

VPMpc = parvocellular component of the ventroposterior medial nucleus

WST = water swallowing test

Online Resources

The following videos and clinical forms are accessible on the PluralPlus companion website (instructions are included on the inside front cover of this book):

Chapter 6. The Clinical Swallowing Examination: The Evaluation of the Oral Mechanism

Dysphagia in Stroke Protocol (DiSP) Form

Cough Reflex Test—Video Example

Chapter 7. The Clinical Swallowing Examination: Assessment of Oral Intake

Sample of a Clinical Swallowing Examination (CSE) Form

CSE—Video Example

Chapter 9. Adjuncts to the Clinical Swallowing Examination

Timed Water Swallowing Test—Video Example

Test of Mastication and Swallowing Solids—Video Example

Chapter 10. Videofluoroscopic Swallowing Study

Sample of a Videofluoroscopic Swallowing Study (VFSS) Evaluation Form

VFSS—Video Example of a Normal Swallow

VFSS—Video Example of Delayed Onset of the Pharyngeal Swallow with Pre-Swallow Pyriform Sinus Pooling and Aspiration During the Swallow

VFSS—Video Example of Decreased Base of Tongue to Posterior Pharyngeal Wall Contact with Valleculae Residue

1 Introduction to Dysphagia and Stroke

OVERVIEW OF STROKE

Epidemiology of Stroke

The yearly incidence of new stroke, either ischemic or hemorrhagic, is approximately 17 million worldwide (Krishnamurthi et al., 2013; Naghavi et al., 2015). Incidence of stroke and stroke-related mortality has decreased over time in high-income countries but has remained unchanged or increased in low- and middle-income countries. In the United States, the yearly incidence of stroke is 795,000 (Mozaffarian et al., 2016). While the incidence of stroke and stroke-related mortality has shown an overall decline, the risk of first-time stroke and stroke-related mortality remains higher for other races and ethnicities compared with non-Hispanic whites.

Approximately 90% of strokes are secondary to ischemia, whereas hemorrhage accounts for 10% (Mozaffarian et al., 2016). Ischemia implies reduced blood flow to the brain and generally is caused by atherosclerosis, which is a buildup of plaque along the lining of the artery. The buildup of plaque leads to stenosis, narrowing of the artery, and formation of a thrombosis, or stationary clot. Thrombotic infarction generally involves large vessels but can also occur in small vessels (lacunar infarction). The plaque may dislodge, yielding an embolism, which travels in the bloodstream until it becomes lodged and disrupts blood flow. Embolisms frequently arise from the heart. Hemorrhagic strokes may result from hypertension that weakens the wall of a blood vessel, ruptured aneurysm, or bleeding from an arteriovenous malformation. Risk factors for stroke include increased age, hypertension, heart disease, diabetes mellitus, hypercholesterolemia, family history of stroke, physical inactivity, smoking, alcohol abuse, and cocaine use.

Neurologic Evaluation

Assessment of the patient with acute stroke begins when the individual presents to the emergency department. The neurologist will obtain a history from the patient (or family if the patient cannot respond) concerning previous medical conditions, medications, and the nature of the stroke event: time of onset, activity surrounding event, initial deficits, progression and duration of deficits, and other related events. A neurologic examination is completed to determine the exact deficits and consists of evaluation of elemental and higher cortical functions. Elemental functions include examination of cranial nerves, reflexes, and motor and sensory systems. Higher cortical function assessment involves evaluation of attention and memory, affect, language, praxis, visuospatial processing, and neglect. Table 1–1 presents an example of a neurologic examination. Diagnostic testing is completed within the first few days of admission in an attempt to uncover the source of the stroke, that is, cardiac embolism or carotid stenosis. Carotid vertebral duplex ultrasound and/or angiography may be completed to identify arterial stenosis. Evaluation for potential cardiac sources of an embolism may include 2D and transesophageal echocardiography.

Neuroimaging

Computed tomography (CT) scanning is completed upon admission to identify the presence of a hemorrhagic stroke. If the stroke is an acute ischemic event and the lesion is relatively small, the CT scan will initially be normal, as X-ray transmission depends on tissue density, and tissue density is without change in acute stroke. Figure 1–1 shows a large acute ischemic stroke. Diffusion-weighted imaging (DWI) acquisition as part of the magnetic resonance imaging (MRI) scan allows identification of small acute infarcts. Within minutes of symptom onset, DWI detects water diffusion changes related to cytotoxic edema and represents the anatomic extent of the lesion (Figure 1–2). Another MRI sequence is perfusion-weighted imaging (PWI). PWI details areas of the brain that are hypo-perfused, that is, brain regions with restricted blood flow. These early changes in the brain correspond to the full functional extent of the lesion. If blood flow can be restored with therapeutic intervention in a timely fashion, the brain tissue identified on PWI can be salvaged.

Table 1–1. Neurologic Examination

I. Mental Status
  A. Appearance and Behavior
  B. Mood and Affect—depression, anxiety, paranoid, vigilant, distracted, circumstantial, tangential, suspicious
  C. Level and State of Consciousness
    i. Level of consciousness—alert, lethargic, obtunded, stuporous, comatose
    ii. State of consciousness—normal, manic, minimally reactive
  D. Orientation—person, place, time, event
  E. Memory—can be assessed in terms of time course and/or function
    i. Time course
      1. Immediate (digit span, serial 7's, immediate recall of three objects)
      2. Short-term (three objects recall at 5 minutes)
      3. Long-term (presidents 5/5, autobiographical)
    ii. Function
      1. Declarative
        a. Episodic (questions relative to recent/remote event: most recent meal, current events in the news, major life events)
        b. Semantic (general knowledge, e.g., capital of Louisiana)
      2. Procedural (describe/demonstrate overlearned tasks such as swinging a golf club)
      3. Working (digit span backwards, serial 7's, oral arithmetic)
  F. Frontal Lobes
    i. Dorsolateral (verbal fluency: F-A-S, categories; abstract reasoning)
    ii. Medial frontal (energy level-apathy, anxiety, depression)
    iii. Orbitofrontal (response inhibition-tactile, visual; social inappropriateness)
  G. Language
    i. Spontaneous speech (fluency)
      1. Nonverbal aspects of language-aprosodia
    ii. Naming (confrontation-high frequency and low frequency words)
    iii. Repetition (single words, phrases)
    iv. Comprehension
    v. Reading/Writing
  H. Praxis (ideomotor, ideational, limb-kinetic, buccofacial)
  I. Constructional Ability/Neglect
    i. Visuospatial
      1. Copy complex figure (intersecting pentagon)
      2. Mapping (topographic abilities)
      3. Clock drawing (spontaneous, copy)
    ii. Neglect
      1. Anosognosia (awareness of deficits)
      2. Hemispatial neglect (cancellation, line bisection)
      3. Extinction (auditory, visual, tactile)
      4. Emotional-Affective processing (expressive, receptive aprosodia)

continues

Table 1–1. *continued*

J. Calculations

II. Cranial Nerves (CN)
  A. CN I—Olfactory (tested only when indicated by history)
  B. CN II—Optic (visual acuity, visual fields, pupil size, regularity, equality, reaction to light, optic fundi)
  C. CN III, IV, VI—Extraocular muscle function (tracking, saccadic eye movements)
  D. CN V—Trigeminal (jaw movement against resistance, jaw jerk reflex, facial sensation, corneal reflex)
  E. CN VII—Facial (symmetry at rest and with movement, corneal reflex, taste anterior 2/3 of tongue, lacrimation and salavation)
  F. CN VIII—Auditory (Webers and Rinne tests, vestibular)
  G. CN IX, X—Glossopharyngeal, Vagus (palatal elevation, uvula position, gag reflex)
  H. CN XI—Spinal Accessory (sternocleidomastoid and trapezius muscle strength)
  I. CN XII—Hypoglossal (symmetry of tongue protrusion, lateralization)

III. Somatosensory
  A. Pain and Temperature
  B. Touch, Position, Vibration, Romberg sign
  C. Cortical Sensory (graphesthesia, stereognosis, double simultaneous stimulation)

IV. Motor
  A. Bulk (atrophy, fasciculations)
  B. Tone (hypotonia, rigidity, spasticity)
  C. Strength—Gross Motor
    i. Formal testing (grading 0–5)
    ii. Localization of deficits (flexor-extensor, proximal-distal)
    iii. Drift
  D. Strength—Fine Motor
    i. Pincer, grasp
    ii. Finger tapping
  E. Adventitious (involuntary) Movements
    i. Localization (axial-appendicular, distal-proximal, symmetric-asymmetric)
    ii. Type of dyskinesia
      1. Hypokinetic (parkinsonism)
      2. Hyperkinetic (dystonia, chorea, athetosis, tremor, myoclonus, hemiballism)
    iii. Presence (at rest, suspension, intention)
  F. Cerebellar
    i. Finger-to-nose (dysmetria, past-pointing), heel-to-shin
    ii. Rapid alternating hand movement (dysdiadokinesia)
    iii. Ataxia-axial/appendicular

Table 1–1. *continued*

G. Gait and Station
  i. Gait
    1. Spontaneous (base, arm swing, associated movements, posture)
    2. Directed (tandem, on toes, on heels)
  ii. Station (Romberg, retropulsion)

V. Reflexes
  A. Deep Tendon Reflexes—muscle stretch reflexes (normal = +2, clonus = +4, hypoactive = 0,1)
  B. Superficial Reflexes
    i. Signs of increased reflexes (Hoffman's crossed adductor, triple flexor, clonus, Babinski response)
    ii. Abdominal reflex, cremasteric reflex, bulbocavernosus, anal wink)
  C. Frontal Release Signs (Glabellar, root, suck, snout, grasp)

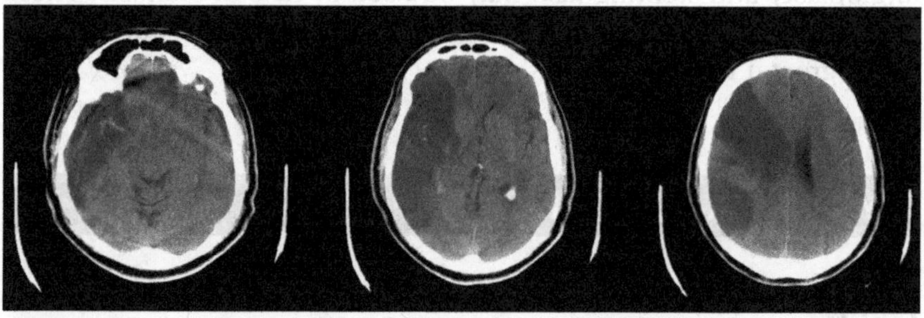

Figure 1–1. Computed tomography scan of a large right middle cerebral artery stroke. The right hemisphere is on the reader's left side.

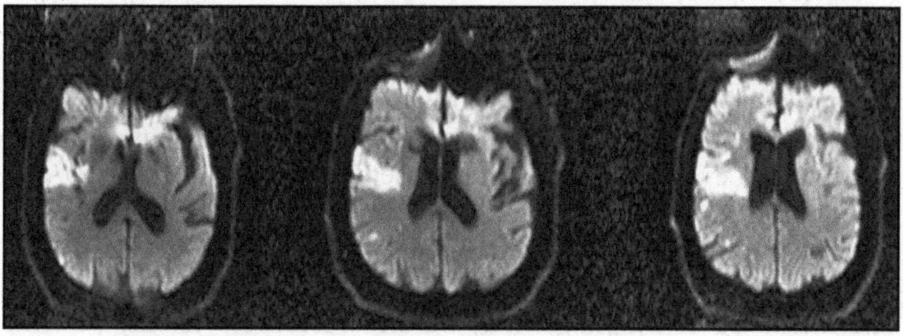

Figure 1–2. Diffusion-weighted imaging scan of an acute right hemisphere stroke. The scan was obtained within 72 hours of admission. The right hemisphere is on the reader's left side.

Medical Management

Identifying the exact time of stroke onset is critical, as it will determine if the patient is eligible for thrombolytic therapies such as tissue plasminogen activator, which may break up or dissolve blood clots. If administered within the first three hours of symptom onset, these therapies may help limit the stroke damage and severity of disability. Antithrombotic agents, such as aspirin and other antiplatelet drugs and warfarin (Coumadin), are generally used for stroke prevention, but they may also be used in the treatment of acute ischemic stroke. Carotid endarterectomy (CEA) is the primary surgical treatment for stroke prevention. It reduces blockage of the internal carotid arteries, which supply blood to the brain. The greatest benefit of CEA is seen in patients with greater than 70% symptomatic stenosis. Carotid angioplasty and stenting also may be used in case of stenosis. These may be options in patients for whom the surgical procedure of CEA is too great a risk.

DYSPHAGIA IN STROKE

Incidence

Dysphagia is a common morbidity following acute stroke; however, there is wide discrepancy concerning incidence, ranging from 25% (Gottlieb, Kipnis, Sister, Vardi, & Brill, 1996) to 81% (Meng, Wang, & Lien, 2000). This variability in the incidence of dysphagia following stroke is due, in part, to patient selection methods (e.g., consecutive stroke admissions, referrals for suspected dysphagia), evaluation methods (e.g., questionnaire, clinical swallowing examination (CSE), instrumental evaluation), time post-onset (e.g., 1 week, 1 month), and definition of dysphagia.

The study of consecutive patients with acute stroke provides a more robust inclusion pool from which to determine epidemiology. The incidence of dysphagia may be underestimated if only patients who have complaints of dysphagia or patients referred to speech pathology are evaluated, or that only those patients with overt signs or symptoms[1] of aspiration risk, such as cough, are referred to speech pathology. Identification of dysphagia based on results from the CSE generally may also underestimate the incidence. As discussed in later chapters, the CSE frequently focuses on overt signs of aspiration—for example, cough or wet voice, which may miss silent aspiration as well as dysphagia without aspiration. Use of these results to determine the incidence of dysphagia is problematic, as patients may have dysphagia without aspiration. Conversely, the incidence of dysphagia may be overestimated if signs and symptoms are used as the outcome measure without confirmation of the underlying swallowing impairment with instrumental assessment. A cough with swallowing may be unrelated to dysphagia. Even with an instrumental evaluation, the incidence of dysphagia may be overestimated if the identification of dysphagia is based on laryngeal penetration or single occurrences of aspiration (e.g., Daniels & Foundas, 1999), as healthy adults may exhibit laryngeal penetration and infrequent occurrences of aspiration (e.g., Butler et al., 2010; Butler, Stuart, Markley, Feng, & Kritchevsky, 2018; Robbins, Coyle, Rosenbek, Roecker, & Wood, 1999).

In determining the incidence of dysphagia, Mann, Hankey, and Cameron (2000) provide the most detailed account for the CSE and videofluoroscopic swallowing study (VFSS) and include fairly descriptive operational definitions. However, they did not utilize a group of healthy participants with whom to compare results from the patients with stroke. As discussed in Chapter 3, increasing knowledge of the variability in swallowing, particularly in regard to aging, has greatly expanded our definition of "normal." Thus, without a control group on which to base an acceptable range of what is normal for transit times, structural timing and movement, and airway invasion, the incidence of dysphagia may be inflated.

One additional factor that may prove important in determining the incidence of dysphagia following stroke is race and ethnicity; however, there are few studies in this area. Two previous studies conducted using various U.S. medical databases demonstrated increased incidence of stroke-related dysphagia in minority groups, particularly Asians, as compared with whites (Bussell & Gonzalez-Fernandez, 2011; Gonzalez-Fernandez, Kuhlemeier, & Palmer, 2008). Characteristics

[1]A sign is defined as an observed, objective indicator of impairment; a symptom is defined as subjective patient complaint.

of dysphagia, however, were not identified, as data were captured retrospectively using ICD-9 codes. In individuals with stroke, higher oral impairment scores have been identified in African Americans compared with whites (Daniels et al., 2017). While these studies suggest minorities may be at higher risk of dysphagia, higher Penetration-Aspiration Scale scores in whites compared with African Americans have also been reported (Cola, Daniels, et al., 2010; Daniels et al., 2017). Further research is required to determine if these findings are stable and reflect true risk effects related to race.

The best determination of the incidence of dysphagia and recovery of function would involve: (1) consecutive patients with acute stroke followed longitudinally, (2) a cohort of age-matched healthy participants, (3) instrumental swallowing assessment, (4) a reliable definition of dysphagia from multiple measures (e.g., bolus flow, structural movement, patient perception), (5) stability in findings over multiple trials, consistencies, and volumes, and (6) analysis of race and ethnicity. Development of a standard method to define dysphagia and recovery of swallowing in patients using VFSS has been initiated with a small sample of patients with stroke and healthy age-matched participants (Daniels et al., 2006; Daniels et al., 2009) as well as with a larger heterogeneous population (Martin-Harris et al., 2008). However, until studies are rigorous in implementing all six of the aspects listed above in a large cohort, determining the incidence of dysphagia and recovery of function will remain elusive.

Lesion Location

Initial notions concerning the occurrence of dysphagia following stroke were based on the assumption that either brainstem or bilateral supratentorial (i.e., cerebral hemisphere and/or subcortical area) infarcts were required to produce disturbances in swallowing. The advent of in vivo brain and swallowing imaging techniques has allowed for expansion of our understanding of dysphagia following stroke. It is now widely understood that a single cortical or subcortical infarct may produce dysphagia (Daniels & Foundas, 1999; Robbins, Levine, Maser, Rosenbek, & Kempster, 1993). Lesions anterior to the central sulcus are associated with dysphagia and risk of aspiration more than posterior lesions (Daniels & Foundas, 1999; Robbins et al., 1993). Strokes involving large vessels (e.g., middle cerebral artery) are associated with aspiration more than small vessels (e.g., deep white matter disease). Specific sites that have been associated with dysphagia in patients with stroke include the brainstem, premotor and primary motor cortices, primary somatosensory cortex, and the insula, as well as white matter tracts which disrupt cortical-subcortical connectivity when lesioned (Alberts, Horner, Gray, & Brazer, 1992; Cola, Daniels, et al., 2010; Daniels & Foundas, 1997, 1999; Daniels, Foundas, Iglesia, & Sullivan, 1996; Galovic et al., 2013; Galovic et al., 2016; Gonzalez-Fernandez, Kleinman, Ky, Palmer, & Hillis, 2008; Robbins et al., 1993, Suntrup, Kemling, et al., 2015). While the astute clinician should have knowledge of neuroimaging tests, CT or MRI results cannot be used in isolation to predict the occurrence or severity of dysphagia.

MULTIDISCIPLINARY MANAGEMENT OF DYSPHAGIA IN STROKE

Given the complexity inherent in swallowing and the vast range of skills involved in meticulous diagnostics, a multidisciplinary approach to identification, diagnosis, and management of swallowing impairment is imperative. The diversity in background provided by various medical disciplines is required to illuminate the multidimensional picture of swallowing pathophysiology. Although the lead clinician in the dysphagia management team is frequently a speech pathologist, assumption of the lead role does not imply that the contribution of the speech pathologist is of greater value to dysphagia management than others.

This text cannot define specific roles or responsibilities; that task lies within the individual medical facility and may be driven by professional practice guidelines. However, caution is expressed that the establishment of a team without recognition of input from all related specialties is to the detriment of patient care. A dysphagia management approach that relies only on patient screening by nursing without the expertise of speech pathology is not in the best interest of the patient. Likewise, an approach by speech pathology without the expertise and contributions of nutritionists or others is shortsighted.

2 The Neural Control of Swallowing

From Central to Peripheral

Swallowing is mediated by a distributed neural network that includes cortical and subcortical structures with descending input to the brainstem. This neural network is composed of multiple levels along the neural axis (cortical, subcortical, brainstem). Specific neural systems (sensory, motor) that cross these levels and interconnect with cortical, subcortical, and brainstem regions are involved in swallowing. Based on anatomic and functional imaging studies, as well as animal models, a neuroanatomic model of swallowing is proposed (Figure 2–1).

It is important that clinicians understand the complexities of the neural network involved in swallowing and appreciate that an infarct, when strategically occurring along this neural axis, can produce acute and protracted dysphagia. In order to advocate for prompt consultation and evaluation of patients with stroke, the clinician must understand basic fundamentals of the neural control of swallowing. With further research, we may be able to determine specific stroke locations or combinations of stroke locations, neurocognitive deficits, and/or comorbidities that more accurately predict acute and protracted dysphagia. Until that time, based on our current understanding of the neural control of swallowing, clinicians have a strong argument to promote the evaluation of swallowing in all patients with acute stroke. Moreover, an understanding of innervation patterns is paramount when completing a clinical swallowing examination (CSE) or interpreting biomechanics from imaging. Specific sensory or motor impairment observed on the cranial nerve (CN) examination can assist in identification of swallowing dysfunction. Following is an overview of the neurology of swallowing, which is particularly relevant in the stroke population.

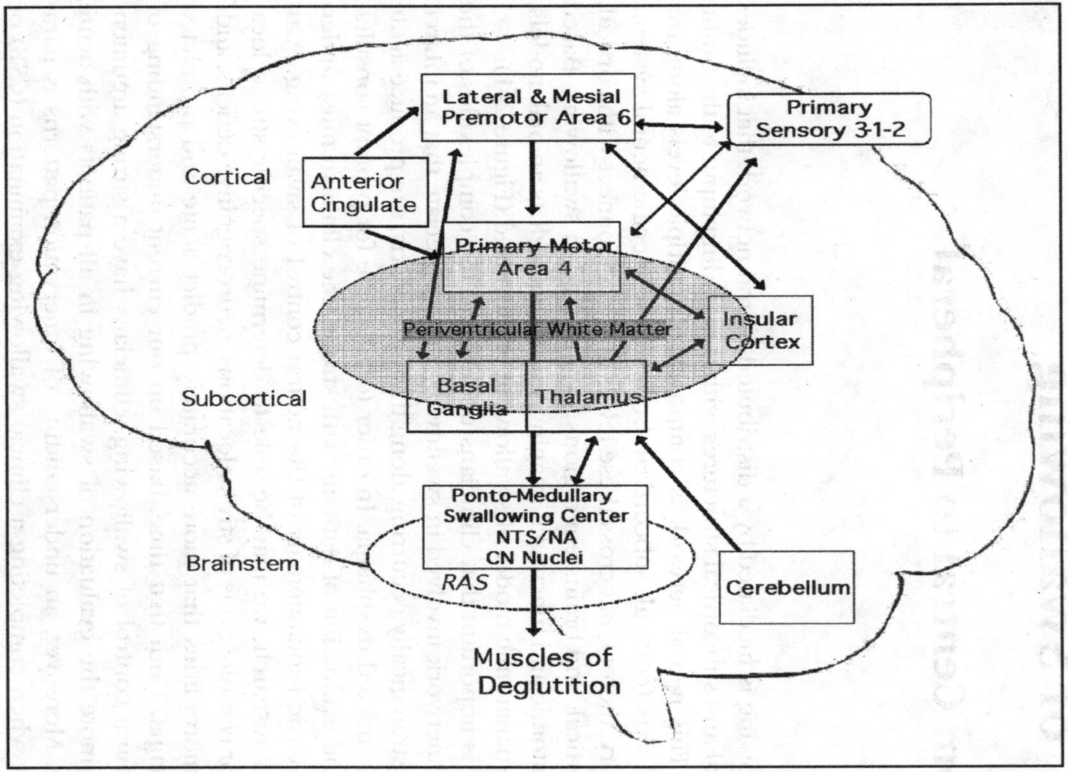

Figure 2–1. Proposed model of the neural networks of swallowing. CN = cranial nerve nuclei, NA = nucleus ambiguus, NTS = nucleus tractus solitarius, RAS = reticular activating system.

METHODS FOR UNDERSTANDING NEURAL CONTROL

Various paradigms have been employed to facilitate our understanding of the neural organization of swallowing. Interestingly, even though methodologies are different, results from studies in animals, healthy adults, and patients with stroke have been generally uniform in suggesting a distributed neural network for swallowing.

Animal models formed our initial basis of knowledge concerning deglutition. Reciprocal translational research, that is, research that moves from animal models to humans and vice versa, continues to play an important role in our understanding of normal and abnormal swallowing. This research is particularly relevant in developing our understanding of potential neural reorganization following stroke. Animal research has included direct stimulation of specific parts of the brain, ablation (lesioning) of specific brain regions, and neuroanatomic tracing with anterograde and retrograde labeling that is used to identify neural pathways in the central and peripheral nervous systems. These techniques have facilitated identification of specific regions of the brain involved with swallowing as well as neural pathways in the central nervous system (CNS) that are related to deglutition.

In humans, localization of swallowing has been based on naturally occurring ablation paradigms, which utilize anatomic imaging (computed tomography, magnetic resonance imaging) of focal lesions in patients with stroke and functional imaging studies that detail activation of brain regions during the actual act of swallowing. Table 2–1 provides a summary of the various techniques used to study the neural control of swallowing.

Functional imaging studies have focused primarily on swallowing in healthy adults. It is evident that, based on neuroimaging, the number of cortical centers involved in swallowing is substantial but somewhat non-specific. With this broad level of activation, it becomes critical to analyze the specific methodology in each study and understand limitations of the various imaging techniques. The use of positron emission tomography and functional magnetic resonance imaging (fMRI) to study patients with stroke-related dysphagia has proven challenging as patients must swallow with minimal extraneous movement while lying flat on their back. Further, imaging studies using measures dependent on blood-oxygen level, such as fMRI and functional near-infrared spectroscopy, can measure activation but

Table 2–1. Techniques to Study the Neural Control of Swallowing in Humans

Technique	*Procedure*	*Results*	*Advantages*	*Disadvantages*
Anatomic Imaging				
Computed tomography (CT) Magnetic resonance imaging (MRI)	Brain images obtained while a person is lying quietly performing no activity. Best if contiguous thin slices.	Lesions are identified and mapped out to determine specific sites. Relationship between lesion size and dysphagia can be made if scans are obtained with limited to no gap between slices.	If obtained at the same time as the instrumental swallowing study, can correlate stroke location with dysfunction.	Patient cannot perform any activity. The CT scan does not immediately show ischemic infarction.
Functional Imaging				
Positron emission tomography (PET)	Radioactive tracers are injected into the bloodstream. They circulate and diffuse in cerebral tissue. Generally a block design is used where subjects repeatedly swallow (water, saliva) for a specified time alternated with rest periods.	Identifies areas activated during swallowing.	Low susceptibility to motion artifact.	Radiation exposure. Expensive. Reduced temporal resolution.
Functional magnetic resonance imaging (fMRI)	Blood oxygenation level dependent effects are mapped.	Identifies areas activated during swallowing.	Excellent spatial resolution.	Reduced temporal resolution.

Technique	*Procedure*	*Results*	*Advantages*	*Disadvantages*
Functional magnetic resonance imaging (fMRI) *continued*	That is, a task (swallowing) yields increased neuronal activity and metabolism in specific brain regions that yield increased blood flow and volume. Generally an event-related paradigm is used where multiple single swallows are completed over multiple trials.		No radiation exposure.	Susceptible to motion; this is mitigated by event-related paradigm.
Other Functional Methods				
Transcranial magnetic stimulation (TMS)	Focal magnetic stimulation of specific cortical surfaces is completed using an external coil. Stimulation of these regions yields contraction of specific swallowing musculature that is measured with electromyography. Areas yielding activation are reconstructed on anatomic templates.	Identifies neural circuitry in swallowing with good temporal resolution.	Cortical regions involved with normal swallowing, and recovery of function can be identified.	The effect of stimulation is limited to superficial cortical structures. An actual swallow cannot be stimulated due to risk of seizure.
Magnetoencephalography	Similar to electroencephalography except that a magnetic versus electric signal is recorded during an activity (i.e., swallowing). Similar to transcranial magnetic stimulation as areas yielding activation are reconstructed on anatomic templates.	Detects postsynaptic magnetic fields generated by neurons activated with swallowing.	Excellent temporal resolution that allows for determination of the onset of activation of specific brain regions during swallowing.	Easy to overinterpret isolated tongue movement as swallowing related movement.

cannot differentiate between activation that is excitatory versus that which is inhibitory (Leopold & Daniels, 2010). Although other imaging methodologies can be obtained with a person seated, they each have their own advantages and disadvantages in the study of dysphagia in clinical populations (Malandraki, Sutton, Perlman, Karampinos, & Conway, 2009).

HIGHER NERVOUS SYSTEM CONTROL

The cerebral cortex and subcortical structures are important in swallowing with evidence that supratentorial regions modulate swallowing (Miller & Bowman, 1977; Sumi, 1969). Historically, it was thought that a stroke must involve the brainstem or both cerebral hemispheres; however, research over the last three decades has revealed that a single unilateral stroke can produce dysphagia. It is important that clinicians have a good understanding of the role of cortical and subcortical regions in swallowing in order to advocate for obtaining a clinical swallowing examination in all acute stroke patients, not just patients with brainstem or bilateral strokes.

The supratentorial network for swallowing involves a sensory system, motor system, and white matter pathways. In research evaluating the temporal sequences of activation during swallowing by healthy volunteers ($n = 16$) on fMRI, Mihai, Otto, Platz, Eickhoff, and Lotze (2014) report successive activation from the premotor cortex, supplementary motor area (SMA), and thalamus, followed by the primary sensorimotor cortex, the posterior insula, and cerebellum and culminating with activation in the pons. Despite methodological differences, anatomic and functional imaging studies have identified similar areas critical for swallowing. These regions include the primary motor cortex, premotor cortex, SMA, primary somatosensory cortex, insula, thalamus, basal ganglia, and anterior cingulate gyrus (e.g., Daniels & Foundas, 1997, 1999; Hamdy, Mikulis, et al., 1999; Hamdy, Rothwell, et al., 1999; Huckabee, Deecke, Cannito, Gould, & Mayr, 2003; Kern, Jaradeh, Arndorfer, & Shaker, 2001; Martin, Goodyear, Gati, & Menon, 2001; Mosier & Bereznaya, 2001; Rangarathnam, Kamarunas, & McCullough, 2014; Suntrup, Kemling, et al., 2015; Toogood et al., 2005; Vasant et al., 2014).

More recently, in a review of 160 patients with stroke, Flowers et al. (2017) used imaging, clinical, and demographic information to develop a comprehensive model to predict dysphagia after first-time stroke. Consistent with prior research, results indicate dysphagia involves a substantial neural network, with predictors of dysphagia greatest for medullary, pontine, insular, and internal capsule lesions. Further, there was increased risk of dysphagia in individuals with at least moderate brain atrophy and increased age. In a study by Li and colleagues (2014), patients with stroke-related dysphagia ($n = 12$) have been shown to demonstrate differences in resting-state connectivity in the sensorimotor-insula-putamen circuits as compared with patients with stroke but no dysphagia ($n = 12$) and healthy controls ($n = 12$). Together with the Flowers et al. (2017) work, this may indicate that swallowing neural control relies heavily on both local and global sensorimotor integration.

Sensory input has parallel ascending and descending input affecting brainstem pathways and cortical pathways. Ascending sensory input is processed by the thalamus (subcortical level), then proceeds to the primary somatosensory cortex (Brodmann's area [BA] 3-1-2, cortical level). Tactile and intra-oral afferent information, such as taste and temperature, can be integrated in regions such as the parietal cortex, posterior cingulate cortex, precuneus, and somatosensory cortex, serving an association role in integrating sensory information (Hamdy, Mikulis, et al., 1999; Miller, 2008; Steele & Miller, 2010). Research has indicated that the sensory strip is somatotopically mapped to represent regions corresponding to the upper aerodigestive tract, including the face, tongue, and pharyngeal regions (Mosier et al., 1999; Rangarathnam et al., 2014; Vasant et al., 2014). The provision of temporary oral anesthesia has been associated with a reduction in somatosensory and motor area activation with magnetoencephalography (Michou & Hamdy, 2009; Teismann et al., 2007). This cortical synthesis of sensory information has implications for patients after cortical stroke, in that patients may exhibit impairment in appropriately modulating a swallowing response to accommodate for various bolus types (Michou & Hamdy, 2009).

Corticocortical connections run along an anterior-posterior axis with sensory input feeding forward to the primary motor cortex (BA 4) and lateral and mesial premotor cortices (BA 6). The lateral premotor cortex integrates input from the prefrontal cortex and cerebellum and is critical for the selection of appropriate movements (Passingham, 1993). The mesial premotor cortex, also referred to as the SMA, is the main cortical target of the basal ganglia (Wise & Strick, 1984) and is critical in the preparation and programming of voluntary movement sequences (Roland, Larsen, Lassen, & Skinhoj, 1980). The anterior cingulate gyrus is important for attention as well as the selection of volitional actions and sends output to the primary motor and premotor cortices. The primary motor cortex has descending connections through subcortical regions to sensory and motor cranial nerve nuclei (Kuypers, 1958a, 1958b). Descending input proceeds through subcortical regions. The periventricular white matter (PVWM), which is the white matter adjacent to the body of the lateral ventricles, is important in these swallowing pathways, as it is composed of ascending somatosensory and descending motor fibers as well as intrahemispheric corticocortical connections (Schulz, 1994). Descending corticobulbar fibers from the mouth/face representation within the ventrolateral precentral gyrus (motor cortex) are located anterolaterally in the PVWM. The anterior insula, in addition to being the primary gustatory cortex (Benjamin & Burton, 1968), has parallel connections with many cortical and subcortical regions that mediate swallowing. These regions include motor and premotor cortices (Mesulam & Mufson, 1985) and the parvocellular component of the ventroposterior medial nucleus (VPMpc) of the thalamus (Mufson & Mesulam, 1984). The VPMpc contains the sensory representation for the face and oral cavity and receives projections from the nucleus tractus solitarius (NTS) (Beckstead, Morse, & Norgren, 1980).

The lateralization of swallowing is a controversial notion. Using various imaging modalities, results thus far are inconclusive as to whether swallowing is preferentially mediated by the left or right hemisphere at the cortical level. Some anatomic imaging studies have suggested that oral stage dysfunction is associated with left hemisphere damage and that pharyngeal stage dysfunction and aspiration are associated with right hemisphere damage (Robbins & Levine, 1988, 1993; Robbins, Levine, Maser, Rosenbek, & Kempster, 1993; Suntrup, Kemling, et al., 2015), whereas others have suggested no difference in dysfunction between hemispheres (Alberts, Horner, Gary, & Brazer, 1992; Daniels & Foundas, 1999; Galovic et al., 2013). These same discrepancies in results have also been noted with functional studies. Bilateral activation of the sensorimotor cortex has been suggested by some studies (Hamdy, Mikulis, et al., 1999; Martin et al., 2001; Zald & Pardo, 1999). It has been suggested that lateralization may be dependent on the task (Martin et al., 2001), with right hemisphere activation associated with volitional swallowing and left hemisphere activation with reflexive swallowing (Kern et al., 2001). Conversely, others have noted left hemisphere dominance with volitional swallowing (Dziewas et al., 2003). A third hypothesis has been put forth and suggests bilateral but asymmetric activation of swallowing (Hamdy et al., 1996, 1997; Hamdy, Rothwell, et al., 1999). That is, both hemispheres are involved in swallowing, but one hemisphere is more dominant and varies across individuals. This notion suggests that dysphagia will occur only if the more dominant hemisphere for swallowing is affected by a stroke, thus perhaps explaining why dysphagia may be present in some stroke patients but not in other patients with lesions of similar size and location. Using this model, it has been suggested that recovery of swallowing function is associated with cortical reorganization of the nondominant hemisphere (Hamdy et al., 1998).

In addition to the debate regarding lateralization, neural plasticity and potential maladaptive cortical plasticity are receiving increased attention (Humbert & German, 2013; Kleim & Jones, 2008; Malandraki, Johnson, & Robbins, 2011; Martin, 2009; Robbins, Butler, et al., 2008; Takeuchi & Izumi, 2012). Neural plasticity refers to the adaptive capacity of the CNS to reorganize its neural circuitry as a result of experience, discussed further in Chapter 19 (Kleim & Jones, 2008). This is critical when considering cortical response to neural impairment and subsequent rehabilitation. The foundational literature regarding neural plasticity arises from animal and limb studies. For example, it has been demonstrated in patients following unilateral stroke that rehabilitation constraining the unimpaired, ipsilesional upper limb not only improves the function of the impaired limb but stimulates activation in the remaining cortex of the injured hemisphere (Kleim & Jones, 2008). However, there are marked differences between swallowing neural control and control for corticospinal limb systems. Swallowing relies on a vastly different musculoskeletal framework, further complicated by uncertainty regarding lateralization of cortical representation for swallowing (Martin, 2009). Nevertheless, there is growing evidence that swallowing-related cortical centers can experience neural plasticity as a result of injury and plasticity associated with behavioral rehabilitation, similar to the limb literature (Martin, 2009). Results from non-invasive brain stimulation techniques, such as transcranial magnetic stimulation and transcranial direct current stimulation, indicate the possibility for cortical reorganization of the swallowing system after injury, as discussed further in Chapter 21.

Fundamental in the discussion of neural reorganization is mention of the potential for maladaptive plasticity and neural changes in the aging brain. Contrary to the positive effects of plasticity, cortical reorganization has also been found to reduce motor recovery after stroke, especially in patients implementing compensatory strategies or experiencing a period of non-use, such as patients deemed unable to eat safely by mouth (Takeuchi & Izumi, 2012). Additionally, as stroke more frequently occurs in the elderly, it is important to consider neural changes in the aging brain. There is evidence that cortical representation and laterality associated with swallowing change as a function of age, with reports of decreased (Malandraki, Perlman, Karampinos, & Sutton, 2011) as well as increased but more diffuse (Humbert et al., 2009) cortical representation. Diminished cortical representation may underlie subclinical changes in swallowing in the aging population that would potentially predispose to impairment in the event of neurological injury. Increased and more diffuse cortical representation may reflect a compensatory mechanism that allows sustained function in the presence of declining peripheral motor function and sarcopenia. This mechanism of increasing brain activation associated with unchanged motor performance in older subjects has also been identified in the limb movement literature (Mattay et al., 2002).

BRAINSTEM MECHANISMS

Whereas supratentorial regions are critical for the modulation and initiation of ingestive swallowing, brainstem structures are recognized as providing the basic motor plan for the pharyngeal response. These more primitive phylogenic structures have been extensively evaluated through early research by Jean, Doty, Car, and others (Amri & Car, 1988; Amri, Car, & Jean, 1984; Car, 1970, 1973; Car & Amri, 1982; Car, Jean, & Roman, 1975; Doty, 1968; Doty, Richmond, & Storey, 1967; Jean, 1984a, 1984b, 1990) who have outlined the critical role of medullary circuitry in the regulation of pharyngeal and esophageal swallowing. Additional work has highlighted the importance of this circuitry in the coordinative interactions between swallowing and respiration (Bautistia & Dutschmann, 2014; Dick, Oku, Romaniuk, & Cherniack, 1993; Saito, Ezure, Tanaka, & Osawa, 2003; Shiba, Satoh, Kobayashi, & Hayashi, 1999). The compact clustering of bilateral CN nuclei and interneuronal connections in this region are considered to be responsible for the complex sequencing and execution of the neuromuscular events involved in swallowing.

The first evidence of a central swallowing center was provided by Miller and Sherrington (1915). These researchers provided electrical stimulation to the exposed cortex and brainstem to identify which regions would result in observable swallowing behavior. Although many cortical and subcortical regions elicited swallowing upon stimulation, a study of decerebrated animals revealed that the medullary brainstem appeared to be the lowest common denominator, with stimulation of this area eliciting pharyngeal and esophageal swallowing in the absence of cortical input. Additionally, Miller (1972) reported that stimulation of specific brainstem cranial motor nuclei would not elicit the complex neuromuscular process of pharyngeal swallowing, although the muscles supplied by these motor nuclei are involved in swallowing. This suggests that there is a more complex interdependent circuitry for the act of deglutition.

Central to our current understanding of brainstem mechanisms is the construct of a *central pattern generator* (CPG). Rossignol and Dubuc (1994) define this term as "an operational expression to designate an ensemble of neural elements whose properties and connectivity can give rise to characteristic patterns of rhythmic activity in the absence of external feedback" (p. 895). A CPG can be thought of as a functionally connected pool of neurons capable of producing a rhythmic, predictable output in the absence of afferent sensory input (Harris-Warrick, 2010). CPGs are found in other systems as well, such as mastication (Morquette et al., 2012), locomotion (Guertin & Steuer, 2009), and respiration (Abdala et al., 2009). Many components of the swallowing network are not dedicated to swallowing alone but can also serve other networks. Therefore, the patterned swallowing response is completed in close conjunction with coordination of associated functions, such as respiration and mastication, through shared pools of interneurons (Jean, 2001). The construct of a CPG for swallowing was initially posed by Doty (1968) subsequent to a study by Doty and Bosma (1956), which documented that swallowing was a sequential and repeatable activation of muscles that occurs even in the presence of impaired peripheral feedback mechanisms.

There are two bilateral regions of the brainstem medulla that are considered to represent the anatomic foundation for the swallowing CPG (Kessler & Jean, 1985). The dorsal region of the medulla is anatomically located 1.5 to 4 mm rostral to the obex and consists of the area surrounding and including the NTS and adjacent reticular formation (Jean & Car, 1979). The NTS is the primary sensory nucleus for the facial, glossopharyngeal, and vagus cranial nerves; afferent pathways from the pharynx and larynx, specifically those from the superior laryngeal nerve, travel to the NTS via these cranial nerves (Carpenter, 1978). Additionally, the NTS region receives input from the trigeminal sensory nucleus of the pons. Mucosal receptors in the pharynx respond to touch, pressure, chemicals, and water and facilitate the initiation and repeated activation of pharyngeal swallowing. Muscle spindle receptors, which are embedded in muscles involved in pharyngeal and esophageal swallowing, are considered to trigger interneurons that modify motor output to muscles. Finally, the specific cortical site that evokes swallowing when activated by electrical stimulation sends fibers to synapse in this dorsal medullary region. Subsequently, according to Miller, Bieger, and Conklin (1997), lesions of the dorsal region prevent electrical stimulation of the cortex from evoking swallowing. This suggests that the dorsal region is the initial neural entrance or afferent portal for input that modulates swallowing (Miller et al., 1997). The dorsal group neurons lack direct connection with hypoglossal and trigeminal motor neurons and connect directly only to the nucleus ambiguus (NA) and associated reticular formation. Thus, neurons in the dorsal region are considered the programming interneurons (Amri, Car, & Roman, 1990) that set up the sequential preprogrammed patterns of neuronal activation that are then transmitted to the ventral regions for motor activation.

The second major component of the medullary swallowing center, the ventral region, consists of the area surrounding and including the NA, located 3 to 6 mm rostral to the obex (Jean & Car, 1979). Structurally, the NA is the primary motor nucleus for the glossopharyngeal, vagus, and spinal accessory nerves and has extensive interconnections with other medullary motor nuclei, such as the hypoglossal, facial, and trigeminal motor nuclei (Amri et al., 1990; Jean, Amri, & Calas, 1983). Thus, the neurons and interneurons in this region send out neural commands that control the muscles of the pharynx, larynx, and esophagus (Roman, 1986). Axons in the NA connect with contralateral brainstem regions involved in swallowing (Jean et al., 1983).

The ventral efferent medullary region receives direct input from the dorsal afferent medullary region. Thus, sensory information entering the brainstem via the NTS is integrated into a swallowing motor plan and then transmitted to the motor nucleus for execution. Interestingly, sensory inputs from the superior laryngeal nerve (vagus), which are known to elicit swallowing upon electrical stimulation, travel to both the dorsal region and directly to the NA in the ventral region. However, synaptic pathways to the ventral region are longer than those to the dorsal region, suggesting that the superior laryngeal nerve can directly modify motor output during swallowing and provide reflexive laryngeal control for a cough response (Miller et al., 1997). With the exception of connections from the NTS to the NA, there are no other ventral medullary connections to sensory nuclei, supporting the role of a tightly encapsulated neural network underlying swallowing. Functionally, direct stimulation of the ventral region does not evoke pharyngeal swallowing despite direct motor neuron connection to the muscles of swallowing.

Individual contraction of the muscles involved in swallowing occurs, but the organized, patterned motor response is absent without the intervening sensory input and consequent motor plan provided by the dorsal region. Amri and Car (1988), therefore, suggest that the ventral neurons serve to link the sensory input from the dorsal neuron group to the motor neurons involved in swallowing. Given this important link, the ventral neuron group may be referred to as the "command interneurons."

The cerebellum and the pons are not traditionally considered integral to the execution of the basic swallowing response, with predominant theories of deglutition focusing on control arising from the medulla (Lang, 2009; Miller, 2008). However, the pons, which is the most rostral section of the hindbrain, is intimately connected with the medulla, the cortex, and the cerebellum, as well as being home to numerous cranial nerves, such as the trigeminal (CN V), abducens (CN VI), and facial (CN VII) (Brodal & Bjaalie, 1992, 1997). CPGs for other systems such as respiration and mastication are well represented in the pons (Abdala et al., 2009; Lund & Kolta, 2006a, 2006b; Molkov, Bacak, Dick, & Rybak, 2013; Morquette et al., 2012; Quintero et al., 2013; Rybak et al., 2004; St.-John & Paton, 2004). Electrical stimulation in rabbits has revealed that regions in the pons and the pontine reticular formation are able to induce a swallowing response (Sumi, 1972).

Similar research highlights the possible role of the cerebellum in swallowing sensorimotor control (Rangarathnam et al., 2014). The cerebellum is connected to the brainstem via three paired cerebellar peduncles and has a role in motor coordination and proprioception (Glickstein & Doron, 2008; Perrini, Tiezzi, Castagna, & Vannozzi, 2013). Efferent information from the cerebellum is primarily communicated through the superior cerebellar peduncle to the red nucleus and the thalamus, which is subsequently relayed to the cerebral cortex. The middle cerebellar peduncle is an afferent projection of pontine cells to the cerebellar cortex. Lastly, the inferior cerebellar peduncle consists of crossed efferent and afferent fibers arising from the posterior medulla (Glickstein & Doron, 2008). In early work, Mussen (1927) was able to elicit a swallow response following stimulation of the cerebellum, specifically the ventral vermis, in a cat model. Cerebellar elicitation of swallowing has been replicated in further studies (Berntson, Potolicchio, & Miller, 1973; Hockman, Bieger, & Weerasuriya, 1979; Martner, 1975). More recently, cerebellar activation has been evidenced with imaging of swallowing in healthy participants (Malandraki et al., 2009; Malandraki, Perlman, et al., 2011; Mosier & Bereznaya, 2001). However, in a meta-analysis of neuroanatomic predictors of dysphagia following stroke, Flowers, Skoretz, Streiner, Silver, and Martino (2011) found no incidence of dysphagia following cerebellar infarct from a total of 656 subjects. While it is highly likely that the cerebellum plays a role in control or feed-forward/feed-back monitoring of swallowing due to its connectivity and anatomic proximity to critical swallowing-related centers, further research is needed to clearly specify the role and importance of these associated structures (Rangarathnam et al., 2014).

In summary, bilateral peripheral afferents from the glossopharyngeal, facial, and vagus nerves enter the afferent portal of the dorsal medullary group. This sensory information is paired with cortical inputs that synapse on the pontine relay nuclei (cortical-subcortical loop), and afferent input from the sensory fibers of the trigeminal nerve. All sensory information is integrated, and the appropriate programmed motor response is sent back out to the periphery via the ventral medullary group. The primary structure of this group, the NA, consequently activates sequential efferent cranial nerve fibers from the spinal accessory, vagus, and glossopharyngeal nerves as well as the motor nuclei for the hypoglossal and trigeminal nerves. At its most primitive level of functioning, this functional "central pattern generator" allows for sequential muscle activation in the absence of sensory feedback. However, for ingestive swallowing, interaction between sensory and motor nuclei via modulation of interneuronal fibers facilitates a patterned motor response specific to the incoming sensory input. Further, it is believed ponto-cerebellar pathways provide feed-forward/feed-back monitoring of swallowing, although this is still being clarified in ongoing research. In functional terms, this allows for differential but safe swallowing of a variety of textures, temperatures, and bolus sizes.

PERIPHERAL NEUROMUSCULAR MECHANISMS

As discussed in the prior section, two regions of the medulla and a host of supramedullary structures and neural circuits are involved in the coordinative efforts of accepting incoming sensory input in preparation for swallowing, organizing a swallowing response that is differentiated to that specific sensory input and engaging a unique motor plan to execute efficient bolus ingestion. Incoming and outgoing inputs from the brainstem are dependent on activation and efficient transfer of neural information through afferent and efferent CN pathways. Thus, elucidation of swallowing neural control demands knowledge of the complex patterns of excitation and inhibition of the cranial nerves that contribute so substantively to swallowing motor control. More importantly, as discussed in Chapter 7, interpretation of CN findings can guide the clinician to more reliable inferences about pharyngeal swallowing behavior. In order to aid clinical application, this section highlights the location of CN nuclei and places CN excitation and inhibition within the context of neuromuscular contributions to swallowing physiology. Three caveats for the clinical reader are:

1. Although the following text is accurate based on the authors' reading, the clinician is advised that there are discrepancies in the literature regarding some aspects of CN constitution and innervation. These are highlighted for consideration in footnotes.
2. The nuclei, nerves, and consequently innervated muscles that control the swallowing process are bilaterally present. In many, but

not all, processes involved in the oral stage of swallowing, and in the entirety of the normal pharyngeal response, these neural structures are activated bilaterally and symmetrically in an intricately timed manner. As such, to avoid redundancy in language, much of the discussions regarding swallowing tend to refer to these structures in singular form; that is, the trigeminal nerve innervates the mylohyoid muscle. Unless specifically stated, this implies that the right and left trigeminal nerves innervate the right and left mylohyoid muscles. Exceptions to this may include some processes of oral bolus manipulation where lateral orolingual movements are required to control the bolus and will be stated as needed.

3. The sequence of innervation, muscle activation, and biomechanical effects listed below should be considered approximate in sequence rather than a hard-wired sequential response. Our ever-evolving research continually challenges the neural and biomechanical execution of swallowing events.

Although generally considered peripheral organs, the CNs have their respective nuclei within the CNS. The motor nerves emerge from these nuclei and synapse peripherally at the neuromuscular junction. Sensory nerves initiate in sensory receptors, traverse from the peripheral system, and synapse on CN nuclei in the CNS. In stroke, knowledge of site of lesion may provide clues for differential diagnosis of swallowing impairment if the clinician has knowledge of the origin of CN nuclei. CN nuclei involved in swallowing are primarily housed in the lower brain regions, with the exception of the nuclei for the olfactory (CN I) and optic (CN II) cranial nerves, both of which are contained within the cerebral cortex. The trigeminal motor and sensory nuclei (CN V) and the facial motor nucleus (CN VII) are situated in the pons. Further down the neural axis, the brainstem houses the remainder of the important nuclei for swallowing. The NTS is the primary sensory nucleus for the facial (CN VII), glossopharyngeal (CN IX), and vagus (CN X) cranial nerves; all afferent information from the pharynx and larynx travel to the NTS via these cranial nerves. Additionally, the NTS receives secondary input from the trigeminal sensory nucleus of the pons. The NA is also housed in the brainstem and is the primary motor nucleus for the glossopharyngeal (CN IX), vagus (CN X), and spinal accessory (CN XI) nerves and has extensive interconnections with other motor nuclei involved in pharyngeal swallowing, such as the hypoglossal (CN XII), facial (CN VII), and trigeminal motor (CN V) nuclei.

Prior to the bolus entering the oral cavity, an individual sees the bolus, which activates CN sensory inputs from the optic nerve (CN II). In addition, a person may smell the bolus, which activates similar receptors from the olfactory nerve (CN I). Input from these peripheral receptors travel via their respective CNs to the primary visual and olfactory cortices before moving on to their respective association cortices for recognition and cognitive processing. This phase of swallowing is often underappreciated in clinical settings—for example, when a patient who is dependent on others for feeding has reduced input from the sight, smell, and tactile manipulation of food inherent in self-feeding (Kayser-Jones & Schell, 1997). At this early point in the pre-ingestive process, and dependent on the stimulus, the individual may have activation of motor fibers of the chorda tympani branch of the facial nerve (CN VII) to initiate salivary flow from the submandibular and sublingual glands; activation of fibers of the glossopharyngeal nerve (CN IX) will assist in production of saliva from the parotid glands. Salivary production is critical for bolus preparation of more viscous textures and initiates the digestive process. Additionally, dependent on the characteristics of the bolus, there may be very early activation of the motor fibers of the recurrent laryngeal branch of the vagus nerve (CN X), which initiates early onset of vocal adduction for airway protection occurring through contraction of the interarytenoid and cricoarytenoid muscles.

Bolus entry into the oral cavity requires paired inhibition and excitation of several muscle groups. Mouth opening generally requires inhibition of facial nerve (CN VII) fibers that contract orbicularis oris muscles. However, for larger volumes swallowed, there may be activation of other fibers of the facial nerve (CN VII), which retract accessory facial muscles (such as the risorius, zygomaticus, and quadratus labi superioris), thus allowing greater spread of the lips. Jaw opening is dependent on excitation of some fibers of the mandibular branch of the trigeminal nerve (CN V), resulting in active contraction of the jaw openers (anterior belly of the digastric and mylohyoid); this movement is further facilitated by activation of the superior root of the ansa cervicalis (fibers of CN XII and cervical spinal nerve 1)[1] for

[1]Discrepancies exist in the published literature on components of the ansa cervicalis. The reader is referred to Chhetri and Berke (1997).

contraction of the geniohyoid muscle.[2] Jaw opening is dependent on relaxation of the jaw closers (temporalis and masseter) and stabilization of the hyoid bone via contraction of the collective strap muscles, also through the ansa cervicalis.

As the bolus enters the oral cavity, the base of the tongue approximates the palate to contain the bolus orally. This is accomplished primarily via excitation of the pharyngeal plexus (CN IX, X), which results in contraction of the palatoglossus muscle. Additional fibers of the facial nerve (CN VII) may result in contraction of the stylohyoid and posterior belly of the digastric; the hypoglossal nerve (CN XII) also contributes to this movement via innervation and subsequent contraction of the styloglossus. This is an excellent example of redundancy in the neuromuscular system that facilitates airway protection even at this very early stage in the swallowing process.

Bolus acceptance requires excitation of the hypoglossal nerve (CN XII), to activate the intrinsic lingual muscles (verticalis, transverse, and longitudinal) to contour the tongue surface and the extrinsic muscles (genioglossus, hyoglossus, and styloglossus) to change the position of the tongue within the oral cavity. These muscles work collectively to groove the tongue with midline drop to collect the bolus. These same neuromuscular substrates consequently elevate the midline to transfer the bolus to the dental surfaces and manipulate the bolus for cohesive formation. Unlike some other biomechanical movement, bolus manipulation is heavily dependent on a single cranial nerve for neural control; all muscles that change the configuration of the lingual surface are innervated by the hypoglossal nerve (CN XII). Lingual position in the oral cavity is similarly controlled but may be secondarily facilitated by facial nerve (CN VII) innervation of the posterior belly of the digastric and stylohyoid to provide some compensatory function in the event of injury.

For semisolid and solid bolus textures, mastication requires reciprocal jaw opening via the anterior belly of digastric, mylohyoid, and geniohyoid muscles and jaw closing via the masseter and temporalis muscles with minor contribution from the medial pterygoid; rotary movement of the mandible is accomplished via reciprocal contraction of right and left pterygoids. As described previously, all muscles of mastication are innervated by the trigeminal nerve (CN V) with

[2]Discrepancies also exist regarding innervation of the geniohyoid muscle. The reader is referred to Curtis, Braham, Karr, Holborow, and Worman (1988).

the exception of the geniohyoids, which are innervated by the ansa cervicalis. The bolus mixes with saliva for breakdown and increased lubrication (Matsuo & Palmer, 2015; Taniguchi et al., 2013).

The motor tasks described above are completed under the guidance of sensory feedback from the maxillary branch of the trigeminal nerve (CN V) for the palate and teeth, the mandibular branch of the trigeminal (CN V) for the mucosa of the mouth, gums, and anterior two-thirds of the tongue. The glossopharyngeal nerve (IX) provides tactile sensory innervation for the soft palate and adjacent pharyngeal wall, the faucial arches and posterior one-third of the tongue. This input facilitates immediate changes in lingual contour and position to contain and form a cohesive bolus. This tactile sensory input pairs with taste input that is mediated through activation of sensory fibers of the facial nerve (CN VII) for the anterior two-thirds of the tongue and the glossopharyngeal nerve (CN IX) for the posterior one-third of the tongue and oral cavity. Cumulative oral sensory information transfers either directly from the facial and glossopharyngeal nerves or indirectly from the trigeminal sensory nucleus in the pons to the NTS of the dorsal medulla to contribute to motor planning for pharyngeal swallowing.

Throughout bolus preparation, the base of the tongue is relatively more elevated than the tongue tip, primarily through activation of the pharyngeal plexus (CN IX, X), which maintains tone in the palatoglossus muscle for glossopalatal approximation. Once the bolus is ready for transfer, the tongue base must drop to allow bolus transfer; this is accomplished passively via terminated activation of the pharyngeal plexus for palatoglossal relaxation, paired with excitation of fibers of the hypoglossal nerve (CN XII) for active contraction of the genioglossus and hyoglossus, which pulls the base of the tongue inferiorly. As the tongue base drops, the hypoglossal nerve (CN XII) also transmits the command to the collective intrinsic lingual muscles to pull the tip of the tongue to the palate and then "squeeze" the bolus from the oral cavity. The tongue tip and blade approximate the hard palate, pressing the bolus posteriorly out of the oral cavity. This serves to increase intra-oral pressure with systematic progression of pressure across the tongue surface (Matsuo & Palmer, 2015). Interestingly, Ali, Cook, Laundl, Wallace, and De Carle (1997) placed a splint in the mouth of healthy adults ($n = 15$), creating a temporary tongue deformity. Results indicate that the presence of an altered lingual position and contour affected pharyngeal swallowing, with reduced peak pharyngeal pressure, reduced intrabolus pressure, and delayed hyolaryngeal excursion. This highlights the importance of lingual propulsive action to the initiation of the pharyngeal phase.

Onset of the pharyngeal response for deglutitive purposes requires three types of input into the NTS: cognitive cortical processing of the food to be ingested via descending corticobulbar pathways, sensory perception of bolus characteristics via trigeminal, facial, and glossopharyngeal nerves, and perhaps some component of deep muscle receptor input linked to depression of the tongue base for bolus transfer. This information converges on the NTS as a series of graded potentials, which summate until they reach an electrochemical threshold to trigger an action potential, which presents as the pharyngeal response. The dorsal nucleus then sends the motor command to the ventral nucleus or the NA for execution. Inconsistency in onset of pharyngeal swallow may represent variable contributions from these three sources of sensory input.

With onset of the pharyngeal response, many CNs and muscles activate in rapid and overlapping succession to produce the complex movements required for ingestion. Hyoid movement is considered to represent the leading complex of the pharyngeal response; velopharyngeal closure is another early event in the pharyngeal swallow. Activation of the pharyngeal plexus (CNs IX, X) results in innervation of the levator veli palatini to facilitate velopharyngeal closure. Hyoid movement is more complex. Superior, and somewhat posterior, hyoid movement is a component of the broader biomechanical shortening of the pharyngeal cavity as a whole. The facial nerve (CN VII) activates the posterior belly of the digastric and the stylohyoid. Additionally, the pharyngeal plexus (CNs IX, X) initiates activation of the middle pharyngeal constrictor, which wraps from a posterior raphe and inserts into the cornu of the hyoid bone to biomechanically pull the hyoid back and up. As the hyoid is pulled up and back, there are concomitant forces pulling this bone forward. Specific anterior hyoid movement is accomplished via excitation of the trigeminal nerve (CN V) for contraction of the anterior belly of the digastric and mylohyoid muscles, and the superior root of the ansa cervicalis (fibers of CN XII and cervical spinal nerve 1) for contraction of the geniohyoid muscle. With the importance of anterior hyoid movement to subsequent biomechanics, the redundancy in neural input is of significance. Research using fine-wire electromyography (EMG) in healthy participants (n = 14) has revealed that the geniohyoid has highest peak-adjusted EMG amplitude compared with the other submental musculature (Inokuchi et al., 2014). Maximum EMG amplitudes for the anterior belly of the digastric varied according to bolus texture, which likely reflects modulation based on sensory responses originating in the oral cavity. For example, the geniohyoid may have primary activation across textures, but increased activation in the anterior belly of the digastric may play a role in greater anterior displacement of the hyoid bone with firm textures.

A delicate balance must exist between neuromuscular forces acting on the hyoid to allow for anterior movement required for deflection of the epiglottis and opening of the upper esophageal sphincter (UES). As a nonmuscular structure, the epiglottis requires external forces for deflection. As the hyoid moves forward, it effectively pulls the base of the epiglottis anteriorly, thus resulting in a functional deflection. Without this anterior movement, innervated by the trigeminal (CN V) and ansa cervicalis (fibers of CN XII and cervical spinal nerve 1), the epiglottis will simply elevate and thus fail to occlude the airway entrance, requiring other mechanisms to protect the airway. Excitation of fibers of the ansa cervicalis (cervical spinal nerves 1 and 2) also will result in contraction of the anterior strap muscles, particularly the thyrohyoid muscle.[3] Both muscle groups result in supraglottic shortening, which consequently allows for compression of the quadrangular membrane over the anterior aspect of the airway entrance, thereby "corking" the laryngeal inlet. Vocal fold adduction via the vagus nerve (CN X), which innervates the interarytenoid and cricoarytenoid muscles, may have already occurred depending on bolus characteristics. Sensory mechanisms within the pharynx and larynx are critical for airway protection during swallowing and airway clearance immediately afterward. The pharyngeal plexus (CNs IX, X) provides sensory innervation to the oropharynx and hypopharynx. The superior laryngeal nerve of the vagus (CN X) receives sensory input from the larynx and trachea, whereas the recurrent laryngeal nerve of the vagus accepts afferent information from the carina, or tracheal bifurcation. Importantly, sensory input from the superior laryngeal nerve not only transmits to the NTS as the primary sensory nuclei, but also transfers directly to the NA, the motor nucleus controlling swallowing, in order to facilitate reflexive cough within milliseconds

[3]Thyrohyoid muscle innervation is inconsistently reported in the literature. Refer to Curtis et al. (1988).

of sensory receptor activation at the larynx. In summary, although the vagus nerve most directly influences the multilayered levels of airway protection, excitation of the trigeminal (CN V) and ansa cervicalis may facilitate closure in the case of impairment.

Bolus transfer through the pharynx is accomplished via contribution from the pharyngeal plexus, hypoglossal, and facial nerves. As the bolus is volitionally transferred into the oropharynx, the hypoglossal nerve innervates the styloglossus muscle to retract and elevate the tongue base. Additional contributions to this movement occur via excitation of the facial nerve (CN VII) for contraction of the stylohyoid and posterior belly of the digastric. The pharyngeal plexus (CNs IX, X) innervates the glossopharyngeus muscle, part of the superior pharyngeal constrictor, which pulls the tongue base directly back to the posterior pharyngeal wall for positive pressure on the bolus. These same nerves and muscles contribute to pharyngeal shortening and are further facilitated in this movement by the glossopharyngeal (CN IX) activation of the stylopharyngeus and pharyngeal plexus activation of the salpingopharyngeus and palatopharyngeus muscles. As base of tongue to posterior pharyngeal wall movement provides the primary pressure on the descending bolus and the pharynx shortens to bring the UES to meet the oncoming bolus, the pharyngeal plexus innervates the superior, middle, and inferior constrictor muscles sequentially to clear the tail of the bolus from the pharynx.

The UES comprises the cricopharyngeus muscle, the thyropharyngeal portion of the inferior pharyngeal constrictor, and rostral esophageal musculature (Jones, Hammer, Hoffman, & McCulloch, 2014). The rostral branch of the superior laryngeal nerve of the vagus (CN X) maintains a state of excitation at rest, which results in tonic contraction of the cricopharyngeus muscle. Bolus transport through the UES requires inhibition of this activation to allow the UES to be pulled open. The trigeminal nerve (CN V) activates the anterior belly of the digastric and mylohyoid, whereas superior root of the ansa cervicalis (fibers of CN XII and cervical spinal nerve 1) innervates the geniohyoid to exert the external traction force to open the UES. Lastly, the bolus itself encourages UES opening, with greater distension pressures of larger boluses leading to increased UES opening (Omari, Dejaeger, Tack, Van Beckevoort, & Rommel, 2013).

As all pharyngeal structures are elevating, anterior hyoid movement is critical to provide directional pull for UES opening. As the bolus passes through the UES, the pharyngeal plexus (CNs IX, X) innervates the inferior pharyngeal constrictor to squeeze the tail of the bolus into the esophagus. Post-swallow pharyngeal residual is detected in normal swallowing via mucosal sensory receptors that initiate glossopharyngeal nerve fibers (CN IX). This information relays back to the NTS and subsequently results in initiation of a clearing swallow to manage pharyngeal residual.

Although CNS structures quite literally provide the brains for swallowing by developing and finely adapting the motor sequence necessary for bolus transfer, efficient function of the peripheral nervous system is required for carrying out that plan. Importantly, testing of the peripheral system will allow the astute clinician caring for the stroke patient a basis on which to hypothesize pharyngeal physiology. Thus, clinicians should be fluent in the language and concepts of neuroscience and learn to rely on this information for differential diagnosis.

3 Normal Swallowing Anatomy and Physiology

DEFINING NORMAL AND ABNORMAL SWALLOWING

How does one define normal in the changing landscape of dysphagia research? In early clinical practice in this field, we adhered to a fairly rigorous definition of "normal swallowing," with little recognition of the innate variance in the normal deglutitive process. However, it is important to recognize that as our knowledge base expands rapidly, definitions of normal will expand as well. We have greater information available to us that is described in subsequent sections, including changes in swallowing that occur as a function of the healthy aging process, as well as variations of swallowing in healthy adults due to other factors. Data regarding these factors, including consistency of bolus and type of swallowing (single versus sequential), are addressed. These differences from the perceived norm do not represent pathology, but rather the expected adaptation of a complex physiologic system to accommodate a variety of processes. Therefore, the clinician should be cautious not to base diagnosis on an inflexible definition of impairment and consequently overdiagnose.

The clinician also should be careful not to underdiagnose impairment. Although identification of aspiration risk is critical, this cannot be the only basis for determining impairment and consequently active management. One can have significant dysphagia that generates significant consequences for nutrition and quality of life without aspiration. Avoiding pulmonary compromise in the short term is an obvious and indisputable goal, but consideration must be given to long-term outcomes. Failing to recognize seemingly benign pathophysiology may ultimately result in the development of a more consequential impairment over the long term. Both short-term and long-term objectives for intervention should be addressed.

So, again, how do we define normal? At a minimum, one could argue that "safe and efficient swallowing" is a workable definition of normal, with "unsafe and inefficient swallowing" defining abnormal. But this leads to the inevitable questions of: How do you define safe and unsafe? How do you define efficient and inefficient? These definitions may be shaped by the overall health and history of patients, their perception of disability, overall quality of life, risks associated with variance in swallowing, the type of diagnostic data collected, and the clinician's knowledge of normal. Additionally, our definition is limited or biased by the instrumentation we use for diagnosis. As availability of techniques expands, our understanding of swallowing will expand for greater diagnostic specificity. In the interim, the best one can do is to evaluate the documented range of behaviors and apply this to individual patients with all of their complexities.

An understanding of the fundamentals of swallowing is prerequisite for defining normal and abnormal swallowing. Following is a synopsis of our current understanding of normal swallowing physiology.

PHASES OF SWALLOWING

Swallowing is generally conceptualized as occurring in several distinct phases. Although these phases facilitate a common vocabulary and framework for discussion and definition, the clinician must realize that division by phase is an artificial construct. Swallowing is a continuous process with substantive interdependencies among features across the system. Isolating these features without consideration of other influences may lead the clinician to misdiagnose. As an example, patients with an impaired cricopharyngeal opening may not have a primary abnormality of the upper esophageal sphincter (UES); rather, they may have substantial gastroesophageal reflux that impacts pharyngeal bolus transport. Thus, by limiting focus to the symptomatic phase, the true source of the pathology can be overlooked, and thus treatment will likely be ineffective. However, for purposes of discussion, the delineation of phases certainly facilitates understanding. The three-phase model of oral, pharyngeal, and esophageal is more traditional; however, a more inclusive model that incorporates a pre-oral phase is used as a scaffolding in this text to discuss normal and abnormal swallowing. Given the potential impairment of cognition and attention in stroke, the recognition of preparatory behaviors is considered essential.

Pre-Oral Phase

Current models of dysphagia consider only the movement of the bolus through the aerodigestive tract. Using this traditional model, external influences such as attention, eating behavior, and feeding method, which may impact swallowing efficiency and safety, are not considered. A model of ingestion that considers both pre-swallowing and swallowing behavior has been proposed, as a strong interaction between each has been suggested, particularly in neurogenic populations (Leopold & Kagel, 1997).

Sight and smell heavily influence the perception and enjoyment of food. The mantra, "You eat with your eyes first" is proclaimed by many experienced chefs. Despite the inaccessibility of taste and smell in the medium, the proliferation of cooking programs on television makes a persuasive, albeit anecdotal, argument for the importance of pre-ingestive sensory input. The literature in food science, and increasingly in dysphagia management, provides substantive and fascinating investigation of these issues.

In the preceding chapters, we discussed the role of the cerebral cortex in modulating swallowing behavior. Research has also focused on the evaluation of olfactory input in the modulation of cortical neurophysiology. As an example, an interesting study by Ebihara and colleagues (2006) documented that inhalation of black pepper oil for 1 min before each meal for 30 days resulted in an increase in the number of swallows and a reduction in the latency of swallowing reflex in elderly and stroke patients. These functional changes were associated with increased regional cerebral blood flow in the insula and orbitofrontal cortices on single photon emission computed tomography scans. These brain areas are known to receive information from olfactory cortex. These changes were not observed following inhalation of lavender oil or distilled water, suggesting that the type of stimulus is a critical factor.

Research has also highlighted the importance of visual input in ingestive behavior. An early study by Maeda and colleagues (2004) documented decreased latency and suprahyoid muscle electromyography during liquid swallowing when individuals were first shown an image of a cold beer compared with a pair of scissors. Magnetoencephalography was utilized by Ushioda and colleagues (2012) to evaluate neural activation during the presentation of a visual cartoon of a man drinking water, time-locked to swallowing sounds. During presentation of these paired stimuli, activation of swallowing-related "mirror neurons" was observed, suggesting a key role of visual and auditory input for facilitating neural activation associated with swallowing. A subsequent study by Kober and Wood (2014) used functional near-infrared spectroscopy to evaluate cortical activation during conditions of water swallowing and mental imagination of water swallowing. Changes from resting activity in deoxygenated hemoglobin in the interior frontal gyrus were similar across the two tasks. Perhaps, as with Ebihara et al. (2006), this offers potential for rehabilitation. This also emphasizes the potential for inhibition of neural activation if sensory information is withheld. Sanders, Hoffman, and Lund (1992), in a study of residents in a nursing home who were dependent on others for oral feeding, documented that the meal was placed directly in front of the patient only 13% of the time. With the knowledge that dependency for feeding has a relatively high predictive value for the development of pneumonia (Langmore et al., 1998), clinicians would be well advised to ensure that these pre-oral issues are actively addressed.

At a purely pragmatic level, consider the patient with right hemisphere damage who presents with reduced attention and impulsivity. The patient may not monitor rate of ingestion or amount delivered to the oral cavity; moreover, this patient may not be aware of deficits. Thus, these apparent cognitive deficits that affect pre-oral phase components can significantly impact swallowing events downstream. Furthermore, factors that may be manipulated in the pre-oral phase, such as cued versus non-cued swallow and sequential versus single swallow, may modify swallowing.

Oral Phase

The oral phase begins once food or liquid enters the oral cavity. As the bolus is delivered into the oral cavity, the lips close anteriorly and the tongue contacts the velum to form a seal posteriorly to contain the bolus and prevent bolus loss. For increased consistency of a bolus, oral preparation is initiated to achieve an acceptable consistency for swallowing. This involves mixing the bolus with saliva during rotary and lateral jaw movement as well as rotary and lateral tongue movement. Preparation concludes when a bolus suitable for oral transfer is formed on the tongue.

Two events related to respiration frequently occur prior to onset of oral transfer and often with bolus loading: (1) apnea onset (Hiss, Strauss, Treole, Stuart, & Boutilier, 2004; Martin-Harris et al., 2005) and (2) approximation of the vocal folds and arytenoid cartilages (Ohmae, Logemann, Kaiser, Hanson, & Kahrilas, 1995; Shaker, Dodds, Dantas, Hogan, & Arndorfer, 1990). Although the specific onset of these events is highly variable, they are among the initial events to occur with swallowing.

Oral transfer generally is initiated by posterior lingual movement squeezing the bolus against the palate. Coordinated bolus transfer is critical for normal initiation and execution of pharyngeal events. Physiologically, the oral phase concludes with the onset of the pharyngeal response. However, for purposes of measurement in the case of substantially delayed onset of pharyngeal swallowing, it is prudent to consider termination of the oral phase when the bolus head reaches any point between the anterior faucial arch and the angle of the mandible. Duration of the oral stage is dependent on determination of the starting point (bolus versus tongue movement, bolus head versus bolus tail) and identification of the endpoint (faucial arch versus mandibular angle). However, duration of oral transfer is generally less than 1 second regardless of parameters measured.

With solids, numerous episodes of food processing followed by lingual propulsion of the triturated bolus to the oropharynx and valleculae may occur prior to elicitation of pharyngeal swallowing (Dua, Ren, Bardan, Xie, & Shaker, 1997; Hiiemae & Palmer, 1999; Palmer, Rudin, Lara, & Crompton, 1992). It is not atypical for masticated food to accumulate in the valleculae for up to 10 seconds in healthy adults before initiation of pharyngeal swallowing (Hiiemae & Palmer, 1999). Initiation of lingual propulsion for food transport typically occurs during exhalation (Matsuo & Palmer, 2015); however, during bolus aggregation, there is no consistent respiratory pattern (Matsuo, Hiiemae, Gonzalez-Fernandez, & Palmer, 2008). That is, an individual may inhale, exhale, or pause respiration. Depending on the duration of aggregation, multiple respiratory cycles may occur. Additionally, a liquid bolus may accumulate in the valleculae and/or hypopharynx prior to onset of pharyngeal swallowing during sequential drinking (Chi-Fishman & Sonies, 2000; Daniels & Foundas, 2001). That is, during sequential swallowing via a cup or straw, lingual propulsion of the liquid may occur multiple times until pharyngeal swallowing is elicited. The accumulation of liquid in the pharynx during sequential swallowing may occur with the larynx lowered and epiglottis upright or with the larynx partially elevated and epiglottis inverted (Daniels & Foundas, 2001).

Pharyngeal Phase

Transition from the oral phase to the pharyngeal phase of swallowing occurs with elicitation of pharyngeal swallowing. Elicitation of pharyngeal swallowing can be classified as part of the oral phase (Martin-Harris et al., 2008) or as part of the pharyngeal phase as in this text. As the oropharynx houses shared sensorimotor areas responsible for production of protective reflexes such as gag, swallowing, and emesis, accurate afferent sensory input is critical for the initiation of these varied responses (Capra, 1995; Miller, 1972). Mechanoreceptors widely distributed across the oral cavity and tongue can detect velocity of tissue movement; this mechanical sensation from the posterior oral region can elicit pharyngeal swallowing when paired with input from chemo- and thermosensitive receptors (Miller, 1972, 2002; Steele & Miller, 2010). Sensory input can further modulate the contraction of muscles involved in pharyngeal swallowing, with research indicating that the duration of electromyography (EMG) activity increases as bolus volume and thickness increase (Hrycyshyn & Basmajian, 1972).

Onset of the pharyngeal phase of swallowing is hallmarked by initiation of hyolaryngeal excursion, sometimes referred to as "hyoid burst" (Nam, Oh, & Han, 2015). Initiation of maximum excursion generally occurs when the bolus head is located between the anterior faucial arch and angle of the mandible. Continued research is expanding our traditional concept of bolus location at swallowing onset. As discussed earlier, as the bolus is processed during mastication, a portion of it is propelled into the valleculae until processing of the remaining material is completed, at which point pharyngeal swallowing is elicited (Dua et al., 1997; Hiiemae & Palmer, 1999; Palmer et al., 1992). Stephen, Taves, Smith, and Martin (2005) evaluated the position of the bolus head at initiation of the pharyngeal stage on videofluoroscopic swallowing studies (VFSS) in healthy volunteers (n = 10). The bolus head position at the onset of swallowing was typically below the level of the mandibular angle, with substantial variability across swallows. Furthermore, during sequential swallowing of liquids from either a cup or a straw, the bolus is frequently propelled to the hypopharynx prior to onset of pharyngeal swallowing (Chi-Fishman & Sonies, 2000; Daniels et al., 2004; Daniels & Foundas, 2001). Further research also reveals considerable variability within and across individuals in bolus positioning of single liquid volumes at onset of pharyngeal swallowing (Martin-Harris, Brodsky, Michel, Lee, & Walters, 2007; Stephen et al., 2005). It is not atypical to have the bolus inferior to the angle of the mandible at onset of pharyngeal swallowing, particularly in healthy older adults. This more inferior location of the bolus at onset of pharyngeal swallowing is not associated with airway invasion in healthy adults.

The pharyngeal stage of swallowing involves the complex coordination of six components: (1) velopharyngeal closure, (2) laryngeal closure, (3) hyoid and laryngeal elevation, (4) base of tongue retraction, (5) posterior pharyngeal wall contraction, and (6) UES opening. The temporal coupling of these events in coordination with cessation of breathing is critical for safe and efficient swallowing.

Velopharyngeal closure involves retraction of the soft palate, medial movement of the pharyngeal wall, and anterior bulging of the adenoid pad. This closure provides a seal between the nasopharynx and oropharynx and contributes to the increase in pharyngeal pressure (Perlman, Schultz, & VanDaele, 1993).

Laryngeal valving involves multiple levels, from inferior to superior: true vocal folds (TVFs), false vocal folds, arytenoids, aryepiglottic folds, and epiglottis. Although onset of glottic closure is one of the first events of swallowing (Ohmae et al., 1995; Shaker et al., 1990), complete TVF adduction along the entire length of the fold does not occur until after onset of laryngeal elevation (Ohmae et al., 1995). With regard to posterior glottic closure, the true and false vocal folds adduct through activation of the interarytenoid and lateral cricoarytenoid muscles (CN X). This contributes to a forward and downward tilting of the arytenoids to further close the glottic space (Dodds, Stewart, & Logeman, 1990). Further, as a result of epiglottic deflection, the quadrangular membrane becomes compressed over the anterior glottis, providing yet another layer of protection. Based on 320-row area detector computed tomography imaging, Inamoto et al. (2011) evaluated specific timing of laryngeal closure during swallowing. In healthy swallowing of liquids, it was revealed that closure of the TVFs, closure of the laryngeal vestibule at the arytenoid to epiglottic base, and epiglottic inversion occurred almost simultaneously and was immediately followed by UES opening (Fujii et al., 2011; Inamoto et al., 2011). Entry of material into the pharynx during normal mastication or with pharyngeal water injection in an experimental paradigm is associated with brief partial TVF adduction, which is known as a pharyngoglottal closure reflex (Dua et al., 1997; Shaker et al., 2003). It is suggested that this reflex is preventive of pre-swallow aspiration.

Superior and anterior movement of the hyoid bone and the larynx is achieved through contraction of the suprahyoid muscles and the thyrohyoid muscle. Superior and anterior movement of the hyoid and larynx occurs due to the suprahyoid muscles (anterior belly of the digastric, mylohyoid, posterior belly of the digastric, stylohyoid, and geniohyoid). The superior movement of the hyolaryngeal complex facilitates supraglottic closure, and the anterior motion contributes to the opening of the UES (Jacob, Kahrilas, Logemann, Shah, & Ha, 1989).

Base of tongue contact with the posterior pharyngeal wall is critical to create the dynamic pressure necessary to drive the bolus inferiorly through the pharynx (Cerenko, McConnel, & Jackson, 1989; McConnel, 1988). Base of tongue retraction involves continued posterior movement after passage of the bolus until the tongue base contacts the posterior pharyngeal wall. Base of tongue contact with the posterior pharyngeal wall yields a buildup of pressure to drive the bolus through the pharynx. As the tongue propels the bolus into the pharynx and the tongue base makes contact with the posterior pharyngeal wall, contraction of the pharyngeal constrictors occurs superiorly to inferiorly. The superior, middle, and inferior pharyngeal constrictors are oriented obliquely (Miller, 2002). This allows not only a reduction of intraluminal space but enables superior and posterior movement to maximize pharyngeal shortening. This descending sequence aids in clearing pharyngeal residue but minimally facilitates bolus propulsion (Kahrilas, Logemann, Lin, & Ergun, 1992). Pharyngeal contraction involves two processes: (1) pharyngeal shortening, which decreases the distance the bolus must travel and modifies pharyngeal recesses to prevent residual, and (2) pharyngeal constrictor contraction, which progresses superiorly to inferiorly.

The UES comprises the cricopharyngeus (CP) muscle, the inferior pharyngeal constrictor, and the rostral esophageal musculature (Williams, Pal, Brasseur, & Cook, 2001). When contracted, the CP muscle prevents passage of air into the stomach and prevents flow of esophageal contents from passing into the pharynx. The UES is contracted at rest through a combination of neural input and passive elastic forces

(Cock, Jones, Hammer, Omari, & McCulloch, 2017). Therefore, opening of the UES is multifaceted, requiring brainstem-driven neural relaxation of the CP muscle alongside propulsion forces from the bolus itself and mechanical opening from anterior-superior movement of the hyolaryngeal complex (Omari et al., 2015; Williams et al., 2001). In a recent study of healthy participants (n = 8), Cock et al. evaluated timing of relaxation and mechanical opening of the UES with simultaneous intramuscular cricopharyngeal EMG and high-resolution impedance manometry. Results indicate that UES relaxation and opening increased with increasing bolus sizes, and the relationship in timing between UES deactivation and submental muscle activity differs based on bolus size as well (Cock et al., 2017; Cook, Dodds, Dantas, Massey, et al., 1989; Kahrilas, Dodds, Dent, Logemann, & Shaker, 1988; Williams et al., 2001). As bolus size increased, UES opening occurred consistently earlier, but submental muscle activity changed from occurring before to after peak UES opening (Cock et al., 2017). This may be preliminary evidence that UES relaxation can arise directly from neural input to the CP itself due to sensory feedback of bolus forces manually pushing through the UES, as opposed to occurring as a result of activation of submental muscle mechanoreceptors (Cock et al., 2017; Cook, 1993; Omari et al., 2015; Walczak, Jones, & McCullough, 2017).

As with oral duration, there are varying reference points used to mark onset and offset of pharyngeal transfer. For onset, the points of measure include arrival of the bolus head at the angle of the mandible (Robbins, Hamilton, Lof, & Kempster, 1992) or arrival of the bolus tail at the posterior tonsillar pillar (Shaw et al., 1995). For offset, measurement points may include passage of the bolus tail through the UES (Robbins et al., 1992) or UES closure (Shaw et al., 1995). Regardless of measure used, duration of movement of the bolus through the pharynx is approximately one second.

Breathing and swallowing are structurally linked via the oropharynx. Coordination of breathing and swallowing is exquisitely timed to prevent aspiration. Apnea, or cessation of respiration, occurs during swallowing. The onset of apnea is highly variable. As noted earlier, the onset of apnea frequently occurs prior to onset of oral transfer. If it does not occur prior to bolus transfer, it is suggested that apnea should occur at onset of transfer or immediately following (Hiss et al., 2004). In a study of swallowing-respiratory coordination of 20 healthy participants, Kelly, Huckabee, Jones, and Carroll (2007) found the largest proportion of swallows occurred mid-expiration, with immediate post-swallow expiration in voluntary, spontaneous, and reflexive swallowing conditions. This pattern allows post-swallow expiration to clear any trace penetration, supplemented by further layers of airway protection (Widdicombe, Addington, Fontana, & Stephens, 2011). Resumption of respiration is more specific, occurring with lowering of the hyoid (Martin-Harris et al., 2005). Expiration preceding and following swallowing is the predominant respiratory phase pattern in healthy individuals (Hiss et al., 2004; Martin-Harris et al., 2005). Whereas inspiration after swallowing rarely occurs in healthy adults, inspiration prior to swallowing may occur in 10% to 20% of swallows (Martin-Harris et al., 2005; Perlman, He, Barkmeier, & Van Leer, 2005).

Esophageal Phase

The upper one-third of the esophagus is composed of striated muscle and the lower two-thirds is composed of smooth muscle. The esophagus is bound by the UES superiorly and the lower esophageal sphincter (LES) inferiorly. Both of these sphincters are actively contracted at rest but relax during swallowing, belching, and vomiting. This contracted resting state prevents retrograde flow of material into the upper aerodigestive tract. The esophageal phase of swallowing involves a sequential peristaltic wave that propels food and liquid into the stomach. In contrast to the rapid pharyngeal phase, normal bolus transit time of the esophageal phase of swallowing varies between 8 and 20 seconds (Dodds, Hogan, Reid, Stewart, & Arndorfer, 1973). The esophageal phase consists of a peristaltic wave propagating the bolus along the lumen and is completed when the bolus is propelled through the LES (Goyal & Chaudhury, 2008). Interestingly, the esophagus has little to no EMG activity at rest, which may reflect deglutitive inhibition prior to peristaltic contraction (Jean, 2001).

Just as the oral stage of swallowing can affect timing and amplitude of pharyngeal biomechanics (Ali, Cook, Laundl, Wallace, & De Carle, 1997), esophageal swallowing can affect the pharyngeal response and vice versa (Allen, White, Leonard, & Belafsky, 2012). In patients with a distal esophageal impairment (e.g., ring), 58% of patients localized symptoms in the pharyngeal region (Smith, Ott, Gelfand, & Chen, 1998). Similarly, Scharitzer et al. (2002) reported that of more than 3,000 patients undergoing VFSS for evaluation of pharyngeal dysphagia, 14% (n = 434) presented with primarily esophageal impairment, despite complaints of pharyngeal dysphagia and globus (Scharitzer et al., 2002). As stated by Allen et al. (2012), "up to one third of patients with the sensation of cervical dysphagia will have an esophageal cause for the symptom" (p. 264). As discussed in Chapter 20, O'Rourke et al. (2014) evaluated the effect of voluntary pharyngeal swallowing maneuvers, including the Mendelsohn maneuver and effortful swallowing, on esophageal physiology in healthy volunteers (n = 10). The voluntary maneuvers affected the occurrence of non-peristaltic esophageal swallowing responses, with fewer non-peristaltic swallows during effortful swallowing (33%) compared with an increase in non-peristaltic swallows during Mendelsohn maneuvers (66%). The ability of the pharyngeal phase of swallowing to directly affect the esophageal response highlights synergies in the complex modulation of sensorimotor control for swallowing.

Variability in Swallowing

Although specific events for normal swallowing are described above, there is considerable variability in the system associated with intrinsic (e.g., aging) and extrinsic (e.g., bolus volume) factors. The influences of specific factors on normal swallowing are summarized in Table 3–1.

For example, normal single sip size ranges from 20 to 30 mL (Adnerhill, Ekberg, & Groher, 1989; Bennett, van Lieshout, Pelletier, & Steele, 2009; Lawless, Bender, Oman, & Pelletier, 2003). Older individuals swallow significantly less amounts (average 14 mL) compared with younger individuals (average 32 mL) (Bennett et al., 2009). Moreover, sip size is increased in males (approximately 25 mL) compared with females (approximately 20 mL), with greater cup size, and with cup drinking compared with straw drinking (Lawless et al., 2003). Sip size, however, decreases across sequential swallows. This information on influences that affect sip size can help the clinician distinguish between normal and disordered swallowing patterns and facilitate the establishment of a protocol for clinical and instrumental swallowing evaluations.

Table 3–1. The Influence of Intrinsic and Extrinsic Variables

Increased Age
• Decreased sip size (Bennett, Van Lieshout, Pelletier, & Steele, 2009) • Increased oral transit time (Cook et al., 1994; Shaw et al., 1995) • Increased stage transition duration (Kim, McCullough, & Asp, 2005; Logemann et al., 2000; Robbins et al., 1992; Tracy et al., 1989) • Increased volume required to evoke a pharyngeal swallow (Shaker et al., 1994) • Increased airway invasion (Butler et al., 2010; Butler, Stuart, Markley, Feng, & Kritchevsky, 2018; Butler, Stuart, Markley, & Rees, 2009; Daggett, Logemann, Rademaker, & Pauloski, 2006; Daniels et al., 2004; McCullough, Rosenbek, Wertz, Suiter, & McCoy, 2007) • Increased pharyngeal residue (Cook et al., 1994) • Decreased isometric tongue pressure (Robbins, Levine, Wood, Roecker, & Luschei, 1995) • Decreased onset of submental contraction (Ding, Logemann, Larson, & Rademaker, 2003) • Decreased extent of hyoid movement (Kern et al., 1999; Logemann et al., 2000) • Decreased pharyngeal and laryngeal sensation (Aviv et al., 1994) • Reduced pharyngeal contraction (Tracy et al., 1989) • Decreased pharyngeal wall thickness and increased pharyngeal lumen area (Molfenter et al., 2015) • Delayed onset of upper esophageal sphincter (UES) relaxation (Shaw et al., 1995) • Increased intrabolus pressure (Kern et al., 1999; Shaw et al., 1995) • Increased duration of UES opening (Rademaker, Pauloski, Colangelo, & Logemann, 1998; Robbins et al., 1992) • Decreased diameter of UES opening (Logemann et al., 2000; Shaw et al., 1995; Tracy et al., 1989) • Increased duration of swallowing apnea (Hiss, Treole, & Stuart, 2001) • Increased incidence of inhalation after swallowing (Martin-Harris et al., 2005)
Increased Volume
• Bolus held more posteriorly in the oral cavity (Tracy et al., 1989) • Decreased oral transit time (Rademaker et al., 1998; Tracy et al., 1989) • Decreased stage transition duration (Rademaker et al., 1998) • Earlier onset of palatal elevation (Dantas et al., 1990) • Increased duration of velopharyngeal closure (Rademaker et al., 1998) • Earlier onset of anterior tongue base movement (Dantas et al., 1990)

Table 3–1. *continued*

- Earlier onset of laryngeal elevation (Dantas et al., 1990)
- Increased extent of hyoid movement (Dodds et al., 1988; Logemann et al., 2000)
- Increased vertical hyoid peak velocity (Nagy, Molfenter, Péladeau-Pigeon, Stokely, & Steele, 2014)
- Increased duration of laryngeal closure (Logemann et al., 1992; Molfenter & Steele, 2013)
- Increased intrabolus pressure (Jacob et al., 1989; Kern et al., 1999)
- Earlier onset of UES opening (Cook, Dodds, Dantas, Kern, et al., 1989; Dantas et al., 1990)
- Decreased duration from laryngeal closure to UES opening (Molfenter & Steele, 2013)
- Increased diameter of UES opening (Dantas et al., 1990)
- Increased duration of UES opening (Dantas et al., 1990; Molfenter & Steele, 2013; Rademaker et al., 1998; Tracy et al., 1989)
- Increased pharyngeal transit time (Molfenter & Steele, 2013)
- Earlier onset of swallowing apnea (Hiss et al., 2004)
- Increased duration of swallowing apnea (Hiss et al., 2001)
- Increased occurrence of airway invasion (Allen, White, Leonard, & Belafsky, 2010), in males (Butler et al., 2018)

Increased Consistency

- Increased oral transit time (Dantas et al., 1990)
- Increased stage transition duration (Robbins et al., 1992)
- Increased oral pressure (Pouderoux & Kahrilas, 1995; Shaker, Cook, Dodds, & Hogan, 1988)
- Increased amplitude and duration of contraction of the inferior orbicularis oris, submental, and infrahyoid muscles (Ding et al., 2003)
- Increased duration of velar excursion (Robbins et al., 1992)
- Increased anterior and superior hyoid peak velocity (Nagy, Molfenter, Péladeau-Pigeon, Stokely, & Steele, 2015)
- Increased laryngeal elevation (Shaker et al., 1990)
- Increased duration pharyngeal contraction (Dantas et al., 1990)
- Increased duration of UES opening (Dantas et al., 1990)
- Later onset of swallowing apnea (Hiss et al., 2004)
- Lower quiet breathing lung volumes (McFarland et al., 2016)
- Decreased airway invasion (Allen et al., 2010)

continues

Table 3–1. *continued*

Taste
• Increased lingual-palatal pressure (Abdul Wahab, Jones, & Huckabee, 2011; Nagy, Steele, & Pelletier, 2014; Pelletier & Dhanaraj, 2006; Pelletier & Steele, 2014) • Earlier onset of submental and infrahyoid contraction (Ding et al., 2003) • Increased submental amplitude (Ding et al., 2003; Leow, Huckabee, Sharma, & Tooley, 2007; Pelletier & Steele, 2014) • Increased pharyngeal pressure (Palmer, McCulloch, Jaffe, & Neel, 2005) • Reduced swallowing speed (volume swallowed per second) (Chee, Arshad, Singh, Mistry, & Hamdy, 2005) • Increased number of swallows to drink 50 mL (Chee et al., 2005)
Sequential Swallowing (compared with single swallows)
• Decreased oral transit time (Chi-Fishman & Sonies, 2000) • Increased stage transition duration (Chi-Fishman & Sonies, 2000) • Decreased duration of UES opening (Chi-Fishman & Sonies, 2000) • Repetitive activation and partial deactivation of surface electromyographic waveform patterns (Chi-Fishman & Sonies, 2000) • Reduced amplitude and velocity of hyoid movement (Chi-Fishman & Sonies, 2002b) • Two patterns of hyolaryngeal elevation (HLC) movement: lowering of the HLC with the epiglottis returning to upright between swallows; partial HLC elevation with continued epiglottic inversion between swallows (Daniels et al., 2004; Daniels & Foundas, 2001) • Variable breathing patterns surrounding the ingestion cycle (Dozier, Brodsky, Michel, Walters, & Martin-Harris, 2006; Hegland, Huber, Pitts, Davenport, & Sapienza, 2011) • Increased ventilation after swallowing (Lederlie, Hoit, & Barkmeier-Kraemer, 2012)
Cued Swallows (compared with noncued)
• Bolus held more posteriorly in oral cavity (Daniels, Schroeder, DeGeorge, Corey, & Rosenbek, 2007) • Decreased oral transit time (Daniels et al., 2007) • Decreased stage transition duration (Daniels et al., 2007) • Reduced bolus advancement to the pyriform sinus at swallow onset (Nagy et al., 2013) • Increased pharyngeal transit time (Nagy et al., 2013) • Increased pharyngeal response time (Nagy et al., 2013) • Lower quiet breathing lung volumes (McFarland et al., 2016)

4 Swallowing Screening in Patients with Acute Stroke

BACKGROUND OF SCREENING SWALLOWING IN STROKE

Early detection of aspiration risk in acute stroke is critical as it allows for immediate intervention, thereby reducing mortality, morbidity, length of hospitalization, and health care costs (Hinchey et al., 2005; Martino, Pron, & Diamant, 2000; Odderson & McKenna, 1993). As such, screening of swallowing has become a best practice in the management of patients with acute stroke and is the important first step in the evaluation process for dysphagia in stroke (Figure 4–1). Screening can be defined as a brief assessment that is easy to administer and minimally invasive. No diagnosis is made with a screening. For patients admitted with suspected stroke, the purpose of swallowing screening is to determine who is *at risk* for aspiration and/or dysphagia. During the acute stroke workup, the focus should be on rapidly determining aspiration risk for patient safety in order to quickly provide oral medication and address patient needs such as fluid intake. After the emergent stroke workup, formal swallowing evaluation by the speech pathologist is necessary to fully evaluate oropharyngeal swallowing and determine if an instrumental swallowing evaluation is warranted. Screening results may be either positive or negative. If the screening results are negative (i.e., individual passes), oral intake without any specific modifications can be ordered by other members of the multidisciplinary team. In this case, referral to speech pathology for a formal swallowing evaluation would be dependent on hospital protocol. On the other hand, if screening results are positive (i.e., individual fails), the individual is made nil per os/nothing by mouth (NPO/NBM), including medication, and referral to speech pathology is expedited. It is important to note that compensatory strategies (posture or diet modification) should *not* be implemented based on the results of a screening.

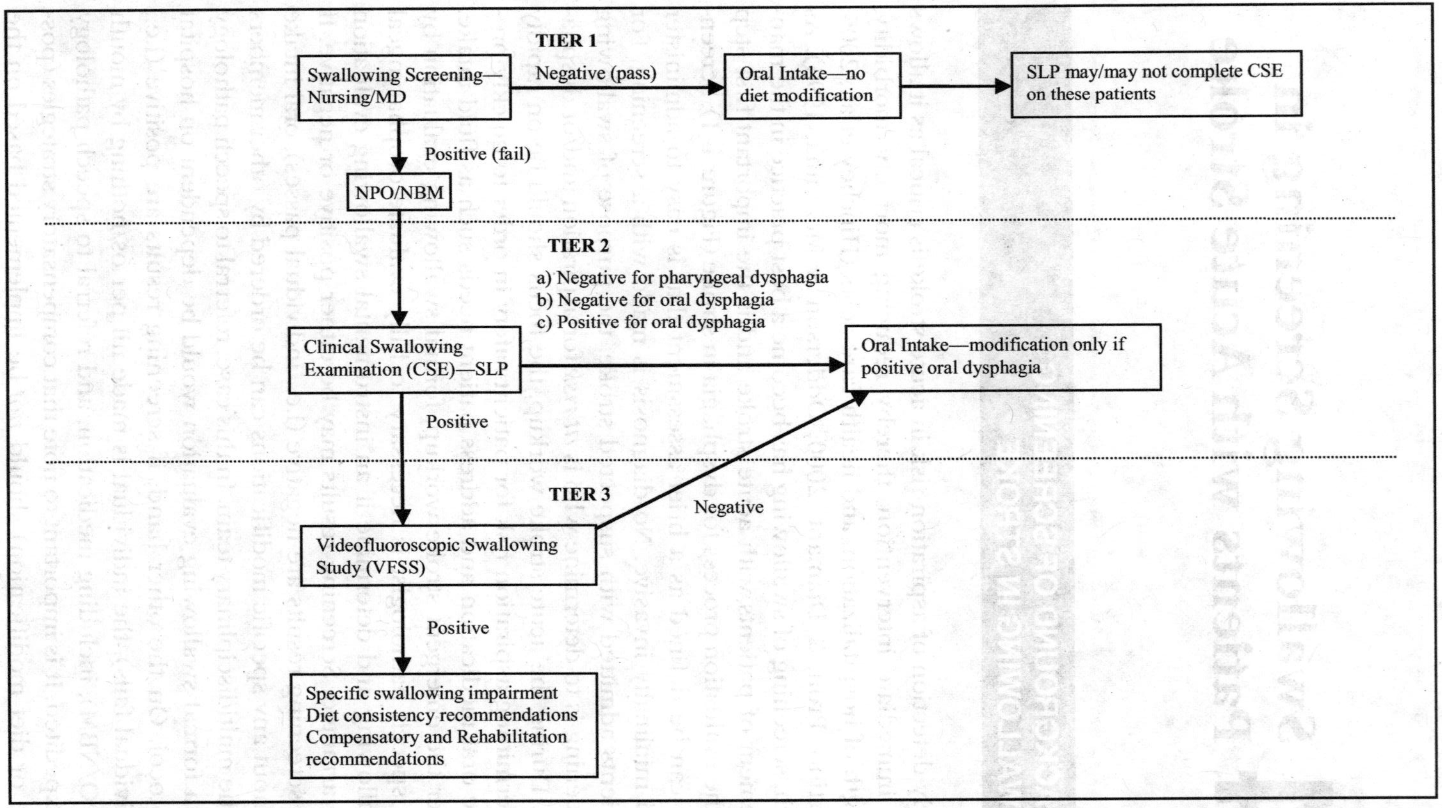

Figure 4–1. Levels of swallowing assessment.

When a consistent swallowing screening is in place, morbidity associated with aspiration decreases (Hinchey et al., 2005; Odderson, Keaton, & McKenna, 1995), health care providers' adherence to screening guidelines is improved (Hinchey et al., 2005), and there is earlier administration of first-dose aspirin (Power, Cross, Roberts, & Tyrrell, 2007). Stroke registry review revealed that individuals were more likely to fail swallowing screening if they were older, had multiple comorbidities, including history of stroke and dementia, demonstrated weakness and/or disordered speech, were more likely to be admitted from long-term care facilities, and had more severe stroke (Joundi et al., 2017). Moreover, failing swallowing screening was associated with pneumonia, disability and dependence, reduced discharge to home, and increased incidence of mortality at 1 year. It is important to note that these findings were equally evident in individuals with mild stroke even though these individuals were less likely to receive swallowing screening. This finding is important in light of previous research demonstrating that health care professionals have a tendency to selectively complete swallowing screening based on stroke severity and not perform screening on patients with low stroke scale scores (Lakshminarayan et al., 2010; Masrur et al., 2013), even though dysphagia and aspiration are evident in individuals with mild stroke (Daniels et al., 2017; Daniels, Pathak, Rosenbek, Morgan, & Anderson, 2016).

The inclusion of swallowing screening prior to the administration of food, liquid, or medication, including aspirin, in individuals presenting with stroke symptoms is part of many national stroke guidelines (Casaubon et al., 2015; Jauch et al., 2013; Nice Guidelines, 2008, updated 2017). While evaluation of swallowing prior to oral intake including administration of oral medication had previously been "recommended" in the American Heart Association/American Stroke Association (AHA/ASA) acute ischemic stroke (AIS) guidelines (Jauch et al., 2013), the initial version of the 2018 AHA/ASA AIS guidelines indicated that it was "reasonable" to complete swallowing screening, but not mandatory (Powers et al., 2018). This less forceful recommendation of swallowing screening implementation was based, in part, on a recent study which reported that there was insufficient information from three randomized controlled trials to determine if swallowing screening reduces morbidity and mortality in patients with stroke (Smith et al., 2018). This change in screening recommendation along with many others in the 2018 guidelines has proven controversial, resulting in the AHA/ASA rescinding the guidelines with many sections, including dysphagia, deleted and with a clarifying work and revision currently in progress.

COMPONENTS OF A GOOD SCREENING TOOL

All good testing tools, whether diagnostic or screening, must be valid, reliable, and feasible. Validity of a swallowing screening tool (SST) is critical; however, since disciplines without expertise in dysphagia may be involved in screening swallowing, issues surrounding education, sustainability of skills, and feasibility become of even greater importance.

Validity

Validity is the degree to which a test measures what it is purported to measure (Sackett, Strauss, Richardson, Rosenberg, & Hayes, 2000; Streiner, 2003). In screening, validity is frequently measured in terms of *sensitivity* and *specificity*. Sensitivity is the probability that a clinical sign (e.g., cough with water) will be present given that an impairment (e.g., aspiration) is present. High sensitivity yields low false negative results; that is, the clinician can be confident that most patients with aspiration are identified. Conversely, if the SST has low sensitivity in predicting aspiration, false negative rates will be high. Patients would have a negative screening, yet they would actually be aspirating. Specificity is the probability that a clinical sign will be absent given that an impairment is absent. A test with high specificity will have a limited number of false positive results; the majority of patients with negative screening results will not aspirate. Low specificity, however, would result in a high false positive result, with a large percentage of patients without aspiration having a positive SST.

Ultimately, high sensitivity appears to be the most important feature in a stroke SST due to increased morbidity and mortality associated with aspiration, which necessitates the requirement for low false negative results. Frequently, specificity will be sacrificed to achieve high sensitivity; however, low specificity cannot be ignored. At a minimum, it can delay the receipt of medication and nutrition and lead to overreferral to speech pathology. At its most severe, if speech pathology evaluation is delayed, it can result in the placement of an unwarranted nasogastric tube (NGT) for feeding, which is associated with medical complications (Ciocon, Silverstone, Graver, & Foley, 1988), particularly in individuals with acute stroke (Brogan, Langdon, Brookes, Budgeon, & Blacker, 2014; Langdon, Lee, & Binns, 2009). Hence, accuracy in identification of individuals with suspected aspiration would logically appear greatest when using a tool with both high sensitivity and high specificity.

If an SST with both high sensitivity and specificity cannot be identified, then these two measures must be balanced with the needs of the hospital. If speech pathology services are readily available on a daily basis, then high sensitivity may be favored over high specificity. If speech pathology services are limited—for instance, weekend coverage is not available—notably reduced specificity would not be acceptable. However, if speech pathologists agree that swallowing screening is an important best practice for stroke and that our subsequent evaluation is critical prior to oral intake with a positive screening, then it is incumbent upon our profession to provide services in a timely fashion in order to prevent prolonged durations of NPO/NBM status and prevent unnecessary insertion of NGTs. In cases of delayed speech pathology evaluation or limited services, telepractice may prove useful. In this model, speech pathologists who are not on site could direct and interpret another health care professional administering a clinical swallowing examination (CSE) via a videoconferencing link. Preliminary research using this model is promising (Morrell et al., 2017). Another option for delayed speech pathology evaluation could be serial screening by the nurse. That is, swallowing is rescreened every shift (approximately every 8 hours) in patients who have an initial positive screening. If a subsequent screening result is negative, oral intake can be initiated, but speech pathology follow-up with this patient would appear warranted. Of course, both notions require further study to determine feasibility and accuracy.

Two other important factors in validity are *positive predictive value* (PPV) and *negative predictive value* (NPV). Unlike sensitivity and specificity, which provide information concerning correct classification of individuals who do or do not present with a positive SST, predictive values deal with the proportion of individuals with or without a positive SST who do and do not have aspiration identified on an instrumental swallowing examination (e.g., videofluoroscopic swallowing study [VFSS]). PPV is the probability of having the condition (e.g., aspiration) if the screening is positive (i.e., fail the screening). Low PPV indicates an increase in false positive results. NPV is the probability of not having the condition (e.g., aspiration) if the screening is negative (i.e., pass the screening). Low NPV indicates an increase in false negative results. Predictive values are highly influenced by the prevalence of the condition (e.g., aspiration) in the studied population. As with sensitivity and specificity, the higher the predictive value, the better. Last, one should consider *likelihood ratios*, primarily positive likelihood ratios greater than 1. A positive likelihood ratio combines sensitivity and specificity to determine if a test result (e.g., positive aspiration screening) changes the probability in the occurrence of a condition (e.g., presence of aspiration on VFSS). Likelihood ratios are not dependent on the population and are thought to be a more stable measure than predictive values.

Reliability

A stroke SST must be reliable. For the purposes of swallowing screening, there are two important components of reliability: *administration* and *interpretation*. In most studies of swallowing screening, generally only one component of reliability is measured or both components are combined when reporting results. It is important to address both components of reliability separately, as each can affect the accuracy of the SST findings. Reliability in administration involves consistent use of directions and procedures to deliver the screening items. This can be measured across or within the individual clinicians. If swallowing 5 mL of water is a screening item, does the health care provider consistently measure out the volume with syringe or use a teaspoon, or does he/she "eyeball" a small amount of water for the patient to swallow or administer the bolus with a syringe? Once a test is administered, patient response must be interpreted. With interpretation, we are asking if the screener can make an accurate judgment as to the presence or absence of a behavior (e.g., the presence of wet voice after swallow). This can be evaluated in terms of the ability of two independent observers to make the same judgment about behavior (interrater reliability) or the consistency of the screener to make the same judgment in the same patient (intrarater reliability). In acute stroke, patients may improve or decline rapidly, thus SST results could change, and it may be difficult to re-administer certain items due to patient safety concerns (e.g., 90 mL water, if a patient coughed during the first screening). These factors make assessing intrarater reliability difficult unless the reliability is tested with audio and/or video recording. Thus, the best method to assess reliability would be to have one person (nurse) administer and interpret the SST and have one or more potential screeners (i.e., speech pathologists and nurses) simultaneously but without discussion also interpret each of the behaviors on the screening tool to determine if interpretation is the same.

If health care providers cannot consistently administer screening items across patients or agree on presence or absence of observations on an SST, the information provided by the tool is invalid and should not be the basis for clinical decision making. Reliability is no easy task to achieve even for speech pathologists who can demonstrate inconsistent reliability on the CSE (McCullough et al., 2000). With swallowing screening, nurses or other health care providers without expertise in dysphagia are the individuals who typically administer the stroke SST. Hence, the simplicity of the SST and the training involved would intuitively appear paramount in facilitating reliability. When these factors are considered, nurses can achieve reliability at the same level as speech pathologists (Anderson, Pathak, Rosenbek, Morgan, & Daniels, 2016; Daniels et al., 2015).

In addition to ensuring initial attainment of reliability, sustainability of accurate administration and interpretation of the SST are imperative. That is, are health care providers able to maintain reliability across a sustained period of time following the initial training? Given the limited training, lack of expertise in dysphagia, and extensive demands on their time and focus, can nurses and/or physicians accurately and consistently administer the SST over time without extensive initial training or subsequent training reviews during the course of the year? Anderson et al. (2016) found that the accuracy rate for the administration and interpretation of swallowing screening items was maximized at 20 screening opportunities. This indicates that with feedback and repeated opportunities to practice, maintenance of skills by nurses is achievable.

Feasibility

Equally important is an SST's feasibility. How easily can it be implemented? This is critical, particularly for a nurse- or physician-administered tool to screen swallowing in individuals admitted with suspected stroke. As noted above, these health care providers are involved in multiple aspects of the patient's care. The most valid and reliable SST is rendered ineffective if it is too time-consuming or complicated to implement, thus leading to low adherence. If these health care providers do not find the SST to be feasible, or they cannot obtain and sustain reliability in implementing and interpreting the SST, or speech pathology identifies that the process of skill training and maintenance requires more time demands than completion of the actual screening, then a speech pathologist may truly be the ideal professional to provide the screening. For a feasible SST, one should consider education requirements, administration time and ease of completing the items, and finally, documentation. A swallowing screening that is completed but not documented is little better than not completing swallowing screening.

MODELS FOR SCREENING IMPLEMENTATION

Several models for the implementation of screening swallowing in patients with acute stroke have been suggested (American Speech-Language-Hearing, 2009). Each model has advantages and disadvantages. Members of the dysphagia team at each medical facility must determine which model is best for their hospital.

Model 1

Trained professionals other than speech pathologists (i.e., nurses and physicians) administer the stroke SST prior to any oral intake, including medication. If the screening results are negative, oral intake without any swallowing restrictions is initiated. Speech pathology is not consulted to evaluate swallowing in these individuals. If screening results are positive, the patient maintains NPO/NBM status, and referral to speech pathology is expedited.

The primary advantages of this model are rapid completion of screening by trained frontline health care providers and no substantial delay of oral intake, including medications such as aspirin, in individuals with a negative screening. The primary disadvantage of this model with patients with stroke is that speech pathology, the discipline with expertise in oropharyngeal dysphagia, is not evaluating swallowing in every patient in this high-risk population. For example, diet adjustments or mealtime recommendations may be required due to cognitive, not swallowing, deficits (e.g., patients with right hemispheric stroke who demonstrate significant impulsive behavior). This would not be identified with a screening. Speech pathology input in this case would be dependent upon a consult to evaluate cognition. Another disadvantage is the potential for delay in speech pathology evaluation in individuals with a positive screening if they are admitted outside the window of time in which speech pathology works, which is frequently an 8-hour shift during the day and no weekend coverage.

Model 2

As in Model 1, the nurse or physician administers the screening tool; however, speech pathology is consulted to evaluate all individuals regardless of the results of the screening. Speech pathology evaluation, generally a CSE, is completed as quickly as possible for individuals with a positive screening; and for individuals with a negative screening, the CSE is completed within a designated timeframe from the screening, e.g., 48 hours. An advantage of this model is that while waiting for the speech pathology evaluation, oral intake is not delayed for individuals with a negative screening, and speech pathology evaluation can be prioritized for individuals with a positive screening. It is important to note that the goal of this model is not to evaluate appropriateness of diet in those with a negative screening result. Rather, this model allows speech pathology to complete a comprehensive evaluation and make the final determination concerning the presence or absence of dysphagia in all patients with stroke, as well as make appropriate recommendations. Thus, the individual with severe cognitive deficits that could affect swallowing safety as described in Model 1 would be evaluated by a speech pathologist. Literature suggests that given the cost of treating pneumonia, completion of a VFSS in all patients with stroke may be warranted (Wilson & Howe, 2012). While this may be extreme, Model 2 does allow for evaluation of all patients by a speech pathologist, regardless of results from the screening administered by a nurse or physician. The primary disadvantage of this model is the use of limited speech pathology resources in patients with a negative screening.

Model 3

All patients admitted with stroke symptoms are automatically referred to speech pathology for screening or assessment, bypassing nursing or physician involvement in the screening process. As is obvious with this model, a significant delay in screening is likely, given that patients are admitted at all hours every day, not just the 8 to 10 hours typically on weekdays when speech pathology works. Needless to say, it would be difficult to keep individuals NPO/NBM prior to speech pathology assessment when using this model.

Model 4

Speech pathology is contacted when individuals with a diagnosis that is high risk for dysphagia and aspiration, such as stroke, are admitted to the emergency department (ED) (Steele, 2002). This model is similar to Model 3, except the nurses use predefined criteria—for example, confirmed cortical stroke—to determine consultation to speech pathology. This model would expedite speech pathology screening/evaluation if the patient arrives to ED during the typical speech pathology shift. Like Models 2 and 3, the advantage is that the dysphagia expert, speech pathology, is the discipline providing screening/assessment of high-risk patients. The primary disadvantage would be delay in speech pathology response for individuals admitted after-hours or on the weekend if no coverage is provided. Even more than Model 1, this model offers no advantages to individuals admitted with stroke symptoms who arrive outside of window-of-service provision. It would result in significant delay in oral intake for *all* patients admitted with stroke symptoms, as NPO/NBM status would need to be maintained until speech pathology screening or evaluation is completed.

IMPLEMENTATION OF A NURSE-ADMINISTERED SWALLOWING SCREENING TOOL

In most settings, it is likely that either Model 1 or Model 2 is the most common framework used for screening in most medical centers, with nursing staff completing the stroke SST. The two key components for implementing an SST by non–speech pathology health care providers are *staff buy-in* and *education*. As noted previously, by adding screening to the list of responsibilities, busy nurses are required to add one more procedure to their list of duties. In order to achieve adherence in screening completion and accuracy of performance, a team concept must be stressed, and potential stakeholders (speech pathologists, nurses, physicians, dieticians, etc.) must be part of the development process. Nurses, or whichever discipline is administering the screening, must understand the importance of early detection of aspiration risk and their critical role in early identification. Without strong support from nursing administration and buy-in from frontline nurses, success of a nursing-administered screening will be limited.

Training in SST Interpretation and Administration

As noted previously, reliability and feasibility in screening are as important as the validity of a stroke SST, particularly if disciplines without dysphagia expertise are completing the screening. Education is critical to obtain adherence in screening completion and accuracy in administration and interpretation. Speech pathology should be the discipline to provide initial training to other health care providers in screening procedures. Training must be comprehensive enough to ensure reliability, but yet it must not be so long that it places an undue burden on the health care provider, thus rendering it not feasible. It must be remembered that swallowing screening is only a small portion of the care these providers deliver to patients. They must undergo continuing education in multiple areas of patient care. Moreover, education cannot result in a burden to speech pathology to continually provide training to ensure sustainable screening skills. Currently, there is no consensus on the duration or type of training required. Review of current stroke SSTs reveals that training may range from a minimum of 10 minutes (Edmiaston, Connor, Loehr, & Nassief, 2010) to a maximum of 4 hours (Martino et al., 2009). Most studies, however, have little to no documentation concerning the education program necessary for nurses or other disciplines to implement a stroke SST. Ten minutes may be too brief to obtain sustainable reliability, whereas 4 hours may be excessively long in the schedule of a busy nurse who is focused on many things in addition to screening of swallowing. Concerning the education of nurses, one must consider timing of education given their frequently rotating schedule and the almost constant addition of new nursing staff. However, it may be that extensive initial face-to-face training by a speech pathologist is required to achieve and maintain screening skills. Booster sessions that briefly review the entire screening process or key components may also be required to augment initial training in order to sustain high adherence and reliability during the course of the year. Follow-up training or booster sessions can be delivered by a speech pathologist or a nursing "champion," who has demonstrated a leadership role in implementing and administering the stroke SST, or they may be web-based, involving didactic training and proxy cases.

Ideally, training would include:

- Incidence of dysphagia and aspiration in stroke
- Health care costs associated with dysphagia and aspiration and related morbidity
- The difference between screening and assessment
- Operational definitions of screening items with examples of the presence and absence of screening items, such as someone with and without dysarthria
- Direct instructions on how to administer and interpret each item
- Opportunity to demonstrate correct administration and interpretation with a patient (actual patients, standardized patient actors, medical simulation mannequins or avatars with preprogrammed responses to screening items, or videotapes of patients with stroke can be used)
- Intermittent assessment of reliability in administration and interpretation with actual patients, or other models as described, which would be necessary with booster sessions on a regular basis to maintain skills
- Documentation of screening results.

Findings from a pilot study on the implementation of a nurse-administered stroke SST in the ED revealed that pocket cards with the screening items and definitions facilitated adherence in completion of swallowing screening before oral intake (Daniels, Anderson, &

Petersen, 2013). Furthermore, a screening template in the electronic medical records facilitated documentation of screening results. Order sets were constructed from the template that automatically placed orders for NPO/NBM status and speech pathology consultation on individuals who failed the screening. Although reliability was not investigated, findings from this study suggest that booster sessions of training may be required for nurses, at least those in the ED, to consistently and accurately complete screening of swallowing in individuals presenting with stroke symptoms.

Anderson et al. (2016) provided a detailed summary of the swallowing screening education provided to nurses. Nurses were provided a 30 minute face-to-face didactic presentation by a speech pathologist with demonstration audiovisual clips. The education included: (1) general information about stroke-related aspiration and dysphagia, (2) an overview on the difference between screening for aspiration risk and formal swallowing assessment, (3) the operational definition for each screening item, and (4) the specific steps for correct administration of each item. The nurse then observed a series of audiovisual clips with real patients with stroke showing the execution and interpretation of the swallowing screening items. The video clips provided nurses visual and auditory reinforcement of the swallowing screening procedure as well as real-life examples of patients who demonstrated normal and disordered responses, e.g., dysarthria, wet voice compared with dysphonia after swallowing. Finally, the nurse had to: (1) correctly interpret a videotape in which the screening items were administered to a patient who had sustained a stroke, and (2) demonstrate correct administration and interpretation of each screening item with a standardized patient actor. In this study, the nurses were re-educated upon observation of an error or incorrect auditory perceptual interpretation. Availability of the same education module as a webinar would ease the burden of the speech pathologist in education and make the training available to nurses around the clock. Additionally, simulation training using medical mannequins can be used to train and evaluate nurses for obtainment and maintenance of swallowing screening competency (Freeland, Pathak, Garrett, Anderson, & Daniels, 2016). While generalization of screening administration and interpretation skills to the standardized patient has been evident after training with the medical mannequin, the use of a standardized patient is recommended as a means to ensure the skills transfer to live patients. The introduction of a standardized patient provides a continued safe environment to practice in areas that the medical mannequin does not support, such as actual administration of water and judging continuous swallowing ability of the patient. The inclusion of this component, or even a supervised practice with real patients, is strongly suggested to bridge the gap between the simulation and clinical practice.

Optimal Setting for Completion of Stroke SST

A stroke SST may be completed in the ED or upon patient arrival to the hospital ward. Ideally, it seems intuitive that the ED would be the best place to complete the SST regardless of the discipline administering the tool, as this is where most patients with stroke symptoms first present for care. Screening in the ED would reduce the chances of inadvertent administration of liquids, food, or medications prior to completion of the SST. However, the ED is an extremely busy and fast-paced environment. It may be difficult for speech pathology to assess patients in the ED given the need to expedite critical tests and procedures, thus nurses or physicians may be the preferred providers to screen in the ED. ED nurses work with a wide variety of acute and critically ill patients, not just individuals with stroke. Depending on the volume of patients with acute stroke admitted in a given month and considering the number of patients with acute stroke admitted during a shift, the opportunity for an individual nurse to administer an SST may be once or twice a month at best. This can significantly affect accuracy of screening as well as the potential for continual addition of new nurses. Conversely, the neurologist is focused on stroke and will have time and numerous opportunities to administer the SST; however, attending physicians rarely evaluate patients in the ED. This responsibility falls upon the neurology resident who rotates between multiple hospitals, suggesting that accuracy in screening administration and interpretation may be difficult to maintain.

If problems implementing swallowing screening in the ED hamper success, it may be better for a facility to screen swallowing once the patient is admitted to the hospital, generally the stroke ward. On the ward, the pace is slowed and the nurse is dedicated to providing care specifically to patients with stroke. Moreover, the attending neurologist is available, thus potentially increasing reliability in screening administration. However, delaying screening until arrival to the hospital ward may increase the chance for oral intake prior to completion of the SST. As is evident, the best discipline and the best location in which to administer screening is variable and dependent on the needs of each hospital.

Once swallowing has been evaluated in acute care by the speech pathologist, screening of previously identified patients does not need to be repeated upon transfer to a rehabilitation unit, long-term care facility, or other type of medical setting. A full assessment by speech pathology, not a screening, in these other settings is required to determine if the patient has improved. The primary reason screening would be completed outside the acute care setting would be a decline in a patient's medical status.

AVAILABLE SWALLOWING SCREENING TOOLS

Items on stroke SSTs should be based on thorough review of the literature. Numerous systematic reviews have been conducted and have graded the quality of research from which to determine items to use for screening (Bours, Speyer, Lemmens, Limburg, & deWit, 2009; Daniels, Anderson, & Willson, 2012; Martino et al., 2000; Perry & Love, 2001; Ramsey, Smithard, & Kalra, 2003). Redundancy of items is evident across the literature (Table 4–1), and items represent both direct and indirect assessment of swallowing (Daniels et al., 2012). While anecdotal evidence may suggest that clinical features such as watery eyes and runny nose after swallowing are associated with dysphagia and aspiration, these findings have not been validated by empiric research and should not be an item on a stroke SST.

Numerous stroke SSTs are available. A few have been validated against instrumental assessment (VFSS, videoendoscopy). The majority, however, are not validated using these standards. We would argue that rigorous methods should be applied with validation; hence, an instrumental swallowing examination, not a CSE, should be the reference standard. Before determining which SST to implement, screenings should be carefully evaluated in terms of quality of study, validity, reliability, and feasibility (Table 4–2).

Table 4–1. Categories of Clinical Items Identified from Systematic Literature Review (Daniels et al., 2012)

Demographic Items

- Age (Mann & Hankey, 2001)
- Gender (Mann & Hankey, 2001)

History Information

- Pneumonia (McCullough et al., 2005)
- Reduced nutrition (McCullough et al., 2005)

Functional Assessments

- Level of consciousness (Smithard et al., 1998)
- Barthel <60 (Mann & Hankey, 2001)
- Right hemiparesis (Yilmaz, Gupta, Mlcoch, & Moritz, 1998)

Oral Mechanism Assessments

- Dysarthria (Daniels, McAdam, Brailey, & Foundas, 1997; Horner, Buoyer, Alberts, & Helms, 1991; McCullough, Wertz, & Rosenbek, 2001)
- Dysphonia (Daniels et al., 1997; Horner et al., 1991; Horner, Massey, Riski, Lathrop, & Chase, 1988; McCullough et al., 2005; McCullough, Wertz, & Rosenbek, 2001)
- Weak volitional cough (Daniels et al., 1997; Horner, Brazer, & Massey, 1993; Horner, Massey, & Brazer, 1990; Smithard et al., 1998)
- Unilateral jaw weakness (McCullough et al., 2005)
- Weak/asymmetrical palatal movement (Mann & Hankey, 2001)
- Reduced secretion management (McCullough, Wertz, & Rosenbek, 2001)
- Reduced pharyngeal sensation (Kidd, Lawson, Nesbitt, & MacMahon, 1993)
- Abnormal gag reflex (Horner et al. 1990; Horner et al., 1993)
- Cranial nerve IX abnormality (Horner et al., 1991)

Swallowing Tests

- Cough after swallow (Chong, Lieu, Sitoh, Meng, & Leow, 2003; Daniels et al., 1997; DePippo, Holas & Reding, 1992; Kidd et al., 1993; Lim et al., 2001; Mann & Hankey, 2001; McCullough et al., 2005; McCullough, Wertz, & Rosenbek, 2001; Nishiwaki et al., 2005; Smithard et al., 1998; Smith Hammond et al., 2009)
- Throat clear after swallow (Daniels et al., 1997; McCullough, Wertz, & Rosenbek, 2001)
- Voice change after swallow (Chong et al., 2003; DePippo et al., 1992; Kidd et al., 1993; Lim et al., 2001; Mann & Hankey, 2001; McCullough et al., 2005; Nishiwaki et al., 2005; Smithard et al., 1998)
- Incomplete oral clearance (Mann & Hankey, 2001)
- Absent swallow (Smith Hammond et al., 2009)
- Reduced secretion control (Smith Hammond et al., 2009)

Source: From "Valid Items for Screening Dysphagia Risk in Patient with Stroke: A Systematic Review," by S. K. Daniels, J. A. Anderson, and P. C. Willson, 2012, *Stroke, 43*(3), Supplemental Table 2. Copyright © 2012 by Lippincott Williams & Wilkins. Reprinted with permission.

Table 4–2. Assessment of Quality of Research, Validity, Reliability, Feasibility (Daniels et al., 2012)

Quality of Research Study*

1. Was the sample representative of patients with stroke (e.g., includes mild, moderate, and severe stroke) who will receive a swallowing screening in clinical practice?
2. Was the instrumental swallowing examination and/or protocol likely to correctly identify dysphagia and/or aspiration?
3. Was the time period between administration of the swallowing screening tool (SST) and the instrumental swallowing examination short enough to be reasonably sure that dysphagia/aspiration status did not change between the two tests?
4. Did the whole sample or a random selection of significant proportion of the sample receive verification of dysphagia/aspiration using an instrumental swallowing examination?
5. Did all patients receive the same instrumental swallowing examination regardless of the results of the SST results?
6. Did the instrumental swallowing examination not include items from the SST and vice versa?
7. Was the instrumental swallowing examination results interpreted without knowledge of results from the SST?
8. Was the SST interpreted without knowledge of results from the instrumental swallowing examination?
9. Was the same patient/clinical data available that is typically available in routine clinical practice?
10. Were uninterpretable results reported?
11. Were withdrawals from the study explained?
12. Was execution and scoring of the SST described in sufficient detail for replication?
13. Was execution and scoring of the instrumental swallowing examination described in sufficient detail for replication?
14. Was patient selection criteria sufficiently described including inclusion and exclusion criteria?
15. Was the sample composed of consecutive stroke patients and not just referrals to speech pathology?

Validity

1. Sensitivity
2. Specificity
3. Positive Predictive Value
4. Negative Predictive Value
5. Positive Likelihood Ratio

continues

Table 4–2. *continued*

Reliability

1. Administration
2. Interpretation
3. Sustainability

Feasibility

1. Training process described in detail
2. Length of training time to obtain reliability
3. Length of training time to maintain reliability
4. Length of time to administer screening
5. Ease of documentation of results

*Items for quality obtained from Reitsma et al., 2009; Sackett, Haynes, Guyatt, & Tugwell, 1991; Whiting, Rutjes, Reitsma, Bossuyt, & Kleijnen, 2003, Whiting et al., 2011.

Source: From "Valid Items for Screening Dysphagia Risk in Patient with Stroke: A Systematic Review," by S. K. Daniels, J. A. Anderson, and P. C. Willson, 2012, *Stroke, 43*(3), Supplemental Table 1.

Five evidence-based swallowing screening tools which were validated against an instrumental swallowing examination and designed for nurses to implement are available and reviewed in Tables 4–3 and 4–4 (Daniels et al., 2016; Edmiaston, Connor, Steger-May, & Ford, 2014; Martino et al., 2009; Suiter & Leder, 2008; Trapl et al., 2007). As with the literature on which these SSTs are based, there is redundancy of items across screenings. All of the screening tools except the 3-oz water swallowing test (WST) (DePippo, Holas, & Reding, 1992; Suiter & Leder, 2008) include both swallowing and non-swallowing items. These SSTs use a tiered system; that is, non-swallowing items are administered first. If any item is present (e.g., tongue asymmetry), the screening is stopped, and swallowing is not directly assessed. If the non-swallowing items are passed, screening proceeds to direct assessment of swallowing. The Yale Swallow Protocol, which was recently developed around the 3-oz WST, does involve a non-swallowing section (Leder & Suiter, 2014); however, the validity of the entire protocol has not been studied. Failure on one of the non-swallowing items does not automatically prevent administration of the 3-oz WST; the clinician is instructed to use his/her judgment.

Table 4–3. Current Validated Stroke Swallowing Screening Tools

SST	Population Tested	Screener	Training Time	Interrater Reliability	Screening	Reference Standard	Outcome	Sens/Spec/ PPV/NPV
ASDS (Edmiaston et al., 2010)	*N* = 300 consecutively admitted	Nurse	10 minutes	Yes: Nurse	2-tiered screen 4 non-swallowing items 3-oz WST	MASA	Aspiration Dysphagia	95/68/44/98 91/74/54/95
BJH-SDS (Edmiaston, 2014)[a]	*N* = 225 consecutively admitted, confirmed stroke DX	Nurse	Not specified	No	Same as above	VFSS	Aspiration Dysphagia	95/50/41/96 94/66/71/93
GUSS (Trapl et al., 2007)	*N* = 50 consecutively admitted first-time stroke, suspected dysphagia	SLP Nurse	Not specified	SLP only	2 tiered screen 2 non-swallowing items and saliva swallow Calibrated volumes of various consistencies	VEES	Aspiration (PAS ≥4–5)	100/69/74/100[b]
RAS3 (Daniels et al., 2016; Anderson et al., 2016)	*N* = 250 consecutively admitted with suspected stroke	Nurse	30 minutes	Yes: Nurse	2 tiered screen 2 non-swallowing items Two 5 mL water, 3-oz WST	VFSS	Aspiration	93/43/18/98

continues

Table 4–3. *continued*

SST	*Population Tested*	*Screener*	*Training Time*	*Interrater Reliability*	*Screening*	*Reference Standard*	*Outcome*	*Sens/Spec/ PPV/NPV*
TOR-BSST© (Martino et al., 2009; Martino et al., 2014)	*N* = 311 consecutively admitted, confirmed stroke DX	Nurse	4 hours	Yes: Nurse	2 tiered screen 2 non-swallowing items Ten 5 mL water volumes, cup sip	VFSS	Dysphagia	96/64/77/93[c]
3-oz WST (Suiter & Leder, 2008; Warner et al., 2014)	*N* = 3000 total; *n* = 468 stroke, retrospective review of patients referred for suspected dysphagia	SLP Nurse	Not specified	No: 2008 Yes: Nurse 2014	3-oz WST	VEES	Aspiration	97/47/31/98[d]

Note. [a]ASDS and BJH-SDS are the same screening tests, [b]Nursing data reported, [c]Acute stroke data reported, [d]Stroke data averaged. SST = swallowing screening tool, Sens = sensitivity, Spec = specificity, PPV = positive predictive value, NPV = negative predictive value, ASDS = Acute Stroke Dysphagia Screen, WST = water swallowing test, MASA = Mann Assessment of Swallowing Ability, BJH-SDS = Barnes-Jewish Hospital Stroke Dsyphagia Screen, VEES = videoendoscopic evaluation of swallowing, VFSS = videofluoroscopic swallowing study, GUSS = Gugging Swallowing Screen, SLP = speech-language pathologist, RAS3 = Rapid Aspiration Screening for Suspected Stroke, TOR-BSST© = Toronto Bedside Swallowing Screening Test.

Table 4–4. Strengths and Limitations of Current Validated Stroke Swallowing Screening Tools

	Barnes Jewish Hospital Stroke Dysphagia Screen
Strengths	• VFSS reference standard • Adequate sample size • 2 hour average time between screening and VFSS ensures no change in patient status • All screened subjects underwent VFSS except for 2 who were explained • Reviewer of VFSS blinded to screening results • Detail to allow for partial replication of screening • Consecutive stroke admissions • Good sensitivity and NPV, moderate specificity for dysphagia • Reliability obtained in nurses • 10 minutes of training and short screening suggest good feasibility
Limitations	• No use of flowchart to document inclusion/exclusion and progression through study • Up to 8 hours between screening and VFSS thus cannot ensure patient status did not change • Operational definition of screening "asymmetry/weakness" was not provided nor how to test for these items which limits replication • No information to allow for VFSS replication • Low specificity for aspiration • Description of nursing education not provided which limits replication • Nursing reliability was not established with "live" patients, nor was it evaluated throughout the study to ensure maintenance; reliability not evaluated in Edmiaston et al. (2014)
	Gugging Swallowing Screen
Strengths	• VEES reference standard • All screened subjects underwent VEES • Reviewer of VEES blinded to screening • Detailed to allow for replication of screening • Good sensitivity and NPV; moderate specificity for nurses

continues

Table 4–4. *continued*

Limitations	• Small sample size, thus underpowered
	• No use of flowchart to document inclusion/exclusion and progression through study
	• Time between screening and VEES not stated
	• Referrals to speech pathology, not consecutive admissions
	• No information to allow for VEES replication
	• Low specificity for speech pathologists
	• No reliability in nurses
	• No information on education nor time to complete entire screening which limits replication and feasibility for nurses
	Rapid Aspiration Screening for Suspected Stroke
Strengths	• VFSS reference standard
	• Patients with suspected stroke recruited
	• Use of flowchart to document inclusion/exclusion and progression through study
	• All screened subjects underwent VFSS except for 2 who were explained
	• <2 hour delay between screening and VFSS
	• Reviewer of VFSS blinded to screening results
	• Adequate details provided to allow for replication of screening and VFSS
	• Consecutive suspected stroke admissions
	• Good sensitivity and NPV
	• Reliability and sustainability obtained in nurses
	• Nursing training described in detail
	• 30 minutes of training and short screening suggest good feasibility
Limitations	• Possibly underpowered given small number of patients with aspiration
	• Patients with more mild to moderate stroke recruited
	• Primarily male participants
	• Large number of patients excluded
	• Low specificity
	• Nurses were volunteers which may inflate reliability
	• Nurses retrained after every error on screening which may inflate reliability

Table 4–4. *continued*

	Toronto Bedside Swallowing Screening Test
Strengths	• VFSS reference standard • Use of flowchart to document inclusion/exclusion and progression through study • Random selection of screened patients underwent VFSS • Reviewer of VFSS blinded to screening results • Consecutive stroke admissions • Good sensitivity and NPV, moderate specificity • Reliability obtained in nurses
Limitations	• Excluded patients with mild stroke, which is not representative of patients admitted who require screening • Did not indicate time between screening and VFSS • Only 19% of subjects screened contributed to validation • Limited information to allow replication of screening and no information to allow for VFSS replication • Reliability not obtained throughout the study • Description of nursing education not provided which limits replication • Questionable feasibility given 4 hours of training
	3-oz WST
Strengths	• VEES reference standard • Screening completed immediately after VEES • Person completing screening blinded to VEES in subsequent studies but not in original Suiter & Leder (2008) study • Good information to allow for replication of VEES and screening • Reliability obtained in nurses (Warner et al., 2014) • Short screening suggests good feasibility
Limitations	• Initially retrospective chart review studies, but later prospective studies • No use of flowchart to document inclusion/exclusion and progression through • Initially included cough after 1 minute and wet vocal quality (Suiter & Leder, 2008); in subsequent studies, no inclusion of these signs and no data to support removal • Referrals to speech pathology, not consecutive admissions

continues

Table 4–4. *continued*

Limitations *continued*	• Time post stroke onset not stated • Low specificity • Nursing reliability not obtained over sustained time period • Description of nursing education not provided which limits replication • Yale Swallow Protocol results reported (Suiter, Sloggy, & Leder, 2014). However, validity based on all 3 aspects of protocol (cognitive screen, oral mechanism screen, 3-oz WST) has not been tested in a single study. No study of nurse-administered reliability for the entire protocol

< = less than, NPV = negative predictive value, VEES = videoendoscopic evaluation of swallowing, VFSS = videofluoroscopic swallowing study, WST = water swallowing test.

Direct swallowing protocols vary with each screening. All use some form of a WST, and one involves administration of various consistencies in addition to water (Trapl et al., 2007). Procedures for administering the water vary across studies. Volumes range from 3 mL (Trapl et al., 2007) to 90 mL (Daniels et al., 2016; Edmiaston et al., 2010; Edmiaston et al., 2014; Suiter & Leder, 2008), and the number of trials per volume differs for each SST.

Utility of incorporating a water swallow section as part of the screening tool has been identified in recent systematic reviews (Brodsky et al., 2016; Chen, Chuang, Leong, Guo, & Hsin, 2016). Brodsky and colleagues (2016) noted that use of calibrated single swallow volumes provided good ability to rule in risk of aspiration when overt clinical signs were present (e.g., cough, wet voice) and that sequential swallowing of large volumes provided good ability to rule out risk of aspiration when clinical signs were not present. Thus, starting with small volumes and gradually progressing to larger volumes appears to be the most reasonable protocol; however, the number of trials and volumes of water administered require continued study to determine the optimal protocol that provides the best validity while maintaining feasibility for a nurse or other health care professional to administer. Health outcomes related to WSTs require further study especially in those protocols that involve administration of large volumes in which the patient is self-regulating the amount. This is important, as research has shown that many patients with stroke are unaware of their swallowing deficits and continue to drink even when coughing (Parker et al., 2004). Clinical findings suggest that some patients may be impulsive following a stroke, which may lead to ingestion of large self-regulated sips. Last, further research is warranted to determine if the inclusion of non-swallowing items improves sensitivity and specificity.

Systematic reviews of various stroke SSTs have been completed (Donovan et al., 2013; Kertscher, Speyer, Plamieri, & Plant, 2014; Poorjavad & Jalaie, 2014; Schepp, Tirschwell, Miller, & Longstreth, 2012). While systematic reviews are important, it is imperative for consumers of swallowing screening research to read the original source in order to fully judge the quality of the research. For example, Schepp et al. (2012) suggested that the Mini Mann Assessment of Swallowing Ability (MMASA) (Antonios et al., 2011) met their quality criteria for a stroke SST. All of the MMASA items, however, were taken directly from the reference standard Mann Assessment of Swallowing Ability (Mann, 2002), a standardized and validated CSE, against which the screening was compared for validation. This violates a key component for validity (Item 6 in Table 4–2) and artificially inflates results. One has to question how thoroughly Schepp et al. (2012) evaluated the reviewed and recommended SSTs given the significant methodological flaw of the MMASA.

There is currently no consensus on a single best stroke SST. This does not mean that swallowing screening in patients admitted with suspected stroke should not be completed. Rather, it suggests that each hospital team should carefully review strengths and limitations of each evidence-based SST to determine which one meets their needs in terms of quality, validity, reliability, and feasibility.

5 The Clinical Swallowing Examination

History, Patient Interview, Informal Cognitive and Communication Assessment

INTRODUCTION TO THE CLINICAL SWALLOWING EXAMINATION

As discussed in Chapter 1, the incidence of dysphagia in stroke is substantial. This, paired with the fact that there is no clear association between site of lesion and dysphagic presentation, makes screening of swallowing in all patients with acute stroke a mandate. Following screening, the clinical swallowing examination (CSE) is the first step in formally evaluating patients with stroke. CSE is not a "screening," as connotations emerge of a cursory, minimalist assessment. Such was eloquently stated by Jay Rosenbek: "it is critical that the CSE not be relegated to the status of screening tool. It is far too powerful" (Rosenbek, McCullough, & Wertz, 2004, p. 449). The CSE involves many components, including: patient interview, observation of gross motor skills, inspection of the oral cavity, cranial nerve evaluation, and swallowing examination involving multiple volumes and textures. An example of a CSE protocol is provided as an online resource.

However, it is important to note that in practice, a thorough CSE is limited in its diagnostic ability. That is, swallowing pathophysiology cannot be defined; thus compensatory and rehabilitative strategies cannot be recommended based on results of the CSE alone. However, the information gleaned from the CSE will clearly contribute to the ultimate diagnosis of dysphagia in the patient when paired with more specific information. The instrumental swallowing examination provides detailed information about biomechanics and ultimately pathophysiology. However, one would be remiss to move directly from screening to instrumental assessment as the multidimensional CSE provides critical information about the patient, including insight into how cognitive and comprehension abilities may affect swallowing. Thus, data from the instrumental assessment are integrated with clinical observation and history and are used to develop a comprehensive and efficacious management approach.

The goals of the CSE are:

- Develop a hypothesis of the pathophysiology of dysphagia.
- Determine if an instrumental evaluation is warranted.
- Formulate ideas concerning a management program.

PATIENT HISTORY

Medical history ideally is obtained from the patient's medical records prior to the CSE. Information obtained from the medical history may help guide the patient interview. If access to the patient's medical record is not available, the clinician should ascertain history information during the interview. For hospitalized patients, the medical chart review may be more detailed, particularly if the patient has had a protracted medical course. For inpatients, the clinician should begin with the history and physical report from the neurologist, whereas for outpatients, the clinician should begin with the note from the referring physician. Stroke onset, characteristics, and complications associated with stroke (if the patient has been in the hospital for a period of time prior to consultation) should be noted. Subsequent notes that may relate to the underlying process or contributors to dysphagia should be reviewed. Moreover, if the patient has a history of dysphagia, any available swallowing evaluation and treatment notes should be reviewed. Table 5–1 provides a focus for medical chart review. Numerous medications can negatively affect swallowing. Specific medications and their effects are too numerous to detail in this book. The interested reader may refer to the book by Carl and Johnson (2006) or other pharmaceutical references for detailed information on this topic.

PATIENT AND FAMILY INTERVIEW

After review of the medical chart and prior to beginning the actual patient assessment, an interview with the patient should be conducted

Table 5–1. Medical Chart Review

- Diseases associated with dysphagia—with each, note if dysphagia was identified
  - Prior history of stroke (note residual deficits)
  - Other neurologic diseases, e.g., Parkinson's disease, myasthenia gravis
  - Head and neck cancer with radiation
- Surgeries associated with dysphagia—with each, note if dysphagia was identified
  - Head and neck resection
  - Anterior cervical spine fusion
  - Carotid endarterectomy
- Pulmonary status
  - Current or prior sustained intubation or tracheostomy tube placement
  - Chronic pulmonary obstructive disease
  - Aspiration pneumonia
- Medications that may affect swallowing
  - Depress consciousness
  - Drug-induced xerostomia
  - Antipsychotic/neuroleptic medications
- Current nutritional intake
  - Nothing by mouth—awaiting swallowing evaluation
  - Nasogastric tube
  - Percutaneous endoscopic gastrostomy tube
  - Intravenous fluids
  - Total parenteral nutrition
- Functional status prior to hospitalization
  - Independent and active
  - Required assistance
  - Totally dependent
  - Bed bound

to determine specific complaints concerning swallowing. The depth of the interview is dependent on the acuteness of stroke and the patient's responsiveness and awareness of deficits. For patients with acute stroke, the interview may be relatively brief, as they may not be aware of any problem or may not be receiving any oral intake due to the results of screening and, therefore, cannot describe any swallowing deficit. The family or patient's nurse, if available, may provide information concerning swallowing for the patient with acute stroke; however, the clinician should not delay initiation of the CSE if family or nursing staff is unavailable. Patients seen in a rehabilitation or outpatient setting will generally warrant a lengthier interview than patients admitted with an acute stroke. For those patients who are seen in outpatient settings but who have limited communication, it is advisable that they be accompanied by a caregiver who can provide information concerning swallowing.

During the initial swallowing evaluation, particularly for patients admitted to the acute care setting, the initial question may be "Are you having any problems with your swallowing?" If the patient indicates no, the clinician should probe further with questions such as "Do you cough or choke when eating or drinking?" If the answer remains no, further questioning may not be indicated, and the clinician should continue with the rest of the CSE. Obtaining limited input from patient questioning does not mean that the clinician should not proceed with the CSE, as patients may not be adequate historians and a great deal of information can be obtained from direct assessment.

It is important that the clinician not equate lack of acknowledgment of a dysphagia with normal swallowing, particularly in patients with acute stroke. Silent aspiration has been identified in 67% of patients with stroke who aspirated during the instrumental swallowing evaluation (Daniels et al., 1998). Furthermore, less than one-half of patients with acute stroke are aware of dysphagia symptoms—for example, coughing, drooling (Parker et al., 2004).

If the patient acknowledges dysphagia or is seeking consultation for a swallowing problem, the initial inquiry may be "Tell me about your swallowing problem." If the patient has adequate communication skills, questions should initially be open-ended. By using open-ended questioning, the clinician will not be directing the patient's response. If communication is impaired or responses are vague, the clinician should ask more direct questions or questions requiring a yes/no response. Questions may be addressed to the caregiver, if available, if the patient is unable to provide adequate information due to communication or cognitive deficits. Table 5–2 provides questions that may be asked during the patient or family interview.

If the clinician evaluates a patient with an acute stroke but there is a history of prior strokes, questions should be asked to determine onset of dysphagia and any prior history of swallowing problems. If

Table 5–2. Specific Questions Concerning Swallowing Ability

- When did your swallowing problem begin?
- Did it begin abruptly or gradually?
- Has your swallowing gotten better, worse, or remained the same?
- How often do you notice your swallowing problem?
  - Specific time of day?
  - Consistently? Intermittently?
- Does it hurt when you swallow?
  - Where?
  - Point to the exact spot where you feel pain
- Do you have problems swallowing a specific type or consistency of food?
  - What happens when you swallow this type of food/liquid?
- Do you cough or choke after swallowing?
- Does food get stuck?
  - Where?
  - Point to the exact spot where it gets stuck
- Do you avoid certain foods/liquids due to your swallowing problem?
  - What are these foods/liquids?
- Have you lost or gained weight since your swallowing problem began?
  - How much?
- Do you do anything that helps your swallowing?

the patient confirms previous dysphagia, the clinician will want to clarify whether swallowing has changed. Additionally, for patients with a history of stroke and dysphagia, it is important to determine whether the patient has undergone previous evaluation and treatment for dysphagia. If the evaluation and treatment reports are not available at the initial interview, the clinician should attempt to discern from the patient the type of evaluation, findings from assessment, type of treatment, and progress made in treatment. If the patient was previously discharged from treatment, attempt to determine the reason why—for example, plateau in progress or discharge from the medical facility.

It is important to determine whether the patient thinks swallowing has changed since discontinuation of prior treatment, particularly if there has been an extended length of time since treatment was terminated. The clinician may benefit by obtaining written consent from the patient to obtain the previous swallowing evaluation and treatment reports.

Upon completion of questioning, the clinician should have an idea of onset of symptoms, progression or resolution of deficits, characteristics of dysphagia, and food type associated with dysphagia. The information obtained from the interview may identify specific areas on which to focus during the clinical and instrumental evaluations. For example, a patient's complaint of right-sided post-swallow residual will alert the clinician to watch for this during the instrumental examination.

Focusing on patient-centered outcomes and improving quality of life (QoL) are of equal importance as goals of dysphagia management, as is rehabilitating physiologic dysfunction. Thus, determining the impact of dysphagia on the patient's QoL and outcomes that are important to the patient are data important to obtain. Numerous QoL and dysphagia self-perception measures are available that can provide insight into the effects of dysphagia on a person's daily life. For outpatients, the QoL questionnaire can be sent home prior to the CSE for completion by the patient, with assistance as needed from family, and reviewed during the CSE. For patients with acute stroke, administration of a QoL questionnaire is not appropriate, as it is too soon to determine the true impact of dysphagia on daily living. These questionnaires are not designed to "screen" swallowing, especially in acute patients who may be unaware of problems or have cognitive and/or communication deficits and thus cannot answer the questions. Likewise, QoL questionnaires should not be substituted for the more open-ended questions concerning dysphagia.

The Swallowing Quality of Life (SWAL-QOL) questionnaire (McHorney et al., 2002) is a standardized 44-item tool designed to measure a patient's perception of quality of life attributable to dysphagia. The questionnaire covers 10 categories (burden, eating duration, eating desire, symptom frequency, food selection, communication, mental health, social, fatigue, and sleep) and requires approximately 15 minutes to complete. Research has shown a modest relationship between SWAL-QOL ratings (McHorney, Martin-Harris, Robbins, & Rosenbek, 2006) and bolus flow measures of oral and pharyngeal transit time and airway invasion. This suggests that the SWAL-QOL contributes unique information about dysphagia, which may be important both diagnostically and therapeutically. Administration of a questionnaire such as the SWAL-QOL prior to and during the course of therapy will allow the clinician to document the effect of improved swallowing on a person's QoL. Patient-centered outcomes and documenting improved QoL is as significant as documenting changes in swallowing biomechanics and may facilitate reimbursement from third-party payers.

Like the SWAL-QOL, the Eating Assessment Tool (EAT-10) (Belafsky et al., 2008), and the Sydney Swallowing Questionnaire (SSQ) (Wallace, Middleton, & Cook, 2000) are designed to assess a patient's perception of his/her swallowing problems. While not as detailed as the SWAL-QOL, the EAT-10 is much shorter, as it consists of only 10 questions and is simple to administer and score. Likewise, the SSQ consists of 17 questions presented in a visual analog rating scale format.

INFORMAL ASSESSMENT OF COGNITION AND COMMUNICATION

Informal evaluation of cognitive, speech, voice, language, and praxis status is important in patients with stroke, as function in these areas may have significant impact on the evaluation and treatment of swallowing disorders. The level to which a patient's cognition and communication are impaired depends on the location and extent of the stroke. A patient with right hemisphere damage (RHD) or a parietal or prefrontal stroke is more likely to present with cognitive impairment than a patient with left hemisphere damage (LHD) or an occipital stroke. Likewise, a patient with LHD is more likely to have aphasia than a person with RHD. A large vessel stroke is more likely to impair cognition and communication versus a single lacunar infarct. Hence, knowledge of the stroke location will provide the clinician with an idea of the levels to which cognition and communication may be impaired.

As the purpose of the CSE is to evaluate swallowing, the clinician cannot complete a prescribed evaluation of cognitive-communication functioning. Rather, the goal is to make an informal assessment of these processes and determine how they may impact swallowing and treatment. Thus, the astute clinician should informally assess cognition and communication based on the patient's ability to comprehend and respond to questions and adequately recall information during the interview, as well as follow instruction and maintain attention during the cranial nerve and swallowing portions of the CSE. The level of cognitive and auditory comprehension deficits will affect the depth to which the CSE can be completed. Table 5–3 details cognitive and communication processes that are generally informally assessed as part of the CSE in patients with stroke.

In addition to informally assessing cognition and communication to determine their potential impact on swallowing and management, the clinician can determine if further evaluation in one or more of these areas is warranted. Physicians may focus on swallowing initially, as this impacts the patient's health and length of stay. By identifying possible communication and/or cognitive deficits early, the clinician can advocate for the patient and obtain the necessary medical orders in order to fully evaluate these areas.

Interpreting Cognitive Findings

The first step of the CSE is to determine if the patient is alert enough to complete the examination. There are five principal levels of consciousness (LOC): alert, lethargy, obtunded, stupor/semi-coma, and coma (Strub & Black, 2000). Each level is described in Table 5–4. The alert patient is awake and interactive when the clinician enters the room. If asleep, the alert patient readily arouses with verbal or light tactile stimulation and easily maintains interaction with the clinician. If the patient is asleep and does not easily awaken, the volume of verbal stimulation and the vigor of tactile stimulation should be increased. If the patient demonstrates lethargy or a reduced LOC, it is important to determine the patient's baseline by conferring with medical staff. It may be that the patient slept poorly the previous night or has been sedated. If possible, determine the optimum time of alertness and proceed with the CSE at that time.

LOC will dictate whether the rest of the cognitive assessment as well as the remainder of the CSE can be pursued. If patients cannot maintain alertness for a sustained period without re-arousal—for example, for 5 minutes—postponement of the swallowing evaluation should be considered.

Deficits in cognition have significance not only for instrumental evaluation and treatment but also for eating and nutritional intake.

Table 5–3. Informal Evaluation of Cognition and Communication

Cognitive and Communication Processes	*How to Informally Evaluate*
Cognition	
Focus/Attention	Maintenance of attention throughout the CSE or requires frequent redirection to task. This can be observed with or without external interference.
Neglect	During the CSE, move to different sides of the patient; note if he/she follows you and makes eye contact regardless of the side. During the swallowing assessment, do not always place food, liquid, or utensils at midline and note if the patient makes use of them given the various locations. If patient is eating from a tray of food, note if one side of the tray or plate is ignored.
Awareness of deficits	Ask about reason for hospitalization, deficits, etc. Observe behavior if coughing during swallowing.
Communication	
Language	
Auditory comprehension	Response to questions during the interview. Ability to follow commands, without visual cues during cranial nerve and swallowing portions of the CSE.
Verbal expression	Response to questions during the interview and throughout the CSE.
Motor speech	Response to questions during the interview and throughout the CSE.
Voice	Response to questions during the interview and throughout the CSE. Sustained phonation and pitch elevation of "ah" during the cranial nerve assessment. Pay particular attention to wet vocal quality, which suggests pooling of secretion on the TVF, and breathy vocal quality, which suggests reduced TVF adduction.
Other	
Buccofacial apraxia	Ability to cough on command, drink from a straw, e.g., the patient says the word "cough," blows versus sucks through the straw.
Limb apraxia	Ability to appropriately use utensils during the swallowing assessment, e.g., the patient uses a knife to eat soup.

Note. CSE = clinical swallowing examination; TVF = true vocal folds.

Table 5–4. Levels of Consciousness

Level of Consciousness	Response
Alert	The patient is awake, fully aware of stimuli, and interactive. If totally paralyzed, interaction can be established with eye contact and eye movement.
Lethargy	The patient requires constant stimulation to maintain wakefulness. Attention is reduced even if eyes are open. Impaired cognitive performance should be interpreted with caution.
Obtunded	This is a transitional state between lethargy and stupor. The patient is difficult to arouse and cannot maintain alertness even with constant stimulation. The patient is confused when aroused.
Stupor/ Semicoma	The patient responds to only persistent and vigorous stimulation. When aroused, the patient responds with groaning or mumbling.
Coma	The patient is completely unarousable.

If the patient cannot maintain focus to task, completing rehabilitation protocols may prove challenging, as the clinician must constantly redirect the patient to task. Likewise, if a chin tuck posture is found to reduce airway invasion, but the patient cannot remember to employ this compensatory strategy, it is of little benefit. Many management approaches, such as super-supraglottic swallow, have multiple, temporally specific levels of instruction that the patient must recall to correctly implement; therefore, intact memory is critical to swallowing treatment.

Neglect is defined as failure to respond or orient to stimuli presented to the contralesional side in the presence of intact elemental sensory and motor functioning (Heilman, Watson, & Valenstein, 2011). Neglect may be evident by sensory inattention, motor neglect (intentional disorders), spatial neglect, and/or unawareness of deficits. Visual inattention impacts eating and swallowing in that the patient may not be aware of food in the contralesional visual field, thus eating only part of the meal and thereby decreasing nutritional intake. Tactile inattention may result in a patient with food remaining in the contralesional lateral sulcus even though sensation is intact. Anisodiophoria, defined as awareness but unconcern of deficits, or anosognosia, defined as unawareness or denial of deficits, may have a significant impact on swallowing safety and compliance in management recommendations.

Although it seems intuitive to the clinician working with patients with stroke that cognitive impairments may impact eating and swallowing, little research in this area has been conducted. Research suggests that patients with stroke who are unconcerned or have poor awareness of their dysphagic symptoms do not modify swallowing behavior, whereas patients who are aware of their dysphagia modify rate and volume of ingestion (Parker et al., 2004). In this study, it also was noted that patients with poor awareness developed more medical complications at three months post-onset compared with a group with good awareness of dysphagia symptoms. Another study found spatial neglect to be associated with initial non-oral intake in patients with acute stroke (Schroeder, Daniels, McClain, Corey, & Foundas, 2006). It may be that patients with RHD or LHD present with similar swallowing pathophysiology, but patients with cognitive deficits—for example, neglect, inattention, or anosognosia—pose a greater risk of aspiration. This may lead the clinician to suggest restricted intake or eventually may lead to increased morbidity and mortality. Moreover, these patients may require greater accommodation to maximize rehabilitation potential as a result of their cognitive deficits. Further research is warranted to determine the relationship between cognitive dysfunction, dysphagia, and recovery of swallowing function.

Interpreting Communication Findings

Language ability will impact interpretation of the cognitive assessment, and thus responses should be analyzed according to language functioning. While expressive aphasia will not affect the swallowing evaluation or treatment other than reduced ability to interview the patient, reduced auditory comprehension will impact the implementation of the CSE, instrumental swallowing assessment, and swallowing management. A patient with reduced comprehension may not understand instructions such as swallowing on cue or volitional cough or the instructions to a rehabilitative strategy. Visual cues and imitation may facilitate comprehension necessary for completion of the CSE and instrumental examination, but they may prove of limited assistance in the actual rehabilitation of dysphagia.

The upper aerodigestive tract is common to speech, voice, and swallowing. Damage to specific cranial nerves may affect one, two, or all three functions. Abnormality in speech and voice has frequently been related to risk of aspiration in patients (e.g., Daniels et al., 1998; McCullough et al., 2005). Although not every patient with a motor speech or voice disorder has dysphagia, the presence of these should alert the clinician to the increased potential for dysphagia in the patient with acute stroke.

Pre-oral behavior such as self-feeding may affect swallowing, particularly in patients with stroke (see Chapter 3 for review), but this has not been empirically studied. It is known, however, that limb apraxia adversely affects activities of daily living (Hanna-Pladdy, Heilman, & Foundas, 2003). Furthermore, severity of limb apraxia has been associated with self-feeding difficulties in patients with stroke (Foundas et al., 1995). Comprehension and motor strength must be intact to make an accurate diagnosis of buccofacial or limb apraxia.

6 The Clinical Swallowing Examination

The Evaluation of the Oral Mechanism

Before beginning evaluation of the oral mechanism, it is recommended that the clinician briefly observe the patient at rest to obtain a global idea of the patient's status. The clinician should note the patient's appearance, alertness, posture, positioning, and respiratory rate. For example, the clinician may note whether the patient is disheveled or neat in appearance, drowsy or alert, sitting upright or leaning to a hemiparetic side, or using rapid mouth breathing or slow nasal breathing. Although it is a widely held belief that aspiration risk is increased if the respiratory rate is over 20 breaths per minute, this has not been empirically confirmed.

STRUCTURAL INTEGRITY

A careful evaluation of oral mucosal integrity is likely underestimated in clinical dysphagia management. The risk of aspiration pneumonia substantially increases when dysphagia coexists with pathogenic oral bacteria and reduced airway clearance (Langmore et al., 1998; Scannapieco, 2006). Altered mastication, salivation, swallowing, and oral hygiene frequently seen in patients following a stroke may place these individuals at high susceptibility for microbial disequilibrium, allowing pathogenic oral bacteria to flourish with an ensuing poor prognosis (Millns, Gosney, Jack, Martin, & Wright, 2003). Although not yet documented for stroke, in other populations interventions that improve oral hygiene have reduced pneumonia rates by 8% to 54% (Quinn et al., 2014; Yoneyama et al., 2002), with cost savings of up to $1.6 million (Quinn et al., 2014).

Executing the Evaluation of Structural Integrity

A brief observation of a patient before entering the room can provide a valuable opportunity to alertness, positioning, respiratory ease at rest, and communication or engagement with family or visitors. Particularly in an acute setting, it also allows the clinician to confirm the presence of any monitoring devices (e.g., oxygen saturation) or tubes (e.g., nasogastric tube, tracheostomy) that would be expected following chart review. Obvious structural deformities or asymmetries of the face or upper torso should be noted, as well as movement of upper limbs, as this will influence independent feeding capacity.

The appearance of the oral mucosa should be evaluated in terms of salivation and color. The mucosa should be moist without evidence of excess saliva or drooling. The color of the oral mucosa should be pink. Any structural abnormality such as sores or lesions in the oral cavity should be identified, and the presence and awareness of food should be noted.

Dentition should be inspected for number and appearance of teeth as well as evidence of dental prostheses. The clinician should note missing teeth and provide a general report of the quality of remaining teeth, such as obvious decay, cracks, and so forth. The presence and fit of dentures should be noted. For inpatients in particular, dentures may be available but not inserted. Not considered a dental assessment, this cursory screening may identify when referrals to dental services are appropriate.

Interpreting the Evaluation of Structural Integrity

Pooling of saliva in the oral cavity generally does not indicate hypersalivation in patients with stroke, rather it may indicate dysphagia. For example, patients with a lateral medullary stroke frequently have severe dysphagia with inability to swallow saliva. This, in turn, may cause collection of saliva in the oral cavity. Sensory deficits may also inhibit intrinsic cuing for the need to swallow secretions. The clinical picture of a patient with an acute stroke expectorating saliva into a cup is frequently evident in individuals with lateral medullary stroke. The presence of drooling should alert the clinician to facial nerve weakness.

Conversely, dry, cracked, or flaking oral mucosa may represent poor neural activation of salivary glands (hypo-salivation) or a more generalized dehydration. Behaviorally, some elderly patients may be reluctant to ingest significant quantities of liquid in an effort to avoid incontinence. Very frequently, dry mucosa is a by-product of any number of medications, particularly tricyclic antidepressants, antipsychotics, atropinics, beta blockers, and antihistamines. Prescription of these drug classes is not uncommon in elderly patients with hypertension or individuals with psychological disorders (Streckfus, 1995).

THE CRANIAL NERVE EXAMINATION: INFERRING PHYSIOLOGY

Basic neuroscience is considered a standard component of professional training programs in speech-language pathology but applying that information to dysphagia management practice eludes many clinicians when faced with the demands of a full clinical load. Astute clinicians will integrate a thorough cranial nerve examination into their clinical swallowing examination (CSE) and use this information to infer aspects of potential pathophysiology. Asking the patient to execute various motor and sensory tasks as clinical indicators of cranial nerve function provides valuable information about the functional status of the task assessed. More importantly, however, a thorough cranial nerve assessment allows the clinician to "see" what they "cannot see"; it allows clinician-inferred insights into unobservable pharyngeal physiology.

Executing the Cranial Nerve Examination

The earlier review of basic neurophysiologic substrates discussed in Chapter 2 provides the foundation for the clinical assessment. Execution of a cranial nerve examination in a patient with neurological impairment will optimally consist of a well-organized protocol of specifically evaluated behavior that allows access to maximal information for the clinician with minimal invasiveness and discomfort to the patient. To accomplish this, it is often more logical to organize the examination not by cranial nerve, but rather by starting at the front of the swallowing system and working to the back of the system. The clinician must be methodical.

- *Face:* Assessment of facial sensation and symmetry with careful observation of differentiation in upper and lower facial movement. Attention to facial grooving/folds (nasolabial fold, forehead, circumorbital, and circumlabial wrinkling) for indication of asymmetry that would suggest unilateral weakness.
- *Lips:* Labial symmetry at rest; range of motion, symmetry, and resistance during functional activity.
- *Tongue:* Observation of lingual structure at rest with careful attention to subtle fasciculations and muscle wasting. Lingual range of motion and symmetry; strength to resistance. Taste and touch perception on lingual surface.
- *Palate:* Assessment of velopharyngeal sensation via touch and symmetry of movement on phonation of non-nasal phonemes. Observation of velar elevation and movement of pharyngeal walls in response to gag elicitation may provide additional information.
- *Pharynx:* Little observation can be made of the pharynx outside of pharyngeal wall contraction during gag. Palpation of the thyroid cartilage will provide the clinician with a subjective marker of laryngeal excursion during swallowing; however, it must be recognized that presence, not adequacy, of hyolaryngeal ascent is provided by palpation. The adequacy of hyolaryngeal ascent can be ascertained only through observation of epiglottic deflection and upper esophageal sphincter opening, thus requiring a videofluoroscopic swallowing study (VFSS).
- *Larynx:* As above, direct evaluation of laryngeal function is not possible from clinical assessment; thorough evaluation of this feature is best accomplished with videoendoscopic evaluation of swallowing (VEES). However, appraisal of phonatory ability can provide clues as to the integrity of laryngeal structure and function. Vocal quality, change in pitch, glottal coup, and cough should be assessed. Data from Malandraki and colleagues (Malandraki, Hind,

Gangnon, Logemann, & Robbins, 2011; Rajappa et al., 2017) documented strong relationships between perceived and measured increase in fundamental frequency and overt/silent aspiration.

- *Speech:* Although speech and swallowing share some common structures and neurophysiologic substrates, and will coexist in some patients, there is not a robust association between these two tasks. Evaluation of speech sound production for isolated phonemes (particularly /g, k/) and connected speech will provide information about overall strength and coordination of muscles as they are recruited for voluntary tasks. Findings may carry over to swallowing tasks in the case of lower motor neuron (LMN) impairment; however, the clinician will need to recognize that upper motor neuron (UMN) pathway activations for swallowing vary from those for speech, and thus may reflect differentially on functional outcomes.
- *Dry swallow:* Initiation of voluntary swallowing and reflexive swallowing for secretion management.

Interpreting the Cranial Nerve Examination

Interpretation of cranial nerve examination findings is outlined in Table 6–1, which provides a summation of cranial nerves primarily involved in swallowing biomechanics. Included are instructions for direct assessment of motor and sensory components, the innervation patterns of those nerves, and a summary of *potential* biomechanical implications of involvement of those muscles. The astute clinician will make every effort to link clinical observations of cranial nerve impairment to suspected pharyngeal pathophysiology. By doing this, the CSE is extended from observed behavior to intelligently inferred behavior and thus may increase sensitivity for detecting pharyngeal swallowing impairment.

Table 6–1. Clinical Testing of Cranial Nerve Function with Potential Pharyngeal Physiologic Abnormalities

Cranial Nerve	*Tested by*	*Muscle Innervation*	*Potential Implications*
V Trigeminal	Motor: • Open jaw to resistance; bite • Jaw lateralization	• Temporalis • Masseters • Medial & lateral pterygoids • Anterior belly of digastric • Mylohyoid • Tensor veli palatini	• Inadequate bolus breakdown and impaired preparation/cohesive bolus formation of semi-solids and solids • Reduced anterior hyoid movement with consequent ∘ Decreased epiglottic deflection resulting in → Intra-swallow penetration/ aspiration 2° impaired supraglottic closure and/or → vallecular residual with post-swallow penetration/aspiration ∘ Decreased UES opening resulting in → pyriform sinus residual and potential for post-swallow penetration/aspiration
	Sensory: • Tactile perception to touch for face, hard palate, oral mucosa, gums, anterior 2/3 of tongue		• Decreased bolus recognition/awareness with consequent inadequate bolus preparation and formation, post-swallow residual • Contribution to delayed pharyngeal response with consequent pre-swallow, or intra-swallow penetration/ aspiration

Table 6–1. *continued*

Cranial Nerve	Tested by	Muscle Innervation	Potential Implications

VII Facial	Motor:
	• Close eyes, wrinkle brow
	• Smile, kiss, whistle
	• Flatten cheeks
	• Lateralize lips
		• Posterior belly of digastric
		• Stylohyoid
		• Submandibular & sublingual glands
		• Muscles of face & lips (orbicularis oris)
			• Reduced elevation of hyoid
			  ○ Decreased pharyngeal shortening
			• Reduced superior, posterior displacement of tongue, hyoid, larynx
			  ○ May have 2° implications for reduced oral containment of the bolus
			    → Pre-swallow pooling and pre-swallow penetration/aspiration
			  ○ Base of tongue to posterior pharyngeal wall approximation
			    → Vallecular residual with post-swallow penetration/aspiration
			    → Pharyngeal residual with post-swallow penetration/aspiration
			• Decreased salivation
			  ○ impaired bolus formation

	Sensory: • Taste perception for anterior 2/3 tongue		• Decreased bolus recognition • Contribution to delayed pharyngeal response with consequent pre-swallow, or intra-swallow penetration/aspiration

continues

Table 6–1. *continued*

Cranial Nerve	Tested by	Muscle Innervation	Potential Implications
IX Glossopharyngeal (in isolation)	Motor: • Gag reflex (high risk of false positive)	• Stylopharyngeus	• Reduced pharyngeal shortening ○ Post-swallow diffuse residual → Risk of post-swallow penetration/aspiration ○ Less likely reduced supraglottic compression → Risk of intra-swallow penetration/aspiration
	Sensory: • Gag reflex (high risk of false positive) • Estimation of onset of swallow (very difficult to assess clinically • Taste and sensation to posterior 1/3 tongue and oral cavity, faucial arches • Observed spontaneous expectoration of pharyngeal residual		• Contribution to delayed pharyngeal swallow ○ Pre-swallow pooling → Pre-swallow penetration/aspiration

Table 6–1. *continued*

Cranial Nerve	*Tested by*	*Muscle Innervation*	*Potential Implications*
X Vagus (in isolation)	Motor: • Vocal quality • Pitch change • Volitional cough • Glottal coup	• Cricothyroid • Interarytenoid • Lateral cricoarytenoid • Cricopharyngeus	• Reduced glottic closure ○ Intra-swallow penetration-aspiration ○ Inability to clear aspirate • Reduced UES opening in width or duration ○ Pyriform sinus residual → Post-swallow penetration-aspiration
	Sensory: • Cough reflex testing		• Recued laryngeal and tracheal sensation ○ Silent aspiration • Reduced distal pharyngeal sensation ○ Failure to elicit a clearing response for residual in distal pharynx
Pharyngeal plexus (IX and X combined)	Motor: • See IX and X above	• Superior, middle, and inferior pharyngeal constrictor • Palatoglossus • Palatopharyngeus • Salpingopharyngeus • Levator veli palatini	• Decreased supraglottic compression ○ Intra-swallow penetration/aspiration • Decreased pharyngeal shortening shortening and contraction ○ Diffuse pharyngeal residual → Post-swallow penetration/aspiration
	Sensory: • See IX and X above (provides sensory feedback to much of pharyngeal mucosa)		• Reduced distal pharyngeal sensation ○ Failure to elicit a clearing response for pharyngeal residual

continues

Table 6–1. *continued*

Cranial Nerve	Tested by	Muscle Innervation	Potential Implications
XII Hypoglossal	Motor: • Lingual movement ○ Superior ○ Lateral ○ Protrusion ○ Retraction	• Intrinsic muscles of tongue • Genioglossus • Styloglossus • Hyoglossus • Strap muscles & geniohyoid when paired with C1-2 to form ansa cervicalis	• Reduced bolus manipulation, preparation, and formation ○ Lack of cohesive bolus for transfer ○ Post-swallow oral residual (buccal and sublingual) ○ Post-swallow penetration/aspiration of oral residual • Reduced active drop of base of tongue ○ Contribution to delayed onset of swallow with pre-swallow penetration/aspiration • Decreased base of tongue to posterior pharyngeal wall approximation ○ Superior pharyngeal/vallecular residual with post-swallow penetration/aspiration

Note. UES = upper esophageal sphincter; 2° = secondary to.

EXTENDING THE CRANIAL NERVE EXAMINATION: THE COUGH REFLEX TEST

A more recent addition to a swallowing assessment provides an option for directly assessing the integrity of the sensory fibers of the vagus nerve. This neural substrate is otherwise very difficult to objectively assess. The inhalation cough challenge, or cough reflex test (CRT), is a simple extension of the cranial nerve examination. Researchers and clinicians in respiratory medicine have utilized cough reflex testing for well over 50 years in the assessment of patients with underlying respiratory disease. First introduced in the 1950s (Bickerman & Barach, 1954; Bickerman, Cohen, & German, 1956), the cough challenge involves the delivery of tussive or chemoreactive agents into the upper airways with a recording of a behavioral response, most readily observed as a cough reflex. The importance of a cough response to airway protection, and consequently pulmonary integrity, has long been acknowledged, particularly in the neurogenic population. Patients with weak cough have an increased risk for developing aspiration pneumonia (Smith Hammond et al., 2001). Absence or delayed recovery of a cough reflex after stroke has been postulated to increase morbidity and mortality (Addington, Stephens, & Gilliland, 1999). Laryngeal cough reflex has been identified in the stroke population to be impaired for up to one month or longer, with permanent impairment in some patients (Kobayashi, Hoshino, Okayama, Sekizawa, & Sasaki, 1994). Despite this, the explicit testing of cough in the dysphagia diagnostic armamentarium has only recently emerged.

The first reported clinical use of inhalation cough challenge in the neurogenic population with dysphagia was published by Addington, Stephens, and Gilliland (1999). A prospective study of 400 patients in the acute post-stroke population was conducted to identify those patients at risk for developing aspiration pneumonia. Participants were administered a single dose of tartaric acid with subsequent cough response scored as normal, weak, or absent. Recommendations for oral feeding were based heavily on outcome of cough challenge testing, with those presenting a normal cough response fed orally and those with absent or weak scores fed either non-orally or on a restricted diet. Incidence of pneumonia was compared with that of a sister hospital that did not employ cough challenge testing in determining management. Results demonstrated that 5 of 400 patients who received the cough challenge ultimately developed pneumonia, whereas in the stroke population of the sister hospital without cough testing, 27 of 204 developed pneumonia, a significant difference. In a subsequent study of 818 consecutive stroke patients, 35 (4.3%) developed pneumonia. Of the 736 (90%) patients who had a normal cough response, 26 (3.5%) developed pneumonia, and of the 82 (10%)

patients with an abnormal cough response, 9 (11%) developed pneumonia despite preventive interventions. These early positive findings are tempered by methodological issues and bias in participant selection. Participants were only included in the cough testing group if they were cognitively able to complete the task of sealing the lips around a nebulizer mouthpiece and fully exhaling and inhaling, thus biasing toward a less impaired population.

In a more recent clinical trial by Miles, Zeng, McLauchlan, and Huckabee (2013), 311 patients with acute, first-event stroke were randomly assigned to either a control group that received "usual clinical assessment" or an experimental group that received a CRT as a component of the CSE. Participants received a 15-second exposure to 0.8 mol/L of citric acid, nebulized at 8 L per minute using a face mask method and passive respiration. Although this study improved on the clinical trial from Addington, Stephens, and Gilliland (1999) by randomizing to well-controlled experimental groups, the researchers did not dictate management practices based solely on results of the CRT, allowing clinicians the flexibility to integrate the results of the test into clinical practice as they deemed appropriate. Analyses of the data identified no significant differences between groups in pneumonia rate or mortality. Results of the CRT were shown to significantly influence diet recommendations and referrals for instrumental assessment; however, the lack of a structured management protocol resulted in anecdotal evidence of disregard for CRT results in determining oral intake.

This research group then followed promptly with a retrospective-prospective-comparison, evaluating the original cohort from the Miles, Zeng, and colleagues (2013) study and a second new cohort at the same facility (Perry, Miles, Fink, & Huckabee, 2018). The prospective cohort received CRT using the same protocol previously described, but a structured protocol to guide interpretation of the CRT results and facilitate appropriate management was added. The Dysphagia in Stroke Protocol (DiSP) required that if cough was absent on CRT, the patient was directed to instrumental assessment prior to any oral intake, including oral trials at bedside. If the patient was identified to silently aspirate on instrumental assessment, oral intake was withheld until documented return of cough. The retrospective and prospective groups were similar on most demographic and health variables with the exception that those in the prospective group had more respiratory comorbidities coming into the study. Incorporation of CRT in this protocol resulted in several statistically and clinically significant findings. A reduction of pneumonia from 28% of the retrospective group to 10% of the control group was documented; within the longitudinal three-month follow-up period for each patient, the two groups also differed in readmission to hospital due to pneumonia (0–5%). This difference in pneumonia rates did not translate to differences in mortality due to pneumonia, reflecting the multifactorial contributions to development of pneumonia and efficiency of medical management. Of interest, at the three-month follow-up, although the proportion of patients on tube-feeding was similar across groups, for those on an oral diet, 81% of the DiSP group had returned to a normal diet, compared with only 55% of the retrospective patients.

Nakajoh and colleagues (2000) evaluated the relationship between cough sensitivity and pneumonia in a cohort of patients with chronic stroke in a nursing home setting. Rather than completing a clinical trial, these researchers identified the dose of inhaled citric acid that produced a cough response. In this study, a significant relationship was identified between cough thresholds, pneumonia rates, and delayed swallowing response to water injected into the pharynx. Those most likely to develop pneumonia had lower cough sensitivity and slower swallowing responses.

Further studies have validated the CRT against instrumental assessment of swallowing. Wakasugi and colleagues (2008) compared results of citric acid–evoked CRT against a VFSS or VEES in 204 patients with suspected dysphagia. When evaluating all 107 patients with documented aspiration, sensitivity of the CRT for detection of aspiration was 0.67 and specificity was 0.97. A similar but expanded validation study was completed by Miles, Moore, and colleagues (2013). In order to determine optimal "dose" of inhaled citric acid, this study derived cough thresholds in 80 patients undergoing VFSS and 101 patients undergoing VEES. Significant associations between CRT result and cough response to aspiration on VFSS and VEES were identified. Sensitivity and specificity were optimized at 0.6 mol/L in patients undergoing VFSS (71% and 60%, respectively) and at 0.4 mol/L in patients undergoing VEES (69% and 71%, respectively). A concentration of 0.8 mol/L had the highest odds ratio (OR) for detecting silent aspiration (OR = 8 based on VFSS; OR = 7 based on VEES). Table 6–2 includes sensitivity and specificity values for all concentrations tested, allowing clinicians the option of selecting a dose of citric acid that best meets their clinical needs. For example, if the CRT is used as a screening tool, the clinician may opt for a dose that produces high sensitivity at

Table 6-2. Sensitivity and Specificity of CRT at Three Concentrations of Nebulized Citric Acid (0.4, 0.6, 0.8 mol/L; when validated to VFSS and videoendoscopy)

			Sensitivity % (95% confidence interval [CI])		***Specificity % (95% CI)***	
			Full Cohort	***Aspirators Only***	***Full Cohort***	***Aspirators Only***
VFSS	0.8		58 (0.36,0.78)	59 (0.43,0.64)	84 (0.78,0.89)	86 (0.47, 0.99)
	0.6		71 (0.47,0.88)	71 (0.55,0.80)	60 (0.54,0.65)	71 (0.34,0.95)
	0.4		77 (0.53,0.92)	77 (0.62,0.88)	35 (0.29,0.39)	57 (0.23,0.86)
Videoendoscopy	0.8	pass vs fail	44 (0.32, 0.54)	44 (0.34, 0.47)	89 (0.82, 0.95)	96 (0.83, 0.99)
		without trace aspirators	59 (0.43, 0.72)	59 (0.46, 0.63)	89 (0.83, 0.94)	96 (0.83, 0.99)
	0.6	pass vs fail	50 (0.37, 0.61)	50 (0.39, 0.55)	85 (0.77, 0.91)	93 (0.78, 0.99)
		without trace aspirators	67 (0.50, 0.80)	66 (0.53, 0.73)	85 (0.78, 0.90)	93 (0.79, 0.99)
	0.4	pass vs fail	69 (0.55, 0.81)	69 (0.58, 0.78)	71 (0.63, 0.77)	81 (0.66, 0.92)
		without trace aspirators	85 (0.69, 0.95)	85 (0.71, 0.94)	71 (0.64, 0.75)	81 (0.67, 0.90)

Source: Reprinted from A. Miles, S. Moore, M. McFarlane, F. Lee, J. Allen, and M. L. Huckabee, "Comparison of Cough Reflex Test Against Instrumental Assessment of Aspiration," *Physiology & Behavior, 118*, 29. Copyright © 2013, with permission from Elsevier.

the cost of low specificity. However, if the CRT is to be used in conjunction with other clinical assessment measures, it may be preferred to select a better balance between the two measures. Although sensitivity and specificity are somewhat low to be used as independent measures, these data compare favorably with other single measures used in swallowing assessment, suggesting that use of the CRT may offer a valuable contribution within the context of a full clinical swallowing assessment.

Of note, another group of researchers is evaluating the phenomenon of "urge to cough," reflecting cortical recognition of the need to cough (Brandimore, Hegland, Okun, Davenport, & Troche, 2017; Hegland, Okun, & Troche, 2014; Troche, Schumann, Brandimore, Okun, & Hegland, 2016). This body of work holds great promise and likelihood for translation to stroke, but at this point, validation is only available in patients with Parkinson's disease.

The preceding work lends support to the inclusion of inhalation cough testing as a valuable adjunct to the clinical assessment. To date, similar research has not been conducted to evaluate the influence of this test on outcomes when it is included as a component of more traditional clinical and diagnostic assessments, rather than used as a sole determinant of oral intake. Swallowing diagnosis is based largely on subjective interpretation of both behavioral presentation and instrumental visualization; there are very few quantitative clinical measures of swallowing-associated behaviors. When a quantitative measure is available and data support that it is effective for identifying patients at risk, it would be wise to integrate it into clinical protocol. One might speculate that outcomes would be substantially improved.

Executing the Cough Reflex Test

A variety of stimuli have been utilized for the CRT, including citric acid (Kastelik et al., 2002), capsaicin (Midgren, Hansson, Karlsson, Simonsson, & Persson, 1992), and tartaric acid (Addington, Stephens, & Goulding, 1999). In a comparison of agents, Morice, Kastelik, and Thompson (2001) documented that only capsaicin and citric acid could be considered reproducible across time and thus were considered reliable for clinical use. Additionally, a number of protocols have been described, including that by Addington, Stephens, and Gilliland (1999). However, given the wide variety of tussigenic agents, concentrations, and delivery methods, universal standards for cough challenge testing are unavailable. The following protocol included in this text is adapted from research by Morice and colleagues (2001) but reflects methods and outcomes of more recent research and is the protocol incorporated into the DiSP.

Citric acid is diluted in 0.9% sodium chloride to prepare samples of stimuli at 0.8 M and 1.2 M concentrations. Clinicians may choose to shift to a single concentration with suppressed cough only at 0.6 M to simplify the test. The clinician will need to consult professionals in the pharmacology department of their facilities for assistance in preparing the stimuli. Delivery of citric acid is presented via nebulized air with an obstructed flow rate of 6.6 L/min, utilizing a full exhalation–full inhalation method (Pounsford & Saunders, 1985). With a nose clip in place, participants are instructed to place the mouthpiece of the nebulizer kit into their mouths to form a good seal. When the nebulizer is turned on, they should fully exhale to functional residual capacity, then fully inhale to vital lung capacity. For the lower concentration, participants are instructed to cough "when you feel the need to cough." Once this is completed, the higher concentration is presented with the instruction to "try to suppress the cough, and cough only when you have to." By using both methods, the clinician is assessing not only the natural cough but also suppressed cough. For this protocol, as described by Morice and colleagues (2001), cough within the first 15 seconds of inhalation is documented. The test is repeated up to three times, and positive cough response is documented when the participant coughs at least twice on 50% of presentations.

The method reported by Addington, Stephens, and Gilliland (1999) prescribes a 20% solution of L-tartaric acid dissolved in 2 mL of sterile normal saline. With a nose clip in place, the single concentration of nebulized stimulus is delivered for a maximum of three trials using a single expiratory-inspiratory method. The test is terminated when a cough response is elicited or no response is generated after all three trials.

The following represents a clinical CRT protocol adapted from the Department of Speech Language Therapy at the Christchurch Hospital (Christchurch, New Zealand) that is based heavily on emerging data from the local research group. This protocol is employed by many hospitals in New Zealand (Table 6–3). Additionally, the DiSP is provided as an online resource.

Table 6–3. Sample Clinical Protocol for Cough Reflex Testing

Clinical Protocol: Cough Reflex Testing

Adapted from Canterbury District Health Board

Who can have a CRT?

Indications for CRT as part of the SLT examination include:

- Patient is alert for assessment
- Medical consent has been given to perform CRT on the patient (stroke patients have blanket consent provided they are alert and able to sit upright)
- CRT would aid management decisions (e.g., patient is a potential candidate for oral diet)
- Airway protection status is a relevant clinical question
- Information about vagus nerve function will aid management/decisions

Contraindications to CRT: requires discussion with medical team

- Medical team is concerned about raised intracranial pressure
- Tracheostomy in situ
- Patients whose management is prescribed comfort cares
- Those patients for whom the medical team deems the test contraindicated
- Pediatrics

Definitions within CRT

Cough reflex PASS:

On 2/3 trials, there are two successive coughs (not interrupted by respiration) within 15 seconds of starting the nebulizer

Strong pass:

On 2/3 trials, there are two successive strong coughs within 15 seconds of starting the nebulizer. The cough is perceived as strong enough to clear material from the airway.

Weak pass:

On 2/3 trials, there are two successive weak coughs within 15 seconds of starting the nebulizer. The cough is perceived as not strong enough to clear material from the airway.

Cough reflex ABSENT:

There is an absence of two successive coughs within 15 seconds of starting the nebulizer on 2/3 trials.

continues

Table 6–3. *continued*

Procedure for administering the cough reflex test

Equipment

a. PulmoMate Compressor Nebulizer System (Model 46501) (DeVilbiss Healthcare LLC, Pennsylvania, US) with a predetermined free flow output of 8 liters per minute. With liquid in the chamber this equals 6.6 L/min.

b. Adult elongated aerosol facemask, tubing, and nebulizer cup

c. Saline solution

d. Citric acid 0.6 mol/L

e. Syringe (2 mL or 5 mL suitable)

NB: This test must be completed using the nebulizer, not piped oxygen, as this will invalidate the test.

Procedure

- Place 3 mL of saline in the nebulizer chamber, connect to mask, and place over patient"s nose and mouth
- Ask the patient to breathe freely for 10–15 seconds after you start the nebulizer to familiarize him/her with the test protocol
- Discard saline
- Using a sterile syringe, place 3 mL of 0.6 mol/L citric acid in the chamber
- Replace mask over patient's nose and mouth
- Instruct the patient to breathe normally while you monitor his/her breathing for up to 15 seconds. "I'm going to have a look at your breathing. [Apply mask] Just breathe through your mouth." Alternatively, tell the patient "Breathe through your mouth and try not to cough." Both sets of instructions are designed to minimize the likelihood of a "placebo cough" or volitional cough to suggestion.
- Stop the nebulizer if the patient coughs **twice successively**. Make a clinical judgment of "strong cough" vs "weak cough."
- Allow the patient to breathe normally for **30 sec to 1 min** to prevent tachyphalaxis
- Repeat the presentation of citric acid a **second time**
    - Stop the nebulizer if the patient coughs **twice successively**.
    - If required the test may be repeated one more time (**a maximum of three trials**) if the above ratings are not consistent.
- If the patient has **two successive coughs on 2/3 trials** mark as **PRESENT**. Please see definitions section regarding rating result as present strong or present weak.
- If the patient has **no or only 1 response on 2/3 presentations**, it is considered an **ABSENT** result.

Table 6–3. *continued*

Infection Prevention and Control

General Infection Prevention Guidelines

- The privacy curtains should be pulled during the cough reflex testing.
- Staff must assess the risk for personal protective equipment (PPE) such as a mask.
- Hand hygiene must be performed before and after the cough reflex test and gloves must be worn when completing CRT.
- Discard nebulizer cough, tubing, and face mask appropriately after use.

Contact Precautions

- Wear the correct PPE as per contact precautions.
- Disinfect any non disposable equipment with a disinfectant.

Equipment

- Any patient shared equipment that touches the patient must be cleaned between uses.
- Routinely clean the nebulizer pump with detergent and water or disposable detergent wipe.
- If scissors are used to cut sterile tubing to insert sterile bleeder (for those using the turbo nebulizer), these should be disinfected with an alcohol wipe.

Interpreting the Cough Reflex Test

Normative data for citric acid cough thresholds are emerging; however, normative data are unavailable for other tussive agents described above. No justification is provided for the selection of stimuli concentrations advocated by Addington, Stephens, and Gilliland (1999). Past research has documented gender differences in cough response, with women having greater sensitivity, hence lower cough thresholds, compared with men (Dicpinigaitis & Rauf, 1998; Kastelik et al., 2002). Children are documented to respond at lower thresholds than adults (Chang, Phelan, Roberts, & Robertson, 1996). Additionally, asthma (Chang, Phelan, & Robertson, 1997) and gastroesophageal reflux disease (Ferrari et al., 1995) lead to increased cough receptor sensitivity, whereas smoking (Dicpinigaitis, 2003) diminishes airway sensitivity. Although these variables may influence outcomes of a CRT, in most respects this does not matter. If patients have any of these comorbidities and cough is either exaggerated or inhibited, this becomes an integral part of their current clinical picture that influences their ability to protect their pulmonary system.

Identification of cough sensitivity may help expand on the diagnostic picture. Addington, Stephens, and Gilliland (1999) advocate a somewhat binary approach, with those passing the test able to assume oral intake and those failing the test being restricted or non-orally fed with no mention of instrumental assessment. Limiting this weighty management decision to a single source of information appears to neglect the importance of other clinically meaningful data. The DiSP requires instrumental assessment for those with absent cough. However, it is important to recognize that patients may very well cough heartily but persist with significant dysphagia that is detrimental to hydration and nutrition as well as quantity of life. Integration of CRT data into the overall clinical picture is critical. As with any diagnostic tool or clinical assessment procedure, its value is seen only with proper integration of results.

Similar to all clinical tools, there are caveats to inclusion of CRT in clinical practice. Considerable research is required before inhalation cough challenge can be fully incorporated into the clinical assessment. Although validity is well established to instrumental assessment in stroke, test-retest reliability and interrater reliability are yet under-evaluated, or concerningly poor, respectively. Although the absence of normative data may be seen as a major limitation to incorporating this as a clinical adjunct, sensitivity and specificity are perhaps more salient to assessment and provide a foundation for adding this test into clinical practice. However, documented sensitivity and specificity are not without complication. This is explained, in part, by methods. The CRT is designed to evaluate presence or absence of cough only. One can only evaluate presence or absence of cough on instrumental assessment if the patient aspirates. Thus, a clinician may identify absent cough on clinical examination and anticipate that the patient may silently aspirate. They then find no cough on instrumental assessment because the patient did not aspirate. In this regard, the test failed to identify silent aspiration, not because cough was inaccurately predicted, but because aspiration was inaccurately predicted. This presents a measurement error of sensitivity and specificity.

Finally, CRT, as described, is designed only to evaluate cough sensitivity, not relative strength or effectiveness of coughing. Cough "strength" as a proxy for effectiveness is known to be different between reflexive coughing and elicited coughing (Addington, Stephens, Phelipa, Widdicombe, & Ockley, 2008; Lasserson et al., 2006; Mills, Jones, & Huckabee, 2017). Despite these lingering issues, given the ramifications of an absent cough response on airway protection and the relatively high incidence of silent aspiration that hinders accurate clinical assessment, emergence of this modality in the diagnostic armamentarium is well overdue.

Specific Comments on the Gag Reflex

The gag response historically has been utilized as a standard test of pharyngeal sensation to aid in prediction of a patient's ability to swallow without risk of airway compromise (Linden & Siebens, 1983). Some suggest that assessment of the gag response in the CSE provides high sensitivity (but low specificity) compared with bedside evaluation alone in identifying aspiration in acute stroke patients (Ramsey, Smithard, Donaldson, & Kalra, 2005). However, other authors report that the presence or absence of gag response does not predict swallowing ability or airway protection (Davies, Kidd, Stone, & MacMahon, 1995; Leder, 1996, 1997). Variability in responsiveness to gag in individuals without swallowing impairment is common (Schulze-Delrieu & Miller, 1997), with as many as 37% in a cohort of 140 healthy adults, young and old, not demonstrating a gag response (Davies et al., 1995). Aviv (1997) points out that assessment of the gag response measures integrity of sensory fibers of the glossopharyngeal nerve; this is valuable information. However, it is the superior laryngeal branch of the vagus nerve that provides sensation to the hypopharynx and larynx and thus is critical for "last chance" airway protection. Due to conflicting reports on association with pharyngeal biomechanics and airway protection, the clinician is left with a conclusion that presence of a gag response indicates integrity of glossopharyngeal sensory fibers; absence of a gag response indicates very little reliable information in isolation but may help to complete the clinical picture when taken in the context of other derived information.

Caveats of the Cranial Nerve Examination

Findings of the cranial nerve examination need to be seen in light of the patient's overall status. A robust patient with adequate cognition and reasonable health may provide clear and unambiguous information. However, patients who are acutely ill and those with substantive neurologic impairment frequently exhibit difficulty in executing the required tasks. It is important to keep in mind that just because patients do not perform the tasks does not mean that neurologically they cannot. Lack of execution does not always implicate a neurologic deficit. If eliciting a response proves difficult, attempts should be made to observe the behavior in spontaneous activity (i.e., volitional cough versus reflexive cough, tongue lateralization versus protrusion versus licking dry lips). Evaluation of the patient at another time, particularly those in the acute post-stroke phase, may yield dramatically different results if their overall status improves.

There are several primary factors to consider in the interpretation of cranial nerve assessment.

- An understanding of direct motor and sensory innervation patterns will allow the clinician to bridge the gap between observed behaviors and inferred physiology. This will prepare the clinician to perform an efficient and well-focused instrumental assessment if deemed appropriate.
- An assessment of laterality of presentation of pathologic findings will provide insights into site of lesion and potential neuromuscular presentation, as well as recovery potential. As the cranial nerves involved in swallowing are bilaterally but asymmetrically represented (with the exception of the lower face and, functionally, the tongue), strong asymmetry of clinical presentation beyond the acute phase would tend to suggest ipsilesional LMN involvement as the bilateral representation softens clinical presentation over time. Lateralizing presentation in the early acute phase can be difficult to specify, as this could reflect either ipsilesional LMN damage or contralesional UMN damage that has not yet softened due to bilateral inputs.
- An understanding of redundancy in the physiologic system will allow for a more realistic reflection of inferred pathophysiology. There are only rare situations in swallowing physiology where a single nerve that feeds a single muscle group accomplishes a task. More often than not, there is redundancy in the system. As an example, apparent damage to the trigeminal nerve may

have significant adverse consequences on anterior hyoid movement as the anterior belly of the digastric and the mylohyoid muscles are innervated by this nerve. However, if the ansa cervicalis remains intact and thus the geniohyoid is likely unimpaired, the clinical inference of impaired anterior hyoid movement may be tempered, leading the astute clinician to suspect impairment of lesser severity.

By taking these factors into account, a clinical picture will emerge that allows the clinician substantial insights into swallowing behavior.

CASE EXAMPLE

A clinician receives a referral on an elderly patient who was involved in a motor vehicle accident 4 weeks prior and had sustained traumatic insult to the base of the skull region. In the emergency department, he experienced acute onset of confusion and dysarthria and was diagnosed with an acute stroke. On examination of the oral mechanism, the patient presents with significant dense, right upper, and lower facial weakness; the patient's smile is asymmetric, with weakness on the right; and the patient is unable to tightly purse his lips. The tongue deviates to the right on protrusion. There is bilateral protrusion of the masseters on biting; however, this is less pronounced on the right, and the jaw deviates mildly to the right when opening against resistance. The gag response is present; volitional cough is strong, with a clear and loud vocal quality. Based on the history and the clinical presentation, the clinician is in a position to query potential physiologic impairments and identify both positive and negative predictors that support the decision-making process. Clinical reasoning for this patient is outlined in Table 6–4.

The ability to make clinical deductions that pair findings of cranial nerve examination with observations of oral ingestion, as described in Chapter 7, will provide the clinician with a more thorough diagnostic picture. This skill characterizes a very strong diagnostician.

Table 6–4. Clinical Problem Solving from Cranial Nerve Findings to Physiologic Probabilities in a Patient with Traumatic Brain Injury and Acute Onset Stroke

CN	***Query***	***Positive Predictors***	***Negative Predictors***
Possible residual effects of UMN lesion of left V or mild LMN of right V	Impairment of mastication (masseters, temporalis)		Not reported from clinical presentation
	Reduced anterior hyoid movement (anterior belly, mylohoid)	Hypoglossal nerve also appears impaired unilaterally, thus implicating involvement of ansa cervicalis and consequently geniohyoid. This increases risk of poor anterior hyoid movement. There was questionable aspiration on solids in clinical assessment which may suggest post-swallow aspiration of pyriform sinus residual that would be consistent with decreased anterior hyoid movement.	Mild impairment overall; aspiration of liquids which would be consistent with poor epiglottic deflection from decreased anterior hyoid movement is not observed on clinical examination.

CN	Query	Positive Predictors	Negative Predictors
Right LMN of VII	Reduced elevation (not anterior) of hyoid 2° involvement of posterior belly of digastric and stylohyoid resulting in decreased pharyngeal shortening and reduced supraglottic compression, May lead to risk of intra-swallow aspiration	With unilateral impairment of hypoglossal and thus implication of ansa cervicalis there would be increased risk of difficulty with supraglottic shortening due to strap muscle involvement.	Pharyngeal constrictors may more directly facilitate pharyngeal shortening and there is no evidence of pharyngeal plexus impairment.
	May have 2° consequences for oral containment of the bolus, and pre-swallow pooling.	Potential impairment of posterior belly of digastric and stylohyoid may be exacerbated by damage to hypoglossal that innervates styloglossus. This may adversely affect elevation of posterior tongue	Palatoglossus muscle is primarily responsible for glossopalatal approximation and there is no evidence of pharyngeal plexus impairment, which would suggest impairment of this muscle.
	Base of tongue to posterior pharyngeal wall approximation with post-swallow vallecular residual	Posterior belly of digastric and stylohyoid may assist with approximation of the tongue to the posterior pharyngeal wall.	This movement is more significantly influenced by fibers of the superior pharyngeal constrictor, of which there is not indication of impairment.
	Decreased salivation: difficulty with bolus prep	Most salivary flow from CN VII	Some salivary flow via CN IX. No clinical reports of dry mucosa.

continues

Table 6–4. *continued*

CN	Query	Positive Predictors	Negative Predictors
Right LMN of XII	Poor bolus manipulation, preparation and transfer resulting in lack of cohesive bolus; post-swallow oral residual (buccal sublingual).	No redundancy in innervation or muscle function for bolus manipulation; fits clinical description. Aspiration of solids that is observed clinically may be from oral residual.	Unilateral involvement.
	Decreased glossopalatal approximation and decreased base of tongue to posterior pharyngeal wall with post-swallow vallecular residual (styloglossus)	When paired with facial involvement (as above), this increases likelihood.	No evidence of difficulty with pharyngeal plexus which would impair contribution of palatoglossus to glossopalatal approximation and pharyngeal plexus to superior constrictor.
	Contribution to delay pharyngeal swallow secondary to inefficient base of tongue transfer of the bolus	Associated cognitive impairment may also inhibit contribution to onset of swallow.	No strong evidence of impaired sensation otherwise in oral cavity CN V and pharyngeal cavity CN IX

Note. CN = cranial nerve; LMN = lower motor neuron; UMN = upper motor neuron; 2° = secondary to.

7 The Clinical Swallowing Examination

Assessment of Oral Intake

As described earlier, completion of a thorough cranial nerve examination will allow clinicians to problem-solve their way to educated deductions regarding potentially impaired features of swallowing. Direct observation of oral intake can provide specific and direct information about observed oral phase swallowing impairments and, through careful observation and *realistic* interpretation, can offer suggestions regarding pathophysiologic features of swallowing in other phases. Integration of cranial nerve function with observed behavior of ingestion should lead the astute clinician to a clinical swallowing examination (CSE) with greater sensitivity and specificity for pharyngeal swallowing impairment.

EXECUTING THE ASSESSMENT OF ORAL INTAKE

Several factors need to be considered in completing the direct swallowing assessment. First, there may be situations where observation of oral intake is not immediately appropriate. Receipt of a referral for swallowing assessment does not necessarily stipulate that the patient must be fed. The overall assessment of cognition, language, and cranial nerve function may suggest that any type of oral intake is premature. A patient who is obtunded may not have dysphagia but would not be a candidate for oral ingestion until consciousness has improved. Likewise, a patient with concomitant respiratory disease who struggles to maintain baseline ventilation also may not be appropriate for initiation of oral intake until respiratory stability is ensured. In the shorter term, a patient who is receiving nothing by mouth (NPO/NBM) and with neglected oral care who presents with unhealthy oral mucosa presents an environment ripe for the proliferation of bacteria. Oral care would be warranted prior to direct assessment of oral intake in order to inhibit the potential aspiration of colonized oral bacteria. If assessment of oral intake is commenced, this should be completed as the patient would normally eat, or in close approximation. The patient should be upright at 90 degrees if possible and should be wearing dentures if this is the norm.

As with the cranial nerve assessment, an organized protocol for evaluation of oral ingestion will ensure efficient and comprehensive observation of a variety of behaviors. No data exist to support that one protocol is more appropriate than another, although certainly clinical biases exist. While the use of standard protocol is beneficial, it is also important to tailor the evaluation for the presenting patient in order to obtain optimal information. For the patient who is NPO/NBM, the clinician may opt for a careful and measured approach of moving through each consistency level. A patient who is currently ingesting a regular diet will require an approach that, while evaluating all consistencies, challenges more difficult consistencies or targets specific foods that are known to the patient to be problematic. One suggested approach to completion of the comprehensive clinical assessment includes:

1. *Presentation of ice chips/crushed ice:* For the patient with significant cognitive or attentional deficits, it may be beneficial to initiate the examination with crushed ice by instructing the patient to chew and swallow promptly. This strong sensory stimulus may assist in directing the patient's attention to the task and lays a foundation for subsequent trials. If a patient fails to respond to this strong stimulus, the clinician may need to reconsider the timing of the assessment and may choose not to proceed with other textures. As a clinical note, in a patient who is NPO/NBM, it is most useful to advise the patient to actively chew and swallow rather than acquiesce to the temptation of holding the stimulus in the oral cavity while it melts.
2. *Thin liquids:* After the patient is attentive and cued to the task, the examination is best continued with evaluation of thin liquids. This consistency should correspond to Level 0 using the International Dysphagia Diet Standardization Initiative (IDDSI) framework, which was recently developed to provide a global framework for dysphagia diet uniformity (Cichero et al., 2017). In the case of the

patient with significant pharyngeal dysmotility and subsequent residual, initiating the examination with heavier textures may consequently "soil" the pharynx such that unbiased evaluation of physiology with liquid is consequently not possible. Although liquids are most frequently aspirated in patients with neurogenic dysphagia (Clavé et al., 2006; Linden & Siebens, 1983), starting with a small measured volume when aspiration is suspected and simply allowing the patient ample time to recover from any discomforting coughing episodes before moving to subsequent trials will ensure that appropriate information is received. For liquids, the clinician may assess drinking directly from a cup, through a straw, or both. It would be important to determine how a patient routinely drinks and mimic the same delivery of liquids in order to obtain the most salient information concerning swallowing ability.

3. *Puree:* Puree consistency may consist of textures similar to applesauce, or other pureed fruit or vegetable, or may extend to a more viscous puree such as pudding or mashed potatoes. This consistency should equal IDDSI Level 4 (Cichero et al., 2017); however, depending on water content, some pureed fruits and vegetables may represent IDDSI Level 3 consistency. Standardized measurement methods should be employed to confirm flow and texture of the foods and liquids tested (http://www.iddsi.org).
4. *Mashable moist solid:* There are likely as many described food consistency levels as there are facilities in which patients with dysphagia reside. A mashable moist solid would represent a bite-sized texture that easily deforms or mashes with a fork or spoon but is able to be picked up with the fingers (IDDSI Level 6). This might be represented by a well-cooked carrot or other vegetable or a ripe banana. Assessment of this consistency level will provide greater information about bolus formation and control.
5. *Firm solid:* This texture level corresponds to IDDSI Level 7. It will challenge the patient for mastication, bolus formation, and control and may also assist in identification of patients with specific impairment of the cricopharyngeus, as transfer through the upper esophageal sphincter (UES) requires substantial deformation of the bolus.

If thin liquids are not well tolerated, some clinicians may elect to proceed to an assessment of thickened liquids (IDDSI Levels 1–4) to evaluate differential effects of viscosity. Although viscosity has been shown to influence both spatial and temporal characteristics of swallowing biomechanics, we would strongly argue against assessing the effects of and making recommendation for thickened liquids or any other compensatory techniques in the CSE without completion of a subsequent instrumental swallowing examination (see Chapter 15, Professional Responsibilities). The rationale behind this thought is the need to accurately determine the specific sign, such as pooling to the pyriform sinus, prior to using a given compensation. Only during an instrumental examination can one confirm the sign and whether a specific compensatory technique is successful (Baylow, Goldfarb, Taveria, & Steinberg, 2009; Logemann et al., 2008). While it may be common to conclude that CSE will underidentify dysphagia and appropriate compensatory strategies will not be recommended, research suggests that the clinical evaluation, at least with water swallow screening protocols, may overidentify dysphagia and unnecessarily recommended restricted diets (Leigh et al., 2016). Moreover, cessation of a cough with the use of a thickened liquid cannot ensure that aspiration is eliminated. As evident on videoendoscopy, some patients who coughed with aspiration of thin liquids did not cough with aspiration of thickened liquids (Miles, McFarlane, Scott, & Hunting, 2018). The compensatory strategy may result in decreased depth or amount of aspiration, thus no cough response is elicited; however, it may not eliminate aspiration and may inhibit the detection of aspiration.

For each bolus consistency, it is important to assess a number of trials. Based on research by Lazarus and colleagues (1993), two to three trials of each evaluated consistency and volume administered are optimal to ensure that a reliable clinical picture is obtained. Certainly, clinical reason will dictate the actual number of trials and the range of textures for a given patient. Circumventing multiple trials and textures would be appropriate in a patient with obvious signs and symptoms of dysphagia who clearly is distressed with oral intake. However, the clinician will need to be aware that results from ingestion of a single bolus of any texture may be misleading, with the potential for inaccurate estimation of risk. Progressive protocols to evaluate increasing volumes and patient's self-regulation ability to mimic more realistic eating situations are described below. How a clinician initiates and progresses through each condition is dependent on the patient.

1. *Controlled ingestion:* For most patients, it is suggested that the examination begin the testing of each viscosity with single sips or

bites that are dictated in size and generally provided by the clinician. This is particularly important for individuals with suspected anosognosia or anosodiaphoria who are unaware or unconcerned about dysphagia and may not properly monitor bolus volume. Bolus size may be precisely measured and provided in increasing increments (5 mL, 10 mL, etc. for liquids) or may be presented as more functional measures (small, unmeasured amount of liquid placed in a cup, a hand-over-hand cup sip, etc.).

2. *Monitored ingestion:* For this condition, bolus size and rate of intake are at the discretion of the patient but are monitored carefully by the clinician to ensure safety. The patient is encouraged to self-feed such that self-monitoring behavior can be observed. For example, a limited amount of liquid is placed in a cup (measured 30 mL or unmeasured), and the patient is asked to take a normal size swallow. Very little is understood about the phenomenon of "apraxia of swallowing" (Daniels, 2000; Daniels, Brailey, & Foundas, 1999); however, if this exists as a component of dysphagic presentation, the ability of the patient to self-feed may significantly influence performance.
3. *Independent ingestion:* Intake rate and bolus size are fully at the discretion of the patient and not restricted but are observed by the clinician. As discussed in Chapter 3, normal liquid bolus sip size is 20 to 30 mL (Adnerhill, Ekberg, & Groher, 1989; Bennett, van Lieshout, Pelletier, & Steele, 2009; Lawless, Bender, Oman, & Pelletier, 2003); however, in testing situations, healthy individuals take significantly smaller sip sizes compared with natural drinking situations (Bennett et al., 2009). Therefore, the clinician should include large volume single swallow trials (20–30 mL) into the evaluation. Independent feeding behaviors may place the patient at significant risk; however, the clinician will want to allow opportunities for observation of these behaviors as they represent typical ingestion patterns.
4. *For liquids only:* Consecutive ingestion of liquids (i.e., sequential swallowing). As discussed in Chapter 3, Table 3–1, continuous swallows create a significantly different biomechanical swallow than single sips (Chi-Fishman & Sonies, 2000, 2002b; Daniels et al., 2004; Daniels & Foundas, 2001; Dozier, Brodsky, Michel, Walters, & Martin-Harris, 2006). Thus, assessment of this type of ingestive behavior will challenge the flexibility of the upper aerodigestive system, with respiration frequently occurring during

sequence (Dozier et al., 2006; Lederle, Hoit, & Barkmeier-Kraemer, 2012). Some individuals who swallow well with single sips may have problems with consecutive liquid ingestion. Conversely, individuals who perform poorly with single sips may demonstrate improved swallowing with consecutive liquid ingestion. In Chapter 9, details are provided for the execution of a specific water swallow test for which normative data are available in the literature.

5. *Full meal:* Following the formal swallowing evaluation, if the decision is made to initiate or continue oral intake without benefit of instrumental assessment, observation of a full meal by the assessing clinician would be appropriate. This final assessment would allow the clinician great insights into the effects of behavior, fatigue, and increased quantity on clinical swallowing presentation.

INTERPRETING THE ASSESSMENT OF ORAL INTAKE

Observation of oral intake can provide substantial information about the efficiency of the oral phase and can allow the clinician, when supported by other data, to infer characteristics of pharyngeal physiology. The assessment of multiple volumes and consistencies is important to maximize the probability of identifying impairment. It is well documented that pharyngeal swallowing adapts to different bolus volumes and consistencies, or may, in the case of neurogenic impairment, fail to adapt. Pathophysiologic features of swallowing will thus be differentially highlighted based on the volume and consistency assessed. As an example, decreased neurosensory input that underlies the abnormality of delayed swallowing will be present regardless of bolus consistency; however, the diagnostic feature of delayed swallowing, or prolonged duration of stage transition, will be more readily detected on liquid or smaller boluses that inherently provide decreased sensory stimulation. Likewise, the weakness that may underlie poor pharyngeal motility will be present regardless of bolus consistency; however, heavier and more viscous consistencies will exacerbate the development of signs secondary to that pathophysiologic feature. Although this may seem a somewhat pedantic distinction, it is important that clinicians understand that they are evaluating swallowing physiology through the use of different consistencies, rather than evaluating ingestion of different textures.

From the initial bolus presentation, the clinician can glean information about pre-oral parameters of swallowing, including awareness of the bolus, attention to task, and problem-solving abilities. Does the patient actively accept the bolus, is the bolus placed in the patient's oral cavity, or does the patient actively refuse the bolus? Regardless of pharyngeal physiology, answers to these questions may supersede all else and ultimately dictate the treatment plan. As the bolus enters the oral cavity, does the mandible actively open and close to accept the cup, spoon, straw, or bolus itself? Is there adequate lip seal to inhibit anterior leakage of liquids and clear a spoon of a more viscous bolus? It will be important to determine if poor abilities at bolus acceptance are reflective of neuromuscular impairment or of impaired cognition and attention and are failing to drive the patient to volitionally participate in the feeding process. Prior assessment of cranial nerve and cognitive function may aid in this differential diagnosis.

Once the bolus is contained within the oral cavity, observation of behaviors becomes more inferential. Requesting that a patient masticate a solid bolus and then allow visualization of the bolus prior to transfer will provide information about bolus preparation and cohesion. Observations of a poorly cohesive bolus would suggest weakened or inefficient neuromuscular function of the intrinsic and extrinsic lingual muscles. This finding should correlate well with evidence of hypoglossal damage on cranial nerve examination through assessment of strength or ease of movement and might be supported by decreased diadochokinetic speech rates. A solid bolus that has not been broken down would suggest either impairment of the masticatory process or an inability of the lingual muscles to position the bolus between the teeth. A pre-existing understanding of cranial nerve function will aid the clinician in making this distinction. Evidence of trigeminal involvement would lead to a clinical speculation of impaired masticatory ability, whereas evidence of hypoglossal nerve involvement supports a speculated diagnosis of impaired bolus positioning. Once the clinician has observed bolus preparation, the patient is allowed to continue with the ingestive process. Reflexive cough or vocal quality changes during the preparatory process *may* suggest inadequate glossopalatal approximation (palatoglossus and styloglossus muscles) that allows for premature spillage of the bolus and the potential for pre-swallow airway compromise. In order to gather supporting evidence for this pathophysiologic feature, the clinician can ask the patient to hold a fairly large liquid bolus in the oral cavity before either swallowing it or expectorating it if intra-swallow aspiration is a substantial concern. An inability to perform this task would support that glossopalatal approximation is insufficient. Post-swallow observation of the oral cavity will provide further information about orolingual control of the intrinsic lingual muscles, as well as the extrinsic lingual muscles if the patient has been unable to transfer a bolus from the oral cavity. Observations of sublingual and buccal residue should be undertaken; allowing a delay before asking the patient to clear with a lingual sweep or finger sweep will provide information about oral sensory perception. Assessment of oral phase pathophysiology often is more apparent on solid or more viscous textures that challenge the neuromuscular system to a greater degree.

Clinical inferences about timing of onset of pharyngeal swallow after transfer of the bolus from the oral cavity are difficult. Although laryngeal palpation may be assistive in identifying onset of pharyngeal swallowing, after the bolus enters the oral cavity and the lips are closed, even the most skilled clinician would be unable to know the location of the bolus within the aerodigestive tract in relation to onset of swallowing. Pre-swallow coughing or vocal changes may reflect the sensory impairment of delayed onset of the pharyngeal swallow after active transfer from the oral cavity, but these observations also may reflect pre-swallow pooling from poor bolus containment. A careful assessment of oral sensation during the cranial nerve examination may be helpful in differential diagnosis. Additionally, delayed onset of pharyngeal swallowing may be more apparent on liquid consistencies because they provide less input to trigger sensory receptors, thus exacerbating the presentation of delay. Although not empirically validated, having the patient implement a "3-second prep" compensatory technique, as described by Huckabee and Pelletier (1999), may help in differential diagnosis as well. Patients with oral phase impairment may demonstrate signs of airway compromise before being instructed to swallow, whereas patients with a pure sensory deficit more likely may present this clinical presentation after the instruction to swallow. Additionally, as described in Chapter 9, cervical auscultation is advocated by some as a means to identify delayed onset of the pharyngeal swallow.

As the bolus moves farther into the lower aerodigestive tract, fewer reliable indicators of swallowing physiology are available. The clinician must then rely heavily on implications from cranial nerve assessment paired with nonspecific symptoms and quite often qualitative judgments to suggest pharyngeal impairment. During swallowing, the clinician can observe the patient for struggling behavior that might suggest discoordination of pharyngeal motility. Palpation of the hyoid and thyroid cartilage often is used by clinicians to identify onset of pharyngeal swallowing; however, as noted earlier, this has limitations. Furthermore, clinicians must be very cautious not to infer adequacy of hyolaryngeal excursion based on laryngeal palpation. The adequacy of hyolaryngeal excursion affects epiglottic deflection and UES opening, and impairment can result in vallecular or pyriform sinus residue. The integrity of these behaviors cannot be observed clinically or determined via laryngeal palpation. Thus, any estimation of hyolaryngeal excursion outside of "presence" or "absence" of movement is speculative at best.

Pharyngeal phase impairment may be detected nonspecifically by presentation of signs after swallowing. Pharyngeal residual may present as a subtle change in vocal resonance or audible breath sounds within the pharynx that can be differentiated from vocal dysphonia, particularly if these signs appear to increase with increasing consistency or quantity of ingested material. Asking the patient to attempt expectoration of pharyngeal residual into a cup will aid in identification of residual and will provide valuable information about the patient's ability to expectorate as a compensatory airway protection mechanism. A pattern of spontaneous multiple swallows, which can be detected with thyroid palpation, may also suggest pharyngeal impairment and residue in the presence of reserved sensation. Clinically, this appears more frequently to be observed in patients with specific UES abnormalities; however, there are no data to support this observation. Multiple swallows also may reflect oral residual that moves into the pharynx post-swallow, or it may be secondary to vallecular residue. The identification of pharyngeal residual as a probable sign is nonspecific; the clinician will be unable to determine whether the residual is due to impaired base of tongue to posterior pharyngeal wall approximation, impaired UES opening, or overall weakened or otherwise impaired pharyngeal motility. Knowledge of cranial nerve findings unfortunately is less helpful in differential diagnosis in the pharynx. Clear evidence of trigeminal involvement in the absence of observed deficits of glossopharyngeal and vagus nerves may lead the clinician to suspect that hyolaryngeal excursion is impaired; thus, pharyngeal sign presentation may reflect impaired epiglottic deflection with post-swallow vallecular residual and impaired UES opening with pyriform sinus residual. Additional facial nerve damage would increase suspicion of vallecular residual secondary to decreased base of tongue to posterior wall approximation. Evidence of cranial nerve damage involving glossopharyngeal and vagus nerves, if trigeminal and facial are intact, would suggest a more likely scenario of overall impaired pharyngeal motility or specific abnormalities of the cricopharyngeus muscle.

Certainly, cough is a visible and audible indicator of aspiration; although once again, it is nonspecific to physiology. Timing of the cough response can provide some additional clues, with pre-swallow coughing suggesting oral phase abnormalities or delayed initiation of pharyngeal swallowing, and intra-swallow or post-swallow coughing suggestive of pharyngeal phase involvement or the possibility of post-swallow aspiration of oral residual. Subtle throat clear or phonatory efforts or wet dysphonia may be detected by careful observation if the cough response is impaired. Some would advocate that detection may be augmented by cervical auscultation. The skilled clinician will want to discriminate between laryngeal dysphonia from vocal fold pathology and wet dysphonia suggestive of penetration or aspiration.

Specific data regarding interpretation of clinical findings are summarized in Chapter 8. The published data focus heavily on the balance between sensitivity and specificity in identification primarily of aspiration. Little data exist regarding the sensitivity and specificity of identifying other pathophysiologic features of swallowing. It is important that clinicians not over-interpret the information they can attain through clinical assessment. Accurate diagnosis is not possible through observation of oral intake. However, by integrating this information with other components of a thorough clinical assessment, the clinician can blend a balance of art and science to increase appropriateness of referrals for instrumental assessment.

8 The Clinical Swallowing Examination

Predicting Dysphagia and Aspiration

THE CLINICAL SWALLOWING EXAMINATION WITH A FOCUS ON CLINICAL FEATURES PREDICTING DYSPHAGIA AND ASPIRATION

Numerous studies have been completed to validate subjective clinical signs and symptoms identified during the clinical swallowing examination (CSE) predictive of dysphagia and aspiration. The clinical features associated with aspiration and dysphagia are presented in Table 8–1. The reader is referred to Chapter 6 for a discussion of objective measures of reflexive cough. Assessing/interpreting responses for each feature is fairly standard to clinical practice, and evaluation techniques for most are discussed in detail in previous chapters. Although many of the research articles concerning validated clinical features do not provide specific detail concerning administration of test items from the CSE (e.g., Horner, Massey, Riski, Lathrop, & Chase, 1988), others provide detailed instruction on administration of items and interpretation of a patient's response (e.g., Daniels, McAdam, Brailey, & Foundas, 1997). Therefore, it is recommended that interested clinicians thoroughly review specific references to obtain detailed information concerning features in which they are interested.

Table 8–1. Summary of Clinical Features Associated with Aspiration and Dysphagia

Study	*Population*	*CSE Focus*	*Instrumental Protocol*	*Outcome Measures*	*Features*	*Sensitivity % / Specificity %*
Daniels et al. (1998)	55 consecutively admitted acute stroke patients	Voice Speech Volitional cough Gag reflex Trial swallows of 5, 10, 20 mL liquid, 2.5 mL semisolid, ½ cookie	VFSS—two swallows each of liquid (volumes 3,5, 10, 20 mL); 2.5 mL pudding	Risk of aspiration: any single incidence of laryngeal penetration with post-swallow residual or actual aspiration	Dysphonia	76/68
					Dysarthria	76/53
					Abnormal volitional cough	48/94
					Abnormal gag reflex	62/82
					Cough after trial swallow	57/85
					Voice change (any type) after trial swallow	38/85
Daniels et al. (1997)	59 consecutively admitted acute stroke patients	Voice Speech Volitional cough Gag reflex Trial water swallows of 5, 10, 20 mL	VFSS—two swallows each of liquid (volumes 3,5, 10, 20 mL); 5 mL pudding; ½ cookie; sequential swallowing	Risk of aspiration: any single incidence of laryngeal penetration with post-swallow residual or actual aspiration	Dysphonia	73/76
					Dysarthria	77/61
					Abnormal volitional cough	39/85
					Abnormal gag reflex	54/67
					Cough after trial swallow	62/79
					Voice change (any type) after trial swallow	31/88
					Any 2 of the 6 features	92/67

Study	Population	CSE Focus	Instrumental Protocol	Outcome Measures	Features	Sensitivity % / Specificity %
Horner et al. (1988)[a]	47 stroke patients referred for swallowing evaluation	Oral motor-sensory assessment	VFSS—not detailed	Aspiration	Unilateral cranial nerve signs	29/61
					Bilateral cranial nerve signs	71/61
					Abnormal vocal quality	91/32
					Reduced sensation	22/48
					Abnormal cough	68/38
					Abnormal gag	60/48
Horner, Massey, and Brazer (1990)[a]	70 bilateral stroke patients who had VFSS	Chart review of specific features	VFSS—½ teaspoon, 1 teaspoon, 1 tablespoon, multiple sips from straw of liquid, ½ teaspoon pudding, cookie	Aspiration	Unilateral neurologic signs	18/69
					Bilateral neurologic signs	82/31
					Abnormal gag reflex	67/73
					Abnormal volitional cough	84/56
					Dysphonia	97/29

continues

Table 8–1. *continued*

Study	Population	CSE Focus	Instrumental Protocol	Outcome Measures	Features	Sensitivity % / Specificity %
Horner, Brazer, and Massey (1993)[a]	38 bilateral stroke patients who underwent a CSE and VFSS	Oral motor-sensory assessment	VFSS—not detailed	Aspiration	Unilateral neurologic signs	37/64
					Bilateral neurologic signs	63/36
					Abnormal gag reflex	74/64
					Abnormal volitional cough	89/64
					Dysphonia	93/09
Kidd et al. (1993)	60 consecutively admitted acute stroke patients	Pharyngeal sensation	VFSS—2, 5, 10 mL liquid, custard, jelly, mince, biscuit	Aspiration	Abnormal pharyngeal sensation	100/60
		Trial swallows—50 mL provided in 5 mL portions			Cough or voice change	80/86

Study	*Population*	*CSE Focus*	*Instrumental Protocol*	*Outcome Measures*	*Features*	*Sensitivity % / Specificity %*
Leder & Espinosa (2002)	53 consecutive stroke patients referred for swallowing evaluation	Voice Speech Volitional cough Gag reflex Trial water swallows via straw	Videoendoscopy—5 mL puree, liquid, solid	Risk of aspiration: any single incidence of aspiration or significant spillage or residue of a bolus into the valleculae, pyriform sinus, or laryngeal vestibule	Presence of any 2 of 6: dysphonia, dysarthria, abnormal volitional cough, abnormal gag reflex, cough after trial swallow, voice change after trial swallow	86/30
Mann & Hankey (2001)[b]	128 consecutive stroke patients	Demographic items and the Mann Assessment of Swallowing Ability	VFSS—5, 10 mL thin liquid, thick liquid, and pudding, 20 mL thin liquid	Dysphagia (defined as a disordered bolus flow)—rated as normal, moderate, severe, complete Aspiration—rated as normal, mild, moderate, severe, complete	Impaired pharyngeal response Male sex Barthel score <60 Incomplete oral clearance Palatal weakness or asymmetry Age >70 Delayed oral transit Incomplete oral clearance	All items listed in features significant based on logistic regression

continues

Table 8–1. *continued*

Study	Population	CSE Focus	Instrumental Protocol	Outcome Measures	Features	Sensitivity % / Specificity %
McCullough, Wertz, and Rosenbek (2001)	60 patients consecutively admitted within 6 weeks of stroke	History—15 items Oral motor—18 items Voice—6 items: speech/"ah" Trial swallows—10 items: 5 mL thin and thick liquid; 5 mL puree, ¼ cookie, 3-oz water	VFSS—two swallow each of 5, 10 mL thin liquid; 5–10 mL thick liquid; 5 mL puree, ¼ cookie	Any single incidence of aspiration	Pneumonia history	32/92
					Poor nutrition	50/76
					Presence of tube feeding	36/95
					Dysarthria	77/55
					Poor intelligibility	73/58
					Poor secretion management	50/84
					Wet voice (speech)	50/78
					Abnormal resonance	46/81
					Dysphonia (ah)	100/27
					Cough after trial swallow	68/82
					Judgment of airway invasion	77/63
					Reduced laryngeal elevation	41/84
					Cough on 3-oz water swallow	86/50
					Clinician rating of dysphagia	91/47

Study	Population	CSE Focus	Instrumental Protocol	Outcome Measures	Features	Sensitivity % / Specificity %
McCullough et al. (2005)	165 consecutive acute stroke patients	History—23 items Oral motor—20 items Voice/Speech praxis—9 items Trial swallows—23 items: 5–10 mL thin liquid thick liquid, puree, ¼ cookie, 3-oz water	VFSS—two swallow each of 5 mL thin and thick liquid, 5 mL puree, ¼ cookie, 3-oz thin liquid	Any single incidence of aspiration	Weak jaw bilaterally*	15/99
					Aspiration 3-oz swallow*	48/95
					Aspiration 10 mL thin liquid	38/96
					Aspiration thick liquid	21/98
					Aspiration 5 mL thin liquid	44/94
					Breathy voice	16/98
					Pneumonia	9/98
					Weak jaw unilaterally	26/96
					Aspiration puree	9/99
					Wet/gurgly voice	22/96
					Poor oral hygiene	14/97
					Aspiration solid	14/97
					Dysphonia*	54/86
					Strained voice	30/92
					Drooling	23/94
					Abnormal velum structure	24/93
					Nonoral feeding	49/84

continues

Table 8–1. *continued*

Study	Population	CSE Focus	Instrumental Protocol	Outcome Measures	Features	Sensitivity % / Specificity %
Smithard et al. (1998)	94 consecutively admitted within 24 hours of symptom onset	Alertness	VFSS—not detailed	Any single incidence of aspiration	Reduced consciousness*	50/92
		Oral motor—3 items			Abnormal tongue movement	40/91
		Voice			Absent gag reflex	45/69
		Trial water swallows 5 mL and 60 mL			Abnormal volitional cough*	45/91
					Cough after trial swallow*	40/93
					Weak/wet voice after trial swallow*	45/74

Note. VFSS = videofluoroscopic swallowing study.

[a]Sensitivity and specificity calculated from data.

[b]Data not available to calculate sensitivity and specificity.

*Regression identified these measures as best for detecting aspiration.

Clinical Features to Predict Dysphagia and Aspiration

When discussing validity, that is, how well a feature predicts aspiration (or dysphagia), the terms sensitivity and specificity generally are used. Sensitivity and specificity, as discussed in Chapter 4, are both important, and ideally a feature would be equally high in both. A clinical feature used to determine aspiration or dysphagia should have a score of at least 70% to be minimally sensitive and specific; scores closer to 100%, of course, are better. When deciding whether to choose measures with high sensitivity or high specificity, clinicians must consider their relative risk tolerance and the environment in which they work. For example, suppose there are two clinicians from two very different facilities who are using specific features from the CSE to determine which patients are at risk for aspiration, thus warranting an instrumental examination. One clinician works in a setting with a large percentage of acute and complicated patients with stroke and has ready access to videofluoroscopic swallowing study (VFSS). This clinician may choose to select features with high sensitivity to identify the majority of patients with aspiration and reduce chances of missing patients with risk of aspiration. In doing this, the clinician must understand the potential for over-recommendation of the VFSS if specificity is low. This may lead to unnecessary expense and radiation exposure as well as the potential for unwarranted diet restriction if there is delay in obtaining the VFSS. The other clinician works in a nursing home where patients are without acute illness and where access to VFSS is limited. This clinician may want to focus on features with high specificity, with the caveat that some patients with dysphagia or aspiration will not receive an instrumental assessment if sensitivity is low. Although this clinician may decrease the expense and burden of travel for VFSS, the potential for increased morbidity and mortality may increase if patients with aspiration are not identified. Again, a balance between both sensitivity and specificity cannot be overly stressed and may be best accomplished by using a cluster of features rather than a single clinical feature, as discussed by Daniels and colleagues (1997) and Logemann, Veis, and Colangelo (1999), reviewed in Table 8–1. While there are many clinical features associated with aspiration, few studies have used dysphagia as the outcome measure by which to evaluate the validity of specific features. The clinician will note that two commonly used features are not included in Table 8–1: runny nose and tearing after swallowing. There is no empirically based evidence supporting either to be associated with dysphagia or aspiration.

Limitations of the CSE

As discussed in Chapter 6 with the cough with reflex test, a focus only on specific features to predict aspiration may result in the clinician ignoring extremely important data collected as part of the global CSE. A focus only on aspiration will miss patients with dysphagia but no airway invasion. A complete CSE will allow the astute clinician to make judgments on swallowing ability, diet, and potential for treatment. With a focus only on a few clinical features, the clinician can address the potential for only aspiration and not other aspects critical to swallowing and recovery of function. Many patients with stroke can have clinically significant dysphagia without aspiration. As noted in Table 8–1, only one study identified clinical features that relate to dysphagia (Mann & Hankey, 2001). More research studies are needed that are highly sensitive and specific in determining patients with stroke at risk for dysphagia, not just aspiration.

Whether using the CSE as a global evaluation of swallowing or extracting specific features to identify aspiration, fewer than 50% of items from the examination have adequate inter- and intrajudge reliability (McCullough et al., 2000). That is, whereas one clinician may identify a patient with dysfunction in one area (e.g., volitional cough), another clinician may assess no dysfunction. In addition, the same judge may have completely different findings between two evaluations completed on the same person. Reliability is critical for an examination to be meaningful. Clinical measures of oral motor functions and voice have proven more reliable than measures of history information or trial swallows (McCullough et al., 2000). It is strongly recommended that clinicians in the same facility determine a definition of normal and abnormal on the clinical measures used to evaluate swallowing and then work together to establish reliability within and across the department.

THE MANN ASSESSMENT OF SWALLOWING ABILITY

If the clinician is uncomfortable integrating findings from a comprehensive CSE, the Mann Assessment of Swallowing Ability (MASA) may be used (Mann, 2002). The MASA is the only standardized clinical swallowing tool that has undergone psychometric testing. The

MASA was designed by the author to be an independent measure of dysphagia and aspiration. It is suggested that results from the MASA should help the clinician identify the pathophysiology of the swallowing problem, facilitate development of a treatment plan, and determine the need for further instrumental assessment.

The MASA provides a relatively good summary of items important in swallowing; however, it is relatively brief, without accounting for further exploration of cognitive, cranial nerve, or swallowing impairment. As with all CSEs, pathophysiology can be only inferred with the MASA; thus, instrumental assessment is required to develop specific management plans.

9 Adjuncts to the Clinical Swallowing Examination

Many of our current practices in the clinical swallowing examination (CSE) rely heavily on qualitative clinical judgment as to the efficiency of movement or safety of swallowing. Inherent in qualitative judgment is the potential for poor reliability and the misinterpretation of observation. Thus, when quantitative measures are identified that are validated and referenced to normative data, inclusion of these into CSE would be well advised. Two clinical tests have been developed that derive quantitative measures of aspects of oral ingestion: the Timed Water Swallowing Test (TWST) and the Test of Masticating and Swallowing Solids (TOMASS). Another quantitative measurement of lingual pressure using the Iowa Oral Pressure Instrument (IOPI) has been addressed in the research and deserves mention as an adjunct to the clinical assessment. Finally, easily accessible instrumentation may be used to augment the clinical assessment, including pulse oximetry and cervical auscultation. Although not all of these adjuncts have passed muster in terms of developing norms and demonstrating reliability and validity, they may have emerged into clinical practice. Execution of these will be discussed with a critique of currently available research.

THE TIMED WATER SWALLOWING TEST

A number of water swallowing tests (WSTs) have been introduced in the literature, primarily as screening tests for aspiration with the assessment based on qualitative observation of cough or wet dysphonia. These measures are covered in Chapter 4. A point of difference was incorporated into a derivative known as the TWST. In particular, a timed component to the basic WST was introduced, allowing for increased objectivity and a quantifiable measure of swallowing efficiency.

Executing the TWST

This very simple test consists of ingestion of either 100 or 150 mL of water from an open cup, with the instruction to drink "as quickly as is comfortably possible" (Hughes & Wiles, 1996, p. 110). Not only are subjective observations such as drooling, coughing, or vocal quality changes noted, but the number of swallows and total time required for ingestion of the liquid are recorded. From these raw data, three quantitative indices are calculated: average volume per swallow (mL/swallow), average time per swallow (sec/swallow), and what the researchers termed swallowing capacity (mL/sec).

Interpreting the TWST

Inter-, intra-, and test-retest reliability of this test was first reported by Nathadwarawala, Nicklin, and Wiles (1992). High levels of agreement were reported within and across clinicians and in patient performance over time, even when variations in flavor and temperature were introduced. Normative data for swallowing speed were established using 101 healthy subjects. The authors further identified that a swallowing capacity of less than 10 mL/sec had a sensitivity of .96 and specificity of .69 for identifying dysphagia in patients across a broad range of neurological conditions. However, presence or absence of dysphagia was defined only by a dysphagia questionnaire.

Hughes and Wiles (1996) completed further research by evaluating the TWST in 181 healthy controls between 18 and 91 years and in 30 patients with motor neuron disease. They compared the impact of age, sex, height, and neurological impairment on swallowing capacity, average bolus volume and average time per swallow. A clearly defined procedure for this assessment was outlined, allowing for this test to be reliably repeated by both clinicians and researchers. A number of bolus volumes were presented, including 150 mL, for which normative data were gained; these data were stratified across sex and four age groups (Table 9–1). Differences in average swallowing capacity were observed across age, sex, and height with greater swallowing capacity documented in younger age, males, and increased height. Those with motor neuron disease who reported the presence of dysphagia displayed reduced swallowing

Table 9–1. Normative Data for the Timed Water Swallow Test

	Water Swallow Test						
	# Swallows	**V/S**		**T/S**		**V/T**	
Time	**Age, y**	**V/S**	**Range**	**T/S**	**Range**	**V/T**	**S/D**
Male	19–34	37.5	25–50	1.2	1.0–1.3	31.9	9.5
	35–55	30	21.4–37.5	1.2	1.0–1.4	24.8	7.8
	56–73	23.2	20.8–30	1.3	1.2–1.4	18.7	5.2
	74+	20	15.7–25	1.5	1.3–1.8	14.6	5.9
Female	19–34	18.8	15–30	1.1	1.0–1.3	18.7	6.0
	35–55	16.7	13.6–21.4	1.3	1.1–1.7	13.6	4.8
	56–73	16.7	13.6–21.4	1.5	1.1–2.1	12.3	4.9
	74+	10.6	9.1–13	1.5	1.4–1.8	7.5	3.3

Note. # = number; V/S = total volume/# of swallows; T/S = time in seconds/# of swallows; V/T = total volume of fluid/time taken to ingest.

Source: Adapted from T. A. Hughes and C. M. Wiles, "Clinical Measurement of Swallowing in Health and in Neurogenic Dysphagia," *Quarterly Journal of Medicine, 89*, 111. Copyright © 1996, by permission of Oxford University Press.

efficiency compared with those who did not report dysphagia and the controls.

Wu, Chang, Wang, and Lin (2004) validated the TWST using 100 mL against the videofluoroscopic swallowing study (VFSS) with 59 patients suspected of having dysphagia (51 with diagnosis of stroke). Reduced swallowing speed on the TWST had a high sensitivity (.85) but reduced specificity (.50) for predicting dysphagia as verified by VFSS. The authors did not report sensitivity and specificity of only swallowing capacity (mL/sec) in predicting aspiration on the VFSS. However, they reported that swallowing capacity, when paired with clinical signs of aspiration, produced a sensitivity and specificity of .85 and .92, respectively.

A benefit of this test is the ease of administration using an internationally accessible material: water. However, the test is limited by the inability of some patients to safely ingest thin liquids and the lack of challenge of the oral phase of swallowing, particularly bolus mastication and preparation. Thus, an accompanying tool that specifically emphasizes oral bolus preparation would be of clinical value, particularly where oral phase deficits predominate and influence the consequent pharyngeal response. Certainly, inclusion of the TWST in patients following stroke would need to be carefully considered in the context of what is known about swallowing impairment. In an acute patient with other signs of dysphagia, the test would likely be deferred until instrumental assessment ensured functional airway protection. It is well suited, however, for patients with high-level dysphagia, those in whom other assessments fail to identify clinical signs or symptoms of impairment despite patient complaints of dysphagia.

THE TEST OF MASTICATING AND SWALLOWING SOLIDS

The TOMASS was developed as a solid bolus swallowing correlate to the TWST presented by Hughes and Wiles (1996). The TOMASS allows a quantifiable measure that is demanding of the oral phase of swallowing which is not challenged by WSTs.

Executing the TOMASS

Completing the TOMASS requires a stop watch, preferably one that includes a lap function, and an appropriate cracker. Individuals are asked to eat a single cracker "as quickly as is comfortably possible and when you have finished, say your name out loud." They are advised not to talk during ingestion. However, speaking their name on completion of the entire cracker is used as a marker of task completion and oral cavity clearance. The clinician quantifies the number of bites by how many discrete segments of cracker the individual placed in his/her mouth, while the number of swallows is recorded based on visual observation of movement of the thyroid notch. The masticatory cycles are counted through observation of jaw movements; a lap function on a digital stopwatch is useful to mark each masticatory cycle and time. Timing is initiated when the cracker passes the bottom lip and is stopped when the individual says his/her name.

Interpreting the TOMASS

A series of studies outlining normative data, reliability, and validity of the TOMASS are available (Huckabee et al., 2018). Initial analyses were not only based on the raw data of time taken to swallow and number of bites, masticatory cycles, and swallows, but extended to include derived measures similar to the TWST (number of masticatory cycles and swallows per bite, and time per bite, masticatory cycle and swallow). Unlike water, crackers are not uniformly available worldwide, thus establishment of normative values must be cracker specific. An initial study of 164 healthy adults, evenly distributed by sex across four age groups ranging from 20 years to over 80 years, compared two commercially available crackers of near identical size, weight, and ingredients. Comparisons between TOMASS performance revealed differences between crackers with the exception of number of bites and time per swallow. Thus, normative data are required for each cracker used, and the authors suggested use of only the raw data rather than derived measures. Additionally, a significant trial effect was identified, likely due to the drying effect of the cracker on oral mucosa. This led the authors to suggest that the first trial should be used for assessment. Age and sex differences were found for all raw data measures across both cracker types with reduced efficiency on all TOMASS raw data measures with increasing age. Thus, normative data are stratified by these two factors. After determining specific measurement guidelines based on early studies, normative data were then collected for the TOMASS from a minimum of 80 healthy adults, stratified by age and sex, for each of seven commercially available crackers from broad regions worldwide. Tables 9–2 and 9–3 contain normative data for the Arnott's Salada™ cracker available within Australasia and the Nabisco Saltine™ cracker available in the United States. Other normative data are available in the original publication (Huckabee et al., 2018). Pediatric data have also been collected and are in press (Frank, et al., 2018).

A further sample of 40 healthy adults was then recruited to establish test-retest and interrater reliability data for the TOMASS (Huckabee et al., 2018). A single cracker (Arnott's Salada™) was evaluated. Participants completed the TOMASS on three consecutive days. Two raters were present during one of these three sessions and each rater independently collected the four raw data TOMASS measures. Interrater reliability, as measured with intraclass correlation coefficient (ICC)

Table 9–2. TOMASS Normative Data Consisting of Mean and 95% Confidence Intervals by Age and Sex for **Arnott's Salada™ Cracker**

TEST OF MASTICATING AND SWALLOWING SOLIDS: Arnott's Salada™ cracker

		Discrete bites per cracker		Masticatory cycles per cracker		Swallows per cracker		Total time (in sec)		Masticatory cycles per bite		Swallows per bite		Time per bite (in sec)		Time per masticatory cycle (in sec)		Time per swallow (in sec)	
Sex	**Age**	**Mean**	**95% CI**	**Mean**	**95% CI**	**Mean**	**95% CI**	**Mean**	**95% CI**	**Mean**	**95% CI**	**Mean**	**95% CI**	**Mean**	**95% CI**	**Mean**	**95% CI**	**Mean**	**95% CI**
Males	20–40	1.76	1.30–2.23	36.53	30.36–42.70	2.35	1.87–2.83	29.22	24.70–33.74	25.13	18.78–31.49	1.54	1.10–2.0	19.63	15.21–24.06	0.82	0.76–0.88	15.08	10.37–19.79
	40–60	1.93	1.44–2.42	41.60	34.60–48.60	3.00	2.11–3.89	36.49	30.74–42.24	23.87	18.93–28.81	1.89	1.15–2.64	21.10	17.09–25.11	0.90	0.82–0.98	13.01	10.73–15.28
	60–80	2.33	1.79–2.87	60.67	50.51–70.82	3.20	2.41–3.99	51.26	40.53–61.99	28.87	21.09–36.65	1.44	1.13–1.76	24.06	17.69–30.43	0.84	0.77–0.92	16.99	14.46–19.52
	80+	3.40	2.65–4.15	89.73	70.52–108.94	4.00	2.73–5.27	84.76	63.13–106.39	28.99	23.04–34.95	1.27	0.88–1.66	28.79	19.33–38.24	0.95	0.80–1.11	24.12	17.15–31.09
Females	20–40	2.71	2.31–3.10	45.94	38.72–53.16	3.18	2.65–3.70	40.84	32.68–49.01	18.37	14.54–22.21	1.30	0.91–1.70	16.44	12.45–20.42	0.89	.079–0.99	13.62	11.87–15.36
	40–60	3.13	2.55–3.72	52.93	45.10–60.77	3.53	2.91–4.16	46.79	36.75–56.83	18.10	15.08–21.13	1.17	1.06–1.27	15.70	13.53–17.88	0.89	0.78–1.00	13.79	11.62–15.97
	60–80	3.27	2.94–3.60	63.33	53.21–73.46	4.07	3.19–4.94	60.37	49.24–71.51	19.89	16.05–23.73	1.28	0.97–1.58	19.04	14.84–23.25	0.95	.85–1.05	14.70	12.59–16.82
	80+	4.33	3.75–4.91	104.33	81.85–126.82	4.67	3.79–5.55	90.08	70.11–110.06	24.51	20.28–28.74	1.09	0.93–1.25	20.92	17.87–23.97	0.85	0.78–0.93	19.44	15.67–23.21

Source: From "The Test of Masticating and Swallowing Solids (TOMASS): Reliability, validity and international normative data" by M. L. Huckabee, T. McIntosh, L. Fuller, M. Curry, P. Thomas, M. Walshe, . . .O. Sella-Weiss, 2018, *International Journal of Language & Communication Disorders*, 53(1), 144–156. Copyright © 2018, by Wiley Online. Reprinted with permission.

Table 9–3. TOMASS Normative Data Consisting of Mean and 95% Confidence Intervals by Age and Sex for **Nabisco Saltine™ Cracker**

TEST OF MASTICATING AND SWALLOWING SOLIDS: Nabisco Saltine™ cracker

		Discrete bites per cracker		*Masticatory cycles per cracker*		*Swallows per cracker*		*Total time (in sec)*		*Masticatory cycles per bite*		*Swallows per bite*		*Time per bite (in sec)*		*Time per masticatory cycle (in sec)*		*Time per swallow (in sec)*	
Sex	**Age**	**Mean**	**95% CI**	**Mean**	**95% CI**	**Mean**	**95% CI**	**Mean**	**95% CI**	**Mean**	**95% CI**	**Mean**	**95% CI**	**Mean**	**95% CI**	**Mean**	**95% CI**	**Mean**	**95% CI**
Males	20–40	1.40	.90–1.90	30.80	25.25–36.35	1.70	0.94–2.46	23.42	17.74–29.09	24.05	20.18–27.92	1.30	0.62–1.98	18.15	13.36–22.74	0.79	0.64–0.95	15.73	12.23–19.23
	40–60	1.40	1.03–1.77	34.30	23.18–45.42	2.20	1.26–3.14	28.04	15.46–40.62	26.20	16.16–36.24	1.65	0.93–2.37	20.70	13.15–28.26	0.81	0.67–0.96	13.22	11.25–15.19
	60–80	2.10	1.69–2.51	41.50	33.94–49.07	2.40	1.90–2.90	30.66	25.22–36.09	21.77	13.18–30.36	1.20	0.90–1.50	16.35	9.29–23.41	0.75	0.67–0.83	13.70	10.43–16.98
	80+	3.70	3.11–4.29	54.30	41.68–66.92	3.40	2.50–4.30	44.29	35.62–52.96	14.65	11.94–17.35	0.91	0.71–1.12	12.08	9.89–14.28	0.83	0.76–0.90	14.17	11.20–17.14
Females	20–40	2.10	1.47–2.72	40.30	30.80–49.80	2.30	1.71–2.89	26.40	21.44–31.35	20.70	16.73–24.67	1.20	0.85–1.55	14.83	9.46–20.20	0.68	0.56–0.81	12.25	9.79–14.72
	40–60	3.20	2.46–3.94	53.40	41.66–65.14	2.50	1.80–3.20	36.41	29.21–43.62	17.37	13.49–21.24	0.81	0.59–1.04	11.80	9.63–13.97	0.69	0.63–0.76	16.36	11.73–20.99
	60–80	2.80	2.50–3.10	39.50	32.75–46.26	2.90	2.49–3.31	37.71	31.52–43.90	13.28	11.97–16.60	1.03	0.96–1.11	13.58	11.38–15.78	0.97	0.83–1.11	13.24	10.92–15.56
	80+	4.00	3.42–4.58	63.60	50.39–76.21	4.00	3.42–4.58	59.50	51.20–67.80	16.08	12.98–19.17	1.00	1.00–1.00	15.23	12.95–17.51	0.99	0.78–1.21	15.23	12.95–17.51

Source: From "The Test of Masticating and Swallowing Solids (TOMASS): Reliability, validity and international normative data" by M. L. Huckabee, T. McIntosh, L. Fuller, M. Curry, P. Thomas, M. Walshe, . . .O. Sella-Weiss, 2018, *International Journal of Language & Communication Disorders*, 53(1), 144–156. Copyright © 2018, by Wiley Online. Reprinted with permission.

was very high (>0.98) for all measures, and test-retest reliability across sessions was also high, with ICC values ranging from 0.83 to 0.98.

The strong reliability data established for the TOMASS reinforces the objective nature of this assessment, and the normative data available for the TOMASS, thus far, presents a normal range to compare patient performance with during clinical use. However, validation of the TOMASS is required to ensure that the TOMASS is a sensitive measure of change in swallowing efficiency and the presence of dysphagia. A final study within this article (Huckabee et al., 2018) validated the clinicians' judgments of number of swallows and masticatory cycles to instrumental measures of the same. The ICC value between objective and behavioral measures was 0.99 for number of masticatory cycles and 0.85 for number of swallows. Additional research into the sensitivity of the TOMASS to identify impairment in specific populations is indicated for establishing predictive validity.

ASSESSMENT OF LINGUAL PALATAL PRESSURE WITH THE IOWA ORAL PRESSURE INSTRUMENT

Lingual palatal manometry measures have been used to quantify aspects of the oral phase of swallowing. The amount of pressure the tongue is able to generate, along with its subsequent movements, plays a key role in masticatory function and allows a cohesive bolus to be manipulated and maintained during transfer from the oral cavity into the pharynx. Although frequently used as an outcome measure in research, this could provide a viable, quantitative adjunct to the CSE given its predictive value for impaired physiology.

Executing Lingual Palatal Pressure Testing

Lingual palatal pressure is most frequently measured using a commercially available device, most often, but not exclusively, reported in the literature to be the IOPI. Measurement of maximal pressure is derived by placing the pressure bulb along the central groove of the tongue, with instructions to patients to push the bulb against the roof of the mouth as hard as possible. Three trials of the movement may be performed; data have been published that represent maximum as either the highest value across trials or an average of the three trials.

A measure of endurance has also been derived by asking patients to sustain a pressure that is 50% of their maximum using the visual display on the device for as long as possible.

Interpreting Lingual Palatal Pressure Testing

Quite a few research groups have investigated aspects of lingual palatal pressure using the IOPI. The reader is directed to a comprehensive meta-analysis of these data by Adams, Mathisen, Baines, Lazarus, and Callister (2013). Reliability of measurement has been reported to be high in prior experimental reports (Robin, Somodi, & Luschei, 1991; Youmans & Stierwalt, 2006); however, more recent research has documented variable reliability, especially with regard to tongue endurance measures (Adams, Mathisen, Baines, Lazarus & Callister, 2015). A further discussion of IOPI reliability can be found in Chapter 20.

Among the published reports, quite a few have reported small sample normative data for lingual palatal maximum pressure and endurance in the context of experimental studies. Vanderwegen, Guns, Van Nuffelen, Elen, and DeBodt (2013) published the largest sample to date, consisting of 420 healthy participants, stratified by sex and age by decade. These results are summarized in Table 9–4. Older participants (age >70) demonstrated lower maximal amplitude than younger participants, although endurance remained stable across the lifespan. Males demonstrated higher pressure and longer endurance than females. Interestingly, the authors point out that their normative values appear to be significantly lower than previously published smaller sample sizes from North America, despite identical methods (Lazarus et al., 2000; Stierwalt & Youmans, 2007). No study is currently available which directly compares pressures across cultures; it is unclear if this difference is statistically significant, and if it is, if the difference is due to methods, participant behavior, or physiology.

In terms of validity, tongue pressure measures are significantly decreased for patients with dysphagia compared with those without swallowing problems (Hamanaka-Kondoh et al., 2014; Hori, Ono, Iwata, Nokubi, & Kumakura, 2005; Stierwalt & Youmans, 2007; Tsuga, Maruyama, Yoshikawa, Yoshida, & Akagawa, 2011). Validity of measurement was extensively studied by Clark, Henson, Barber, Stierwalt, and Sherrill (2003). Specifically, the authors sought to evaluate the relationship between subjective and objective assessment of lingual palatal pressure and oral phase swallowing characteristics.

Table 9–4. Normative Data for Lingual Palatal Isometric Pressure and Endurance Measured with the IOPI (Vanderwegen et al., 2013)

		Male					Female				
			95% CI mean					95% CI mean			
	Age, y	Mean[a]	Lower	Upper	Min	Max	Mean[a]	Lower	Upper	Min	Max
MIP^{b}_{ant}	20–30	58.13	53.37	62.90	30	94	49.93	44.95	52.92	23	65
	31–40	56.03	51.43	60.63	36	78	44.07	39.24	48.89	16	73
	41–50	55.90	50.76	61.04	18	78	47.80	44.11	51.49	31	68
	51–60	50.10	46.19	54.01	26	69	46.73	42.89	50.58	26	75
	61–70	42.90	37.37	48.43	10	68	39.83	35.32	44.34	9	71
	71–80	34.43	29.61	39.25	13	62	33.97	28.81	39.12	11	66
	80+	33.70	29.30	38.10	10	60	28.11	24.07	32.14	6	49
MIP^{b}_{post}	20–30	48.43	43.01	53.86	26	79	44.07	39.49	48.65	19	72
	31–40	48.17	42.83	53.50	17	75	42.80	38.26	47.34	12	63
	41–50	52.23	47.75	56.71	15	69	46.80	42.72	50.88	18	66
	51–60	45.87	41.57	50.16	21	71	44.33	40.67	47.99	27	61
	61–70	41.67	35.47	47.87	10	69	39.33	33.68	44.98	8	74
	71–80	31.83	27.39	36.27	9	49	32.34	27.07	37.62	11	60
	80+	30.73	26.69	34.78	9	50	27.21	22.82	31.61	5	45

		Male					Female				
			95% CI mean					95% CI mean			
	Age, y	Mean[a]	Lower	Upper	Min	Max	Mean[a]	Lower	Upper	Min	Max
End^{c}_{ant}	20–30	28.14	22.90	34.58	7.94	77.62	20.64	16.76	25.43	6.03	64.57
	31–40	29.34	21.64	39.79	7.08	177.83	33.19	26.44	41.68	12.02	199.53
	41–50	33.31	24.75	44.84	7.94	199.53	28.54	21.59	37.73	7.08	199.53
	51–60	24.22	18.85	31.11	5.01	60.26	19.94	15.08	23.36	3.98	67.61
	61–70	26.80	19.53	36.76	3.98	199.53	20.38	15.12	27.47	3.02	144.54
	71–80	21.05	16.73	26.49	7.94	79.43	14.99	11.17	20.11	3.02	87.10
	80+	17.10	12.78	22.88	3.98	77.62	10.90	8.72	13.62	3.98	47.86
End^{c}_{post}	20–30	16.48	14.21	19.11	7.94	33.11	17.82	14.96	21.24	6.03	38.90
	31–40	18.14	15.12	21.76	7.08	45.71	21.01	16.39	26.92	5.01	81.28
	41–50	18.94	15.42	23.27	6.03	48.98	14.70	12.08	17.88	5.01	34.67
	51–60	16.76	12.87	21.83	3.98	67.61	18.41	13.64	24.84	5.01	128.82
	61–70	15.59	11.92	20.39	6.03	128.82	12.84	9.88	16.70	3.98	61.66
	71–80	11.21	9.02	13.93	3.02	39.90	11.96	8.75	16.36	2.00	50.12
	80+	11.75	8.80	15.69	3.02	66.07	8.86	7.08	11.08	3.02	26.92

Note. [a]Mean = geographic mean for endurance measures. [b]Maximum = isometric pressure, anterior or posterior location, expressed as kPa. [c]Endurance, anterior or posterior location, expressed as seconds.

Source: From "The Influence of Age, Sex, Bulb Position, Visual Feedback, and the Order of Testing on Maximum Anterior and Posterior Tongue Strength and Endurance in Healthy Belgian Adults," by J. Vanderwegen, C. Guns, G. Van Nuffelen, R. Elen, and M. De Bodt, 2013, *Dysphagia*, *28*(2), 162. Copyright © 2013 by Springer. Reprinted with permission.

The researchers concluded that oral phase swallowing impairments could be well predicted based on both subjective and objective IOPI measures. Although subjective measures are not norm referenced, clinician judgment appeared to be adequate for judgment of bolus manipulation, mastication, and oral clearance. Of note, experienced raters were, not surprisingly, better at predicting swallowing function than inexperienced raters.

In summary, there is a known association between isometric lingual palatal pressure and swallowing pressure (Robbins, Levine, Wood, Roecker, & Luschei, 1995), and patients with swallowing impairment differ from healthy counterparts. There are further data that support reliability and validity of lingual palatal pressure measures. However, given the availability of the oral cavity to observational assessment and the fact that the technique requires specialized instrumentation and does not directly assess functional ingestive behavior, quantification of these measures may not provide additional benefits.

PULSE OXIMETRY

Executing Pulse Oximetry

It has been suggested that the inclusion of pulse oximetry during evaluation of oral trials on the CSE will increase accuracy of identification of aspiration. This is justified by the hypothesis that aspiration results in reduced oxygen saturation of arterial blood. The device is attached to the earlobe or finger, and oxygen saturation is monitored during oral intake. Pulse oximetry should decrease from baseline by a specific amount if aspiration occurs. The optimal way to evaluate the accuracy of pulse oximetry in an experimental paradigm is to complete simultaneous pulse oximetry and instrumental evaluation. The reviewer coding aspiration on the instrumental examination should be blinded to the pulse oximetry results and vice versa.

Interpreting Pulse Oximetry

Numerous studies have evaluated the reliability of pulse oximetry to identify aspiration in stroke patients; however, contradictory findings are prominent. Some studies suggest that pulse oximetry is accurate in identifying aspiration (e.g., Collins & Bakheit, 1997; Zaidi et al., 1995), whereas others show no association between the occurrence of aspiration identified during the instrumental examination and a decrease in oxygen saturation identified with pulse oximetry (Colodny, 2000; Leder, 2000). A recent study specific to stroke identified no difference in oxygen saturation levels on endoscopically observed swallows with and without aspiration in 50 acute stroke patients (Marian et al., 2017), thus supporting a lack of diagnostic validity.

Desaturation criteria may account for some of the different findings. Many studies set a criterion of greater than 2% change in saturation to suggest a significant compromise, whereas others used a greater than 4% criterion. It is reported that 59% of healthy adults desaturate greater than 2% during swallowing, and 15% desaturate greater than 4% during swallowing (Hirst, Ford, Gibson, & Wilson, 2002). Moreover, many studies did not complete simultaneous pulse oximetry and instrumental swallowing evaluation, which may contribute to differences in findings.

Very recently, Britton et al. (2018) offered a systematic review of the literature relative to the capacity for pulse oximetry to detect aspiration. They summarize: "The majority of studies failed to demonstrate an association between observed aspiration and oxygen desaturation. Current evidence does not support the use of pulse oximetry to detect aspiration" (p. 282).

Pulse oximetry, however, may provide other benefits to the CSE. As it is not uncommon in individuals with stroke to present with concomitant underlying respiratory conditions, monitoring of oxygen saturation may provide valuable clinical information regarding the patient's ability to tolerate the respiratory work of ingestion. Desaturation may not imply aspiration, but it may suggest that the apnea associated with swallowing is taxing to the underlying respiratory system. More research is required to determine additional information that pulse oximetry can provide to the CSE.

CERVICAL AUSCULTATION

Executing Cervical Auscultation

Cervical auscultation to amplify either swallowing sounds or airway sounds during direct oral intake may be employed by clinicians.

Generally, a simple stethoscope is used, but a microphone (Cichero & Murdoch, 2002) or accelerometer (Takahashi, Groher, & Michi, 1994) may be added for improved fidelity and signal recording. Various stethoscope placements have been proposed to monitor the acoustics of swallowing. One suggested placement is the lateral border of the trachea just inferior to the cricoid cartilage (Takahashi et al., 1994), whereas the lateral portion of the thyroid cartilage with the larynx at rest is suggested by others (Hamlet, Nelson, & Patterson, 1990). To amplify breath sounds, the stethoscope is placed on the lateral side of the neck around the laryngeal area (Zenner, Losinski, & Mills, 1995).

Interpreting Cervical Auscultation

When measuring swallowing sounds with auscultation, the clinician is listening for a "double click," which is associated with pressure changes involved in upper esophageal sphincter opening and closing (Hamlet et al., 1990). Although it is suggested that patients with dysphagia will not produce this sound, no data are available to support this. Cervical breath sounds are hollow or "tubular" (Zenner et al., 1995). Normal swallowing has a brief apneic period followed by exhalation after swallowing with clear breath sounds. If the respiratory pattern is deviant from this, impairment in the pharyngeal phase of swallowing is suspected. Aspiration is suspected when a "flushing sound of material" is evident prior to initiation of swallowing or when breath sounds are changed—for example, wet—after swallowing.

Two studies recently evaluated the reliability of cervical auscultation for detecting aspiration in patients with stroke (Borr, Hielscher-Fastabend, & Lucking, 2007; Leslie, Drinnan, Finn, Ford, & Wilson, 2004). In both studies, participants underwent cervical auscultation and a VFSS. Results suggest reduced reliability among raters, which in turn yielded reduced ability to distinguish between patients with and without aspiration. Lagarde, Kamalski, and van den Engel-Hoek (2016) completed a systematic review of auscultation in adults and children. They summarized that "the reliability of cervical auscultation is insufficient when used as a stand-alone tool in the diagnosis of dysphagia in adults. There is no available evidence for the validity and reliability of cervical auscultation in children. Cervical auscultation should not be used as a stand-alone instrument to diagnose dysphagia" (p. 199).

Crary and colleagues have taken a slightly different approach. Rather than evaluating the capacity of auscultation to detect an aspiration event, they have used acoustics to document swallowing frequency only, a quantitative rather than qualitative assessment. An initial study evaluated 62 patients with stroke using a small microphone on the lateral cricoid region (Crary, Carnaby, Sia, Khanna, & Waters, 2013). They report that stroke and swallowing severity was significantly correlated with swallows per minute (SPM) and that patients with dysphagia produced significantly fewer SPM than patients without stroke-related dysphagia. Their data suggest that recording swallowing frequency across a 5- to 10-minute period was sufficient for diagnostic sensitivity. A subsequent study of the data from 62 patients with stroke documented that compared with a typical nurse-administered swallowing screening, the measure of SPM was superior for identifying dysphagia (Crary, Carnaby, & Sia, 2014). The Mann Assessment of Swallowing Ability was considered the researchers' gold standard rather than instrumental confirmation of dysphagia. This binary approach, with a quantitative outcome, may ultimately prove a much more viable use of swallowing acoustics in swallowing assessment.

In the absence of adequate reliability of clinical perception of adequate swallowing acoustics, intensified research has been focused on instrumental detection and analysis of swallowing acoustics to differentiate healthy individuals from those with impairment. Considerable research has been published within the past 5 years in which speech pathologists have joined with engineering colleagues to improve measurement of swallowing acoustics (Dudik, Coyle, El-Jaroudi, Sun, & Sejdić, 2016; Dudik, Coyle, & Sejdić, 2015; Dudik, Kurosu, Coyle, & Sejdić, 2016; Jayatilake et al., 2015; Movahedi, Kurosu, Coyle, Perera, & Sejdić, 2017). A Japanese research group have taken this research to the development of a commercial device—the Swallowscope—for not only detecting and analyzing swallowing but providing biofeedback to patients with dysphagia (Jayatilake et al., 2014, 2015; Kuramoto, Jayatilake, Hidaka, & Suzuki, 2016). Future research on this and applications may support the development of innovative and valid options to augment the clinical swallowing examination.

10 The Instrumental Swallowing Examination

The Videofluoroscopic Swallowing Study

THE NEED FOR DIAGNOSTIC SPECIFICITY

Once the clinical swallowing examination (CSE) has been completed and the need for an instrumental examination is determined, the clinician must decide which procedure will provide the greatest information for a particular patient. In acute stroke, it is currently believed that the videofluoroscopic swallowing study (VFSS) provides the most comprehensive information, as it offers the clearest view of the integration of the different phases of swallowing. Findings from the VFSS will detail bolus flow and biomechanics. However, the VFSS will not provide all of the diagnostic information needed to fully understand the nature of swallowing physiology. This is of significant consequence. By not understanding the specific nature of the swallowing disorder, management of dysphagia may, in fact, exacerbate the disorder rather than facilitate recovery.

It is increasingly clear that diagnostic precision is a mandate of rehabilitative effectiveness. As an example, early research into the technique of thermal-tactile application is not compelling to support its efficacy (Rosenbek, Robbins, Fishback, & Levine, 1991). However, a careful examination of much of that literature reveals that inclusion criteria for those studies were based on signs of pre-swallow pharyngeal pooling. We now understand that this sign can be due primarily to either a motor or sensory-based disorder. It would not be surprising that outcome data for this technique are unconvincing if a proportion of participants possessed primarily a motor deficit, and thus would not demonstrate response to a sensory treatment. Basing rehabilitation on signs is shortsighted; careful definition of pathophysiology is required.

The complexities of swallowing cannot be understood based solely on clinical examination and frequently can defy understanding based on a single diagnostic tool. We want to emphasize the need for multimodality assessment when appropriate and highlight the unique contribution of emerging techniques. Frequently the information obtained from a single examination will provide general information on biomechanics, but a subsequent assessment may be needed to identify the underlying specifics of pathophysiology. Indeed, new information about both compensatory and rehabilitative techniques suggests substantial potential for harm with misidentification of physiology.

Although there are additional tools available to facilitate identification of pathophysiology, such as pharyngeal manometry, further development in diagnostic procedures will facilitate greater understanding and more precise diagnosis. Our understanding of swallowing and the underlying nature of dysfunction is dynamic. What is known has changed considerably over the last 40 years since health professionals have addressed oropharyngeal dysphagia as a diagnostic entity. The process will continue to evolve, and in another 40 years or perhaps even fewer, current diagnostic and management approaches will likely appear inadequate.

The goals of the instrumental examination in the diagnosis of dysphagia in stroke include:

- Evaluation of biomechanical and physiologic function and dysfunction
- Determination of swallowing safety and efficiency
- Identification of effects of compensatory management
- Determination of appropriate diet
- Planning of rehabilitation approaches, as appropriate.

The various types of instrumental evaluations are discussed: the VFSS, VFSS with swallowing-respiratory coordination assessment, videoendoscopic evaluation of swallowing (VEES), low-resolution manometry, high-resolution manometry, impedance, and ultrasound. The advantages and disadvantages of each evaluation method are presented in Table 10–1. It is important to emphasize that the evaluation of swallowing should involve a multidisciplinary team, for example, speech pathologist, radiologist, gastroenterologist, laryngologist, and so forth. Involving experts across various disciplines is critical to fully diagnose dysphagia.

Table 10-1. Advantages and Disadvantages of Each Instrumental Examination Method

Instrumentation	*Strengths*	*Weaknesses*	*When to Use*
Videofluoroscopic Swallowing Study	Direct assessment of oral, pharyngeal, and esophageal stages Evaluate bolus flow, temporal and spatial structural measurements Determine the effects of compensatory strategies	Radiation exposure that limits the length of the examination Difficulty with patient positioning, especially patients with hemiplegia or contractures Non-natural environment—may exacerbate cognitive problems Use of barium as opposed to real food Poor temporal resolution	Preferred evaluation for most diagnostic disorders, particularly neurogenic diagnoses, especially the initial assessment
Swallowing Respiratory Coordination	Completed at bedside No time constraints No radiation exposure Can be used in combination with other imaging modalities Can be monitored during naïve swallowing or during bolus swallowing	Does not visualize anatomic structure or biomechanical movement Hindered by incomplete and/or conflicting normative data	Used as a supportive measure of swallowing impairment and aspiration risk when primary diagnostic tests have already been completed Can aid in training some compensatory strategies (e.g., supraglottic swallow)

continues

Table 10–1. *continued*

Instrumentation	***Strengths***	***Weaknesses***	***When to Use***
Videoendoscopic Evaluation of Swallowing	Completed at bedside Use of real food No time constraints No radiation exposure Direct visualization of the larynx	No visualization of the oral stage No visualization of the actual swallow due to "white out," thus details of oral and pharyngeal motility must be inferred No ability to assess esophageal functioning Limited to no ability to evaluate bolus flow, and analyze structural movement	Physical or cognitive limitations would significantly restrict videofluoroscopic findings Patient is ventilator dependent or in the intensive care unit Follow-up assessments to restrict radiation exposure
Low-Resolution Manometry	Quantification of observed pharyngeal biomechanics No time constraints No radiation exposure Not subjective Can be used in combination with other imaging modalities High temporal resolution	Does not visualize anatomic structure or biomechanical movement Scope of evaluation limited to pharyngeal pressure, only at the points where the sensors are located Intra-swallow movement can alter location of the sensors May not be appropriate for assessment of upper esophageal sphincter function	Differential diagnosis of pharyngeal motility disorders when primary diagnostic tests have been completed Objective measure of change in pharyngeal physiology Follow-up assessments to restrict radiation exposure

Instrumentation	*Strengths*	*Weaknesses*	*When to Use*
High-Resolution Manometry	Same as above, with the exception of measuring the entire nasopharyngeal tract into the esophagus Insertion simple as sensors span the length of the catheter High temporal resolution	Does not visualize anatomic structure or biomechanical movement Scope of evaluation limited to pharyngeal pressure Limited normative data at present	Same as above Gold standard to assess upper esophageal sphincter pressure parameters
Impedance Manometry	No time constraints No radiation exposure Can be used in combination with other imaging modalities Can be used to detect the speed and direction of bolus movement; a surrogate measure of bolus flow	Does not visualize anatomic structure or biomechanical movement Scope of evaluation limited to the relationship between pharyngeal pressure and bolus flow Requires use of a bolus of high conductivity (e.g., added salinity) At present, impedance manometry catheters are large in diameter	For differential diagnosis of pharyngeal motility disorders when primary diagnostic tests have been completed Can be implemented as a screening (e.g., "Swallow Risk Index") when other imaging modalities are unavailable Follow-up assessments to restrict radiation exposure
Ultrasound	No time constraints No radiation exposure Can be used in combination with other imaging modalities Relatively inexpensive; common in many health care settings	Bony structures, such as the hyoid, cannot be visualized directly Maintaining the position of the transducer is crucial to ensure accurate measures	Objective measurement of muscle morphometry and kinematics of oral, pharyngeal and laryngeal structures For differential diagnosis when primary diagnostic tests have already been completed Follow-up assessments to restrict radiation exposure

THE VIDEOFLUOROSCOPIC SWALLOWING STUDY

Executing the Videofluoroscopic Swallowing Study

The Videofluoroscopic Swallowing Study Setup

The ideal setup for obtaining a VFSS is to record the study for later viewing. Swallowing is a rapid event with many features occurring simultaneously or within milliseconds of each other; thus, it is ideal to review the study, preferably with the opportunity to view it in slow motion or frame by frame. Additional options strongly recommended for recording the VFSS are a microphone and a counter timer. By having audio input, the clinician may verbally identify the volumes and consistency provided to the patient and the compensatory strategy employed. A cough response can be identified as well as the strength of the cough. As patients with stroke may have cognitive and/or attentional impairments, the microphone will capture the amount of verbal cuing provided to the patient and any extraneous verbalization by the patient. The counter timer encodes digital time in hundredths of a second on each video frame. This, in turn, allows the clinician to make objective and precise temporal measurements.

Radiation beam rate is an important variable to consider when capturing VFSS images, as multiple swallowing events occur at a very rapid rate. Radiation delivery can be either continuous or pulsed. While lowered pulse rate can reduce radiation exposure, it can result in loss of clinically significant information in terms of identifying aspiration and underlying pathophysiology (Bonilha et al., 2013; Cohen, 2009). Recommendations concerning diet and treatment were different in all VFSS when analyzed at the capture rate of 30 pulses per second (pps) and a simulated 15 pps (removal of every other frame) rate (Bonilha et al., 2013). In order to maintain an efficient study with maximum diagnostic and clinical yield, maintaining a minimum of 30 pps appears to be critical. Equally important is ensuring that the recording equipment acquisition rate is 30 frames per second with either the continuous or 30 pps fluoroscopic sequence. In this manner you can ensure that discrete spatial and temporal measurements can be made without loss of valuable information (Peladeau-Pigeon & Steele, 2013).

Patient Positioning

Obtaining adequate patient positioning for the VFSS can be challenging in patients with stroke, due in part to hemiplegia and cognitive deficits. The advent of specially designed VFSS chairs that can be positioned from stretcher to chair have facilitated patient transfer and positioning. The VFSS is initiated with the patient in the lateral position. This allows a clear view of the upper aerodigestive tract. Ideally, the clinician should be able to view the oral cavity, larynx, pharynx, and cervical esophagus. This allows for documentation of bolus flow and structural movement through the oropharyngeal swallowing system. The clinician may find, however, that the patient with stroke does not maintain optimal positioning and moves out of the fluoroscopic view or cannot be positioned properly due to hemiplegia. In these cases, findings from the CSE are extremely important in identifying the possible area of focus for the VFSS. Moreover, the patient may shift positions throughout the evaluation. As such, it is important that radiology personnel be prepared to move the fluoroscopic tube as the patient moves in order to capture swallowing behaviors. Having the patient hold the bolus in the oral cavity until verbally cued to swallow may assist in obtaining a higher quality view of the swallowing; however, swallowing on cue is not typical swallowing behavior. Research has shown that verbal cue does affect swallowing in healthy adults (see Table 3–1).

Obtaining an anterior-posterior (A-P) view may be routine in some VFSS protocols to evaluate pharyngeal contraction and esophageal clearance (Martin-Harris et al., 2008), or it may be optional and dependent on identification of pyriform sinus post-swallow residue. Fortunately, specially designed VFSS chairs allow for easy rotation of patients into the A-P position. After identifying post-swallow residual in the lateral plane, the patient is turned to the A-P position. The patient's chin is slightly lifted to clearly view the hypopharynx, thereby allowing for identification of post-swallow residual location. By obtaining an A-P view, the clinician can determine whether the residue is unilateral or bilateral. Unilateral pharyngeal hemiparesis frequently results in residue in the contralesional pyriform sinus and often is evident in patients with stroke. It is important to distinguish between unilateral and bilateral residual, as specific management strategies are designed for each. The A-P view also helps identify unilateral vocal fold paresis, which is not uncommon in lateral medullary stroke. In the A-P view, the patient phonates "ah" and movement of the true vocal folds can be seen. If unilateral vocal fold paresis is identified, a referral to otolaryngology should be made.

Nasogastric Feeding Tubes

Many patients with stroke, particularly those individuals evaluated acutely, may have a nasogastric tube (NGT) for feeding present for the VFSS. Changes in bolus flow with an NGT present have been identified in healthy adults and individuals with stroke. In healthy young adults, large-bore NGTs significantly affected durational measures such as stage transit duration (STD) and upper esophageal sphincter (UES) opening, with similar trends evident with small-bore NGTs (Huggins, Tuomi, & Young, 1999). Although most durational measures were increased with the NGT present, STD was decreased. The authors suggested that earlier elicitation of pharyngeal swallowing with the NGT in place may be a result of: (1) anticipatory behavior to avoid pharyngeal discomfort, (2) compensatory behavior yielding earlier hyolaryngeal elevation, or (3) pharyngeal wall stimulation. The presence of a large-bore NGT also has been shown to increase bolus flow timing measures in patients with stroke, although findings were not statistically significant (Wang, Wu, Chang, Hsiao, & Lien, 2006). The presence of both small- and large-bore feeding tubes increased airway invasion, pharyngeal residue, and pharyngeal transit times in healthy older adults (Pryor et al., 2015). Moreover, the presence of a manometric catheter in the pharynx was associated with increased airway invasion in healthy older adults (Robbins, Hamilton, Lof, & Kempster, 1992); however, in other studies of patients referred to speech pathology for swallowing assessment, the NGT was not associated with increased aspiration (Fattal, Suiter, Warner, & Leder, 2011; Leder & Suiter, 2008). Dziewas et al. (2008) identified mechanical interference of the NGT resulting in material adhering to the NGT with post-swallow aspiration in 2 of 25 patients with an acute stroke. Thus, if an NGT is present during the VFSS, the clinician must determine whether the feeding tube is contributing to the dysphagia. In facilities where it is the purview of the clinician to do so, obtaining physician orders for removal of the NGT during the VFSS will allow the clinician the opportunity to remove the feeding tube if there is fluoroscopic evidence suggesting that the NGT may be causing or exaggerating any swallowing problem.

Bolus Presentation Guidelines

Barium is the contrast medium used during a VFSS. While all possible food consistencies cannot be tested due to the need to limit radiation exposure, ideally a thin liquid, semisolid, and solid are evaluated. Standardized Varibar® barium in thin liquid, nectar, thin honey, thick honey, and pudding consistencies is available in many countries. Each of these barium consistencies has been shown to correlate with a thickness classification on the newly described International Dysphagia Diet Standardization Initiative (IDDSI) (Steele, 2017) for those clinicians who adhere to this protocol. They are not designed to be mixed with foods other than using the pudding to coat any solid consistency evaluated. If non-standardized contrast agents must be used, the IDDSI syringe flow test (http://www.iddsi.org) can be used to evaluate thickness characteristics (Cichero et al., 2017) allowing for a uniform consistency administration across VFSS at a given hospital.

There is no set protocol for liquid and food administration for the VFSS; however, in most instances, multiple volumes and consistencies are tested, and if warranted, the effect of compensation on impaired safety and/or efficiency is evaluated. Figure 10–1 provides an example of a VFSS protocol. The VFSS may be defined as protocol-driven or patient driven (Campion, Haynos, & Palmer, 2007). In the protocol-driven assessment, the clinician administers the same volumes and consistency without considering a patient's needs. In the patient-driven assessment, the VFSS is tailored to a patient's specific needs. For patients with stroke, a combination of the two approaches is recommended. Like the CSE, it is ideal to start with small volumes of thin liquid, particularly in the initial evaluation. This limits the amount of aspiration should it occur and any post-swallow residual, which is less with thin liquids, thereby reducing the effects on subsequent swallows. Self-administration with a cup or straw is preferred, to mimic real-life eating situations. The influence of ingestion of liquids via cup versus straw on bolus flow has not been studied empirically in healthy adults or individuals with stroke; thus, it is unclear whether there are either positive or negative aspects of bolus delivery for ingestion of liquid. The use of a cup or straw in which to administer the liquid

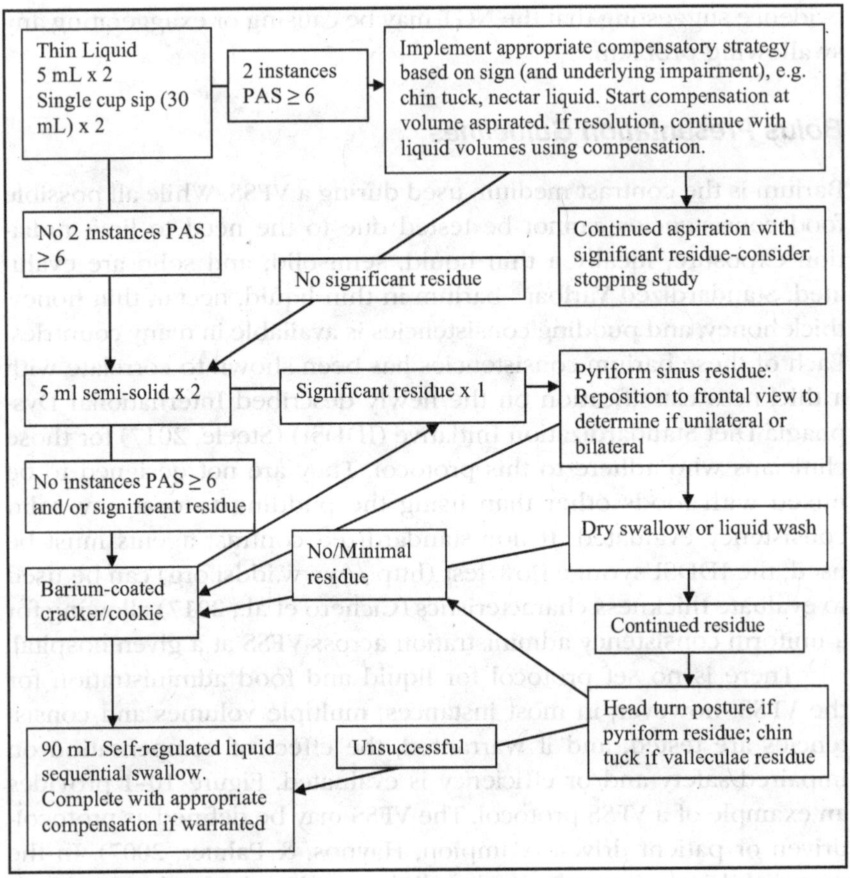

Figure 10–1. Flowchart of an idealized videofluoroscopic swallowing study protocol. PAS = Penetration-Aspiration Scale. Source: From "Cerebro-Vascular Accidents and Dysphagia," by A. R. Gallaugher, C. L. Wilson, and S. K. Daniels, 2012, in R. Shaker, P. C. Belafsky, G. N. Postma, and C. Easterling (Eds.), *Principles of deglutition: A multidisciplinary text for swallowing and its disorders* (p. 389). Copyright © by Springer Nature.

may be determined from the CSE. If the patient has difficulty with oral containment and anterior bolus loss is identified, use of a straw may be preferred.

In addition to considering the effects of method of liquid ingestion, the clinician must consider the impact of verbal cuing on swallowing. Frequently, verbal cue to swallow is arbitrarily applied in the VFSS, yet, as discussed earlier, research indicates that verbal cues affect swallowing in healthy adults (Daniels, Schroeder, DeGeorge, Corey, & Rosenbek, 2007; McFarland et al., 2016; Nagy et al., 2013) (see Table 3–1). Currently, it is unknown whether a cue to swallow has a facilitatory or deleterious effect on swallowing in patients with stroke. Anecdotal evidence suggests that cue to swallow may contribute to "apraxia of swallowing" in patients with left hemisphere damage (Logemann, 1998; Robbins & Levine, 1988; Robbins, Levine, Maser, Rosenbek, & Kempster, 1993); however, this has not been empirically confirmed. Conversely, as cited in Huckabee and Pelletier (1999), Kagel speculated that cue to swallow may increase volition in the act of swallowing by allowing the patient an opportunity to organize and execute bolus transfer, thus facilitating swallowing. The use of a cue to swallow should thus be based on systematic clinical thinking, with interpretation of potential positive and negative effects integrated into treatment planning.

Calibrated volumes may be used for the VFSS, or, as with the CSE, an unstructured but still carefully regulated examination may be undertaken. By using calibrated volumes, the clinician can identify the precise volume in which swallowing difficulty begins. This may prove beneficial when recommending oral intake. For example, if a patient demonstrates a safe and efficient swallow with a 5 mL thin liquid volume but significant aspiration with a 10 mL thin liquid volume, 5 mL thin liquid volumes for pleasure or during treatment may be recommended, albeit translating this measured restriction to practice may be challenging. Furthermore, subsequent re-evaluations can begin at the volume of difficulty. By using specific volumes, at least initially, the clinician can compare patients and results, thereby creating a database in which to report possible clinical research findings. Generally, a clinician may initiate the study with a thin liquid volume (3 or 5 mL) and progress to larger volumes up to 20 to 30 mL, which is the normal single-bolus volume range for thin liquids in healthy adults (Adnerhill, Ekberg, & Groher, 1989; Bennett, van Lieshout, Pelletier, & Steele, 2009; Lawless, Bender, Oman, & Pelletier, 2003). Given that individuals frequently ingest smaller sip sizes in testing situations (Bennett et al., 2009), it would be important for the clinician to ask the patient to drink the larger volumes in a single swallow in order to fully assess typical sip size. Two to three trials of each volume or consistency are recommended to reliably judge swallowing function and account for individual variability between swallows (Lazarus et al., 1993; Lof & Robbins, 1990; Molfenter & Steele, 2011). If dysphagia with resulting aspiration is identified, the examination is not necessarily terminated, but rather, appropriate compensatory techniques are initiated to facilitate swallowing. If aspiration is evident on the first swallow, the clinician should repeat the swallow using the same volume and consistency unless strongly contraindicated. It may be that the patient requires a "warm-up" period, and swallowing improves after the first or second swallow.

If dysphagia and aspiration persist with liquids, compensatory techniques should be employed. Selection of the appropriate compensatory technique is determined by the specific swallowing problem. Compensatory management is discussed in detail in Chapter 18. Generally, it is ideal to begin with compensatory strategies that do not restrict the diet (e.g., cyclic ingestion, postures). If none of the appropriate strategies facilitate swallowing, altering the consistency of the bolus (e.g., thickened liquid) should then be attempted. The patient's comprehension and memory function may dictate the type of compensatory strategy employed. For example, in a patient with a right hemispheric stroke and poor attention and memory who presents with consistent aspiration of thin liquid barium at 10 mL due to a delayed onset of the pharyngeal swallow, the clinician may have the patient attempt a chin tuck posture to determine its benefit. The clinician can determine the extent of cuing necessary for the patient to implement and maintain the posture as well as use information obtained from the CSE to determine whether cognitive deficits will affect consistent implementation during mealtime. Even if improvement is evident in the VFSS, the clinician also should determine the effect of consistency manipulation (e.g., nectar-thick liquid) due to the potential for limited success for consistent implementation and improbability that a caregiver could be present for every meal. If successful, thickened liquid may be the compensatory strategy recommended for this patient due to the extent of cognitive deficits. However, if chin tuck was also successful, in addition to addressing rehabilitative techniques to facilitate elicitation of the pharyngeal swallow, the clinician can train in maintaining the chin tuck posture. It should be noted that thickened liquids are not typically part of the routine VFSS and are administered only as indicated as a compensatory strategy. If a compensatory strategy is successful at a particular volume, the clinician should continue the VFSS protocol using the compensation for the consistency it is intended to facilitate. That is, if consistent pre-swallow aspiration occurs at 5 mL, test the compensation at 5 mL. If successful, liquids should be advanced according to the VFSS protocol using the compensatory strategy. If consistent aspiration occurs at the next liquid volume, attempt another compensatory strategy, if available. Ideally, the clinician is able to test sequential swallowing using the successful compensation. In the event of small bolus liquid aspiration, termination of liquid trials may be indicated if the patient does not respond to typical compensatory techniques, does not produce a protective cough response, and is deemed at significant risk of chest infection. However, bolus size may influence aspiration, and if deemed safe, proceeding to a larger bolus to assess the influence of size and sensory input may be appropriate.

To evaluate ingestion of semisolids, barium pudding is administered. It is optimal to have the patient self-feed; however, for some patients with stroke, particularly those individuals evaluated in the acute phase, the clinician may need to administer the semisolid. To evaluate mastication and swallowing of a solid bolus, a solid such as part of a cookie is coated with barium pudding. If the patient has reported difficulty with a particular food type, it is ideal to mix the barium pudding with that type of food.

As noted previously, all food types cannot and should not be assessed during the instrumental examination due to time constraints imposed by radiation exposure and attentional limitations of the patient with stroke. In addition, the clinician must allow enough time in the VFSS to pursue management strategies. Thus, it is imperative that astute clinicians infer swallowing function across food types from a limited number of consistencies administered during the VFSS.

If large single volumes of liquid can be safely swallowed by the patient, sequential swallowing should be evaluated, as this is a more typical pattern of swallowing compared with single, discrete swallows. For sequential swallowing, the patient is provided with a large volume—for example, 90 mL—and instructed to continually swallow. The patient self-regulates the volume and pace of ingestion. The use of straw or cup delivery depends on the results of the earlier single swallows. If a compensatory strategy was required to safely swallow single volumes, it should be employed during the sequential swallowing trial.

If significant aspiration is not observed, esophageal motility may be screened. Research documenting esophageal motility following stroke is limited, with results indicating that propagation of distal esophageal peristalsis, percent of completed peristaltic events (Aithal, Nylander, Dwarakanath, & Tanner, 1999), and resting pressures of upper and lower esophageal sphincters (Lucas, Yu, Vlahos, & Ledgerwood, 1999) are reduced following stroke. To screen for esophageal motility, a liquid bolus and a semisolid bolus should be followed as each progress through the esophagus to the stomach with the patient viewed in the A-P plane. Although it is important for the clinician to have a cursory understanding of esophageal motility, as esophageal dysfunction may contribute to pharyngeal dysfunction (Martin-Harris & Easterling, 2006), it is equally important to recognize that an esophageal screening is not a valid assessment of esophageal motility. However, evaluation of esophageal clearance using the Modified Barium Swallow Impairment Profile (MBSImP) has demonstrated significant association with abnormal esophageal findings as measured by multichannel intraluminal impedance-esophageal manometry (Gullung, Hill, Castell, & Martin-Harris, 2012), indicating that the VFSS can be used to identify individuals who require further esophageal work-up. As always, consultation with a radiologist concerning results of the esophageal screening should be obtained.

Interpreting the Videofluoroscopic Swallowing Study

The clinician must integrate numerous components of the VFSS in order to obtain a complete and accurate determination of swallowing function and safety. The components of the VFSS include:

- Anatomic abnormalities
- Bolus flow
- Temporal coordination of structural movement relative to bolus flow
- Extent of structural movement
- Response to compensatory strategies and determination of a treatment plan.

Although the VFSS may be interpreted online during the assessment, it is best to record and review the study after the examination is completed. In this fashion, swallowing motility can be viewed at various speeds to facilitate identification of dysfunction. A narrative may be written or an evaluation sheet may be used to document dysfunction, with the narrative taken from the score sheet. An example of a VFSS form is provided in the online resources. As with the CSE, it is strongly recommended that clinicians working on the same case at various sites, such as hospitals or nursing homes, determine specific parameters to define dysphagia and work together as a team to establish inter- and intrarater reliability on these variables within their respective institutions. Until this is completed, diagnosing dysfunction on VFSS will not be consistent across or within individual clinicians (Kuhlemeier, Yates, & Palmer, 1998; McCullough et al., 2001; Scott, Perry, & Bench, 1998; Stoeckli, Huisman, Seifert, & Martin-Harris, 2003; Wilcox, Liss, & Siegel, 1996).

Anatomic Abnormalities

Judgment of the integrity of anatomic structures should be completed with all patients in collaboration with a radiologist. Although anatomic abnormalities such as cervical osteophytes are unrelated to stroke, their incidence, like stroke, may increase with age. The identification of any anatomic abnormality should be noted, as well as its effect on swallowing. Deviation in anatomy may exaggerate the swallowing problem that occurs following stroke. As the VFSS is a test of swallowing physiology and not head and neck structural pathology, completion of the examination without a radiologist present is becoming more common. Ideally, a joint evaluation with both the speech pathologist and radiologist present and engaged is preferred. Without a radiologist present, the speech pathologist must be aware of the potential for anatomic abnormalities and seek consultation from the radiologist if anatomic deviations are suspected.

Bolus Flow

Bolus flow is generally evaluated in terms of timing, direction, and clearance. Timing is discussed in terms of transit times—for example, oral transit time, STD, and so forth. Timing may be characterized in general terms, such as slow or delayed, or it can be objectively quantified. Using the various playback speeds of the recording, the clinician can make subjective judgments of oral and pharyngeal transit times and time to onset of the pharyngeal swallow. Additionally, with a time code generator, the clinician can capture onset and offset points for each timing measure of interest to obtain objective measures of bolus timing (Table 10–2).

Table 10–2. Calculation of Durations for Bolus Timing Measures

Bolus Timing	*Onset*	*Offset*
Oral Transit Time	Beginning of anterior or posterior movement of the bolus head or tail	Leading edge of the bolus at the posterior angle of the ramus of the mandible
Stage Transit Duration	Leading edge of the bolus at the posterior angle of the ramus of the mandible	Initiation of maximum superior movement of the hyoid
Pharyngeal Transit Time	Leading edge of the bolus at the posterior angle of the ramus of the mandible	Bolus tail passed through the upper esophageal sphincter
Pharyngeal Response Time	Initiation of maximum superior movement of the hyoid	Bolus tail passed through the upper esophageal sphincter
Total Swallowing Duration	Beginning of anterior or posterior movement of the bolus head or tail	Bolus tail passed through the upper esophageal sphincter

When determining onset of evocation of pharyngeal swallowing, or STD, it is important that the clinician distinguish between onset of *maximum* hyolaryngeal complex (HLC) elevation and movement of the tongue and HLC in an attempt to initiate the swallow. Onset of maximum HLC elevation is characterized by smooth, continual superior and anterior movement of the HLC toward maximum. Whereas, when pharyngeal swallowing is notably delayed or absent, repetitive oral and base-of-tongue movement is evident producing HLC movements; these movements do not progress toward maximum, and the subsequent pharyngeal events in swallowing do not occur.

Bolus direction is described in terms of laryngeal penetration or aspiration. Direction of bolus flow can be determined using either a global notation of laryngeal penetration and aspiration or the more detailed Penetration-Aspiration (P-A) Scale (Rosenbek, Robbins, Roecker, Coyle, & Wood, 1996). The P-A Scale is a validated ordinal scale to measure bolus direction by focusing on depth of airway invasion, clearance, and the patient's response (e.g., cough) to airway invasion. The scoring system is as follows: 1–no airway invasion, 2–penetration with clearing, 3–penetration with laryngeal residue, 4–penetration to the true vocal folds (TVF) with clearing, 5–penetration to the TVF with laryngeal residue, 6–aspiration with clearing from the trachea, 7–aspiration with unsuccessful attempt at clearing from the trachea, and 8–silent aspiration. As the P-A Scale was developed to capture airway invasion during all points of time during the swallow, VFSS is the instrumentation of choice in which to use the P-A Scale.

Timing of airway invasion is classified as either pre-swallow, during the swallow, or post-swallow. Pre-swallow airway invasion is identified by entry of material into the larynx prior to onset of maximum HLC excursion. Airway invasion during the swallow is determined by entry of material into the larynx during the course of the pharyngeal swallow. Airway invasion during the swallow can be visualized only with VFSS. Post-swallow airway invasion is determined by entry of material into the larynx following return of the structures to rest. If a spontaneous response to aspiration, i. e., cough, does not occur, the clinician should cue the patient to cough in an attempt to clear the aspirated material.

Bolus clearance is judged by post-swallow residual in the oral cavity, valleculae, and pyriform sinuses, as well as along the base of the tongue, aryepiglottic folds, and posterior pharyngeal wall. The clinician should note changes in residue over multiple swallows or with increased bolus consistency. The amount of residue cannot be objectively determined during any instrumental swallowing examination used for clinical purposes. Clinicians, however, can subjectively judge the amount of residue by using a semi-objective rating scale (Eisenhuber et al., 2002; Hind, Nicosia, Roecker, Carnes, & Robbins, 2001; Perlman, Booth, & Grayhack, 1994). An example of such a rating scale would be: 1 = no retention, 2 = coating of a structure or space, 3 = slight collection of residue, 4 = moderate retention encompassing up to half of the oral cavity or pharyngeal space, and 5 = severe bolus retention with residue encompassing over half of the oral cavity or pharyngeal space. More quantitative, pixel-based measures are also available to determine the amount of pharyngeal residue (Dyer, Leslie, & Drinnan, 2008; Pearson, Molfenter, Smith, & Steele, 2013). The Normalized Residue Ratio Scale (Pearson et al., 2013) involves extracting specific VFSS clips (after the first swallow in which the hyoid and larynx have returned to rest and before subsequent dry swallows) and analysis using ImageJ software (National Institutes of

Health, Bethesda, MD) which is available to the public without cost. The freehand tool of the software is used to outline the residue as well as the specific pharyngeal cavity being measured (valleculae, pyriform sinus). Additionally, the distance between cervical vertebras 2 and 4 is measured to obtain an individual anatomic scaler reference. Thus, the amount of residue relative to size of the pharyngeal cavity and proportionate to the size of the person can be determined.

The clinician should identify the occurrence of spontaneous dry swallowing in response to post-swallow residual before the patient is cued to dry swallow. Spontaneous dry swallowing provides important information about oral and pharyngeal sensation. The effect of dry swallowing (clearing of residue or no change in residue) should be noted. If spontaneous dry swallowing does not occur, the clinician should cue the individual to dry swallow to determine if this is effective in clearing residue.

Temporal Coordination and Extent of Structural Movement

Timing and distance of structural movement can be obtained with a VFSS. As with bolus timing, temporal and spatial structural measures can be made subjectively and are traditionally used in the clinical setting, as more objective measures are labor intensive. Objective measurement of timing of structural movement in relation to bolus flow may be calculated when employing the onset and offset of movement of specific structures such as the UES opening duration. Spatial measurement of structural movement can be determined manually employing special software such as ImageJ, which is available to the public without cost, to determine exact distances, such as extent of HLC elevation. Commercial software is now available which automatically calculates a wide variety of spatial and temporal measurements (Swallowtail, Belldev Medical, Arlington Heights, IL). Normative data concerning spatial and temporal measures of swallowing are available (Leonard & Kendall, 2014). Regardless of whether the clinician is employing subjective or objective measures, one should note velar elevation, base-of-tongue retraction, superior and anterior HLC movement, closure of the laryngeal vestibule, and UES opening in terms of coordination of movement relative to bolus flow and extent of structural movement.

Response to Compensatory Strategies and Determining the Treatment Plan

By the end of a thorough VFSS, the clinician should have objective confirmation of the effects of specific compensatory swallowing strategies that were evaluated and should be able to make recommendations concerning diet management, behavioral compensation, and rehabilitation. As discussed earlier, the recommendation for a particular compensatory strategy as well as the types of rehabilitative techniques will depend on the patient's comprehension and cognitive status.

Assignment of Severity

With few exceptions, most of our diagnostic tests for swallowing impairment rely on subjective interpretation of objective information. The VFSS provides a clear representation of swallowing events, but its value in the diagnostic process is dependent on the skill and experience of the clinician. Interpretation of dynamic radiographic data is not simple. Thus, clinicians have sought to develop methods for structuring interpretation of this information.

There is an inherent tradeoff in these methods between specificity and utility. Many scales provide some organization and definition of various parameters of swallowing. The sample VFSS score sheet provided in the online resources is an excellent example. This type of scale covers a lot of ground quickly and can be very helpful to classification and diagnosis. However, scales of this type typically are based on binary assessment (presence or absence) of a pathophysiologic feature and, therefore, do not offer a mechanism for quantifying severity. Thus, they are unable to measure anything but very large increments of change in post-treatment repeated studies. In response, assignment of severity may be included (e.g., perceptually determining mild, moderate, or severe residue). However, these are problematic due to lack of objectivity. What is mild to an experienced clinician may be perceived as quite severe to a less experienced clinician.

When specific and unambiguous definitions are provided, the scales tend to address only a limited number of swallowing features, such as the P-A Scale or a scale developed by Murray, Langmore, Ginsberg, and Dostie (1996) for documenting pharyngeal secretions observed with VEES. Published tools such as these are readily available to clinicians and are very valuable in clinical quantification of the feature under observation and in standardizing the language that clinicians use to communicate regarding swallowing impairment. However, they do not help to define other complex features of impaired swallowing that may not present with aspiration as a sign. Others such as the Dysphagia Outcome and Severity Scale (O'Neil, Purdy, Falk, & Gallo, 1999) pair safety and efficiency as determined by VFSS along with independence and diet recommendations.

The MBSImP is a commercially available, validated, standardized, semi-objective measurement tool developed in an attempt to quantify the underlying swallowing problem by assigning severity levels to the specific biomechanical processes of swallowing (Martin-Harris et al., 2008). Seventeen components are measured (6 oral, 10 pharyngeal, 1 esophageal) using a rank-ordered severity scale. An overall impression (OI) score based on the highest (worst) score for each component across all swallows is recorded. Oral OI scores and pharyngeal OI scores are then calculated to obtain the oral total (range 0–22) and pharyngeal total (range 0–29) impairment scores. Single trials of various consistencies including nectar- and honey-thick liquids are evaluated using this protocol. It is important to note that MBSImP has not been studied in healthy young and older adults, thus specific oral and pharyngeal OI scores have not been identified that distinguish between normal and disordered swallowing.

11 The Instrumental Swallowing Examination

Evaluation of Swallowing Respiratory Coordination—An Auxiliary to the Videofluoroscopic Swallowing Study

As discussed in Chapter 3, the pharynx serves a dual role as a conduit for both ingested food and ventilatory air; therefore, several functional adaptations of the aerodigestive tract have developed to protect the airway during swallowing (Preiksaitis & Mills, 1996). The epiglottis directs an oncoming bolus to the lateral channels, around the entrance to the airway and into the esophagus. Adduction of the true vocal folds and the ventricular folds shields the airway from pulmonary invasion (Hadjikoutis, Pickersgill, Dawson, & Wiles, 2000). This represents one of the earliest airway protection mechanisms and has been reported to precede the onset of hyoid movement associated with onset of pharyngeal swallowing (Martin-Harris et al., 2005; Shaker, Dodds, Dantas, Hogan, & Arndorfer, 1990). The momentary cessation in respiration during deglutition is termed swallowing apnea (SA) and is considered a key feature of airway protection (Palmer & Hiiemae, 2003).

Although SA appears as a biomechanical component of pharyngeal swallowing, there is evidence that a distinct apneic reflex exists during swallowing that is centrally integrated (Bolser, Gestreau, Morris, Davenport, & Pitts, 2013; Bolser, Pitts, Davenport, & Morris, 2015; Broussard & Altschuler, 2000; Miller, 1999; Samson, Praud, Quenet, Similowski, & Straus, 2017; Widdicombe, 1986). Clinical evidence for this central integration is provided through studies of patients who have undergone a total laryngectomy (Hiss, Strauss, Treole, Stuart, & Boutilier, 2003) or who are intubated (Nishino & Hiraga, 1991), where biomechanical apnea is prevented. Regardless, these patients continue to demonstrate measurable SA in the absence of glottic closure, thus suggesting that this apnea is not driven by the biomechanical interruption of respiration but is centrally initiated. This central control mechanism is confounded by biomechanical factors, and thus potentially places the patient with neurologic impairment at significant risk.

As such, research has focused on the importance of swallowing respiratory coordination in airway protection. Although more frequently engaged as a research tool, the development of preliminary normative databases and the substantial implications for swallowing safety in patients with stroke suggest that this evaluation may emerge as a standard adjunct to the instrumental assessment.

Acquisition of instrumental techniques in isolation, as described above, allows us to clinically investigate, and sometimes carefully quantify, features of the deglutitive process. However, these techniques in isolation may bias our view of the complex relationships involved in swallowing. A multimodality assessment may be required to fully grasp the intricacy of relationships among oral, pharyngeal, laryngeal, esophageal, and respiratory structures and functions. This is particularly true for the assessment of swallowing respiratory coordination.

EXECUTING THE EVALUATION OF SWALLOWING RESPIRATORY COORDINATION

Measurement of swallowing respiratory coordination requires instrumentation for monitoring the respiratory waveform, as well as some measure of swallowing onset or execution. Respiration can be monitored using a nasal thermister, which measures temperature at the entrance to the nares, or a respiratrace, which monitors expansion and contraction of the thoracic dimension (Selley, Flack, Ellis, & Brooks, 1989a). Although these techniques provide the information required, they are fairly specialized pieces of equipment and thus not readily available in clinical settings. More often reported in the literature is a system of evaluating nasal airflow by standard nasal prongs, as used to deliver oxygen in health care settings. This plastic tubing is simply placed at the entry to the nares and secured over the ears. The patient must be instructed to breathe through the nose. Those with habitual mouth breathing may require an alternative measure of respiration.

Respiratory tracings can be acquired synchronously with several other types of instrumental techniques. Onset of swallowing can be easily documented with the use of surface electromyography (sEMG) of the floor of mouth muscles. These muscles are chosen as they provide a proxy measure of onset and peak hyolaryngeal excursion, which is considered the leading complex of pharyngeal swallowing. After the skin surface is cleaned to remove any excess oil, makeup, or loose epithelial tissue, standard surface electrodes are placed longitudinally over this muscle group. Outputs from these sensors are fed into any digital recording system that will display ongoing time by amplitude waveform data.

For more detailed information regarding coordination of respiration with specific biomechanical features of airway protection and pharyngeal motility, the clinician may wish to couple the respiratory tracing with either radiographic or endoscopic evaluation of swallowing. To accomplish these integrated evaluations, respiratory recordings are required during the completion of diagnostic protocols described in prior sections of this chapter. Figure 11–1 represents a combined assessment of respiration and swallowing biomechanics using videofluoroscopy.

Once the instrumentation is in place, regardless of the nature of the paired assessment, swallowing respiratory coordination can

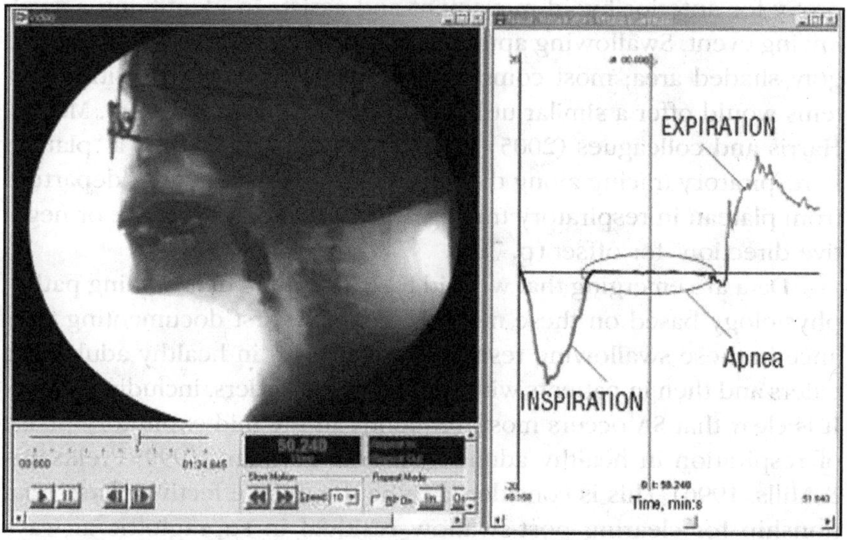

Figure 11–1. Simultaneous diagnostics incorporating VFSS (*left*) and swallowing respiratory coordination (*right*). VFSS = videofluoroscopic swallowing study.

be monitored during naïve swallowing of secretions or during bolus swallowing of increasing size and consistency as are acquired during other assessment protocols. In order to ensure temporal specificity, an integrated hardware/software system that allows for synchronized acquisition from multiple digital data sources is required. This type of system can be custom designed by biomedical professionals.

INTERPRETING THE EVALUATION OF SWALLOWING RESPIRATORY COORDINATION

Interpretation of data from the evaluation of swallowing respiration coordination focuses on the temporal relationships between apnea and other biomechanical features of swallowing and the duration of swallowing apnea. Phase relationships generally are coded using the classification provided in Figure 11–2. In these figures, the downward moving component of the tracing negative to the abscissa represents inspiration, the upward moving component positive to the abscissa represents expiration, and the flat line of the waveform represents SA.

The sEMG tracing (in the lower windows of Figure 11–2) is a proxy for anterior hyoid movement and assists in identifying a swallowing event. Swallowing apnea duration (SAD) is represented by the gray shaded area; most commercially available data acquisition systems would offer a similar utility for waveform measurement. Martin-Harris and colleagues (2005) operationally define SAD as a "plateau in respiratory tracing along the abscissa" for the onset and "departure from plateau in respiratory tracing along abscissa in positive or negative direction" for offset (p. 763).

Data are emerging that will aid the clinician in determining pathophysiology based on these measurements by first documenting variance in these swallowing respiratory measures in healthy adults and elders and then in patients with neurologic disorders, including stroke. It is clear that SA occurs most frequently in the mid-expiratory phase of respiration in healthy adults (Klahn & Perlman, 1999; Preiksaitis & Mills, 1996). This is considered to be the most effective phase relationship for clearing post-swallow residual in supraglottic airways and thus inhibiting post-swallow aspiration (Hadjikoutis et al., 2000). However, reported frequencies vary. For example, Hiss, Treole, and Stuart (2001) reported greater than 62% of apneic periods during

Phase Categorization	Abbreviation	Example
Mid-expiration	E-E	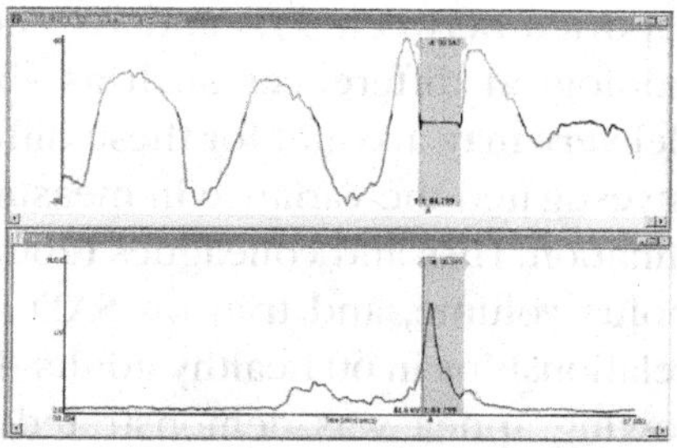
At the transition between expiration and inspiration	E-I	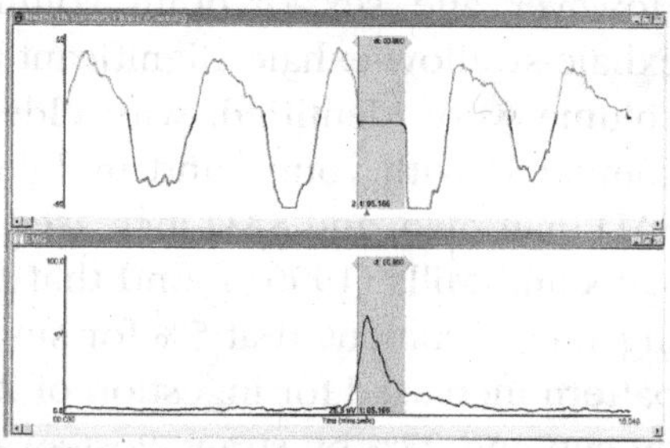
Mid-inspiration	I-I	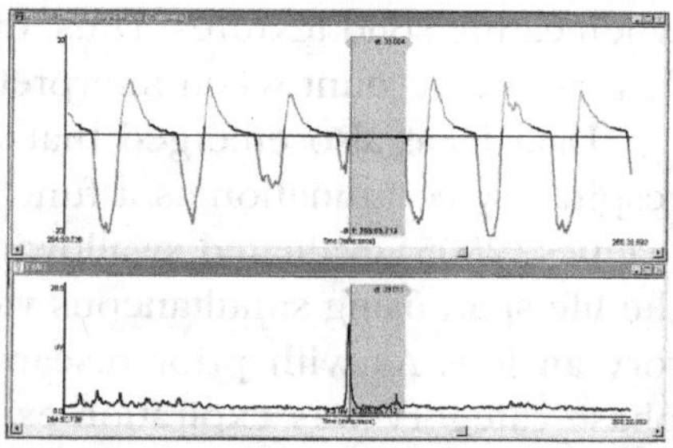
At the transition between inspiration and expiration	I-E	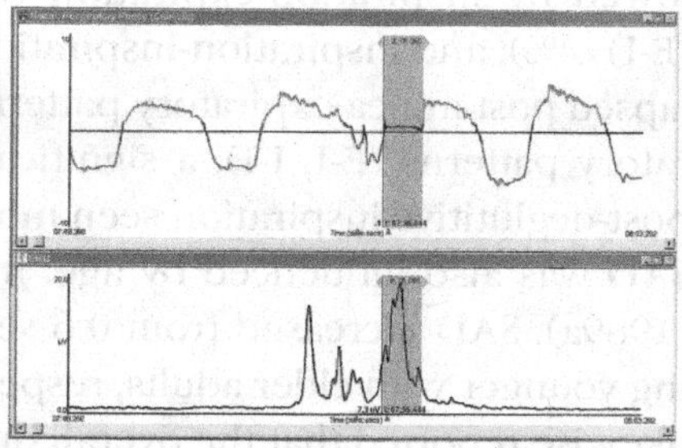

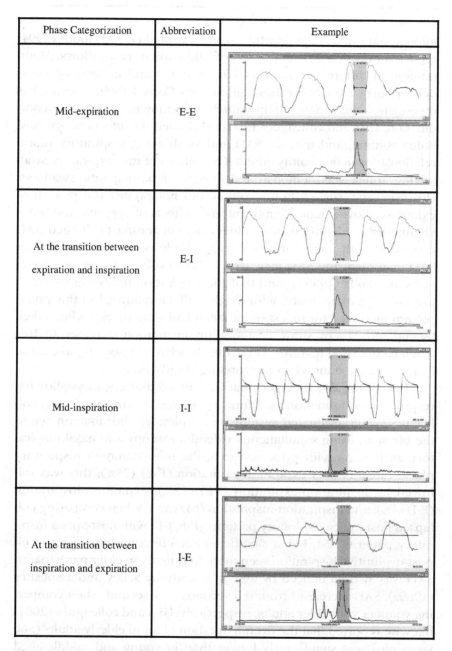

Figure 11–2. Phase categorization descriptions for classifying swallowing respiratory coordination. E-E = expiration-expiration, E-I = expiration-inspiration, I-I = inspiration-inspiration, I-E = inspiration-expiration.

mid-expiration, whereas Martin, Logemann, Shaker, and Dodds (1994) reported between 94% and 100% of mid-expiratory swallows. Methodological differences such as size of bolus and method of bolus delivery may account for these differences. Considerable research has investigated the variance in measures of swallowing respiratory coordination. Hiss and colleagues (2001) evaluated the effects of age, sex, bolus volume, and trial on SAD and swallowing respiratory phase relationships in 60 healthy adults. The pattern of mid-expiratory swallowing apnea was demonstrated in 62% of participants' swallows. However, age, sex, or bolus volume did not predict the pattern of exhale-swallow-exhale. Significant main effects of age, sex, and bolus volume were identified, with elders demonstrating prolonged SAD compared with young and middle-aged adults. Women had longer SAD than men, and SAD increased as bolus volume increased. Preiksaitis and Mills (1996) found that the inspiration following swallowing was documented at 5% for single bolus swallows, but this phase pattern increased for ingestion of 200 mL of fluid to 23% when taken by cup and 27% by straw. Post-swallow inspiration increased to 16% when eating solid textures. Thus, the clinician will need to take these factors into account when interpreting clinical data.

Data have also emerged that document changes in swallowing respiratory coordination as a function of age. Martin-Harris and colleagues (2005) evaluated swallowing respiratory coordination across the life span using simultaneous videofluoroscopy and nasal respiratory airflow. As with prior research, the most common respiratory phase category was expiration-expiration (E-E) (75%); this was followed by inspiration-expiration (I-E) (18%), expiration-inspiration (E-I) (4%), and inspiration-inspiration (I-I) (3%). When comparing collapsed post-apnea expiratory patterns (E-E, I-E) with post-apnea inspiratory patterns (E-I, I-I), a significant age effect was also seen, with post-deglutitive inspiration seen more frequently in elder participants. SAD was also influenced by age. In a study by Selley and associates (1989a), SAD increased from 0.6 seconds to 1 second when comparing younger with elder adults, respectively. Hiss and colleagues (2001) likewise reported that the overall duration of SA in elderly adults (>60 years old) was significantly longer than in young and middle-aged adults (<60 years old). In the study by Martin-Harris and colleagues (2005), SAD during ingestion of a 5 mL water bolus ranged from 0.5 to 10.02 seconds, with a median duration of 1.0 seconds. All outliers were among the oldest participants. As many individuals who are evaluated for swallowing impairment post-stroke are in this age group, recognition that age influences swallowing respiratory coordination is critical.

Aberrant patterns of swallowing respiratory coordination have been reported in patients with neurologic disorders by Selley, Flack, Ellis, and Brooks (1989b). These authors reported that 43% of a population of patients with mixed neurologic disorders demonstrated post-swallow inspiration, whereas Hadjikoutis and associates (2000) reported this finding in up to 91% of their population studied. Specific to stroke, Leslie, Drinnan, Ford, and Wilson (2002) studied a relatively small sample of 18 stroke patients with mixed site of lesion and stroke severity and 50 healthy controls. Individuals with dysphagia subsequent to stroke were found to present fewer instances of post-swallow expiration than those in the control group. SAD was not significantly different in patients with and without stroke, although in both groups, SAD increased with advancing age. Disparate findings for SAD were identified in a study by Butler, Stuart, Pressman, Poage, and Roche (2007), who described swallowing respiratory relationships in patients with dysphagia subsequent to stroke who aspirate and those who do not aspirate, and compared these data with those for healthy elders. Those patients with documented aspiration demonstrated significantly longer SAD than those without aspiration. Additionally, they demonstrated SAD that was twice as long as that in healthy elder adults. In reference to patterns of swallowing respiratory coordination, stroke patients with documented aspiration demonstrated a greater percentage of swallows within mid-inspiration (9%), with an increasing percentage of this pattern with increased dysphagia severity. Non-aspirating patients with swallowing impairment presented this pattern on 3% of swallows, with healthy elders documented at only 0.1%.

As with many of our emerging diagnostic tools, the evaluation of swallowing respiration coordination is hindered by incomplete and/or conflicting normative data. As research in this area continues, clinicians will be in a better position to assign diagnostic criteria to the data gleaned from this assessment. Until that time, the assessment of swallowing respiratory coordination can be cautiously compared with existing data and used as a supportive measure of diagnosing swallowing impairment and aspiration risk.

12 The Instrumental Swallowing Examination

Videoendoscopic Evaluation of Swallowing

The videofluoroscopic swallowing study (VFSS) is generally the evaluation of choice for patients with stroke, as it allows integrated investigation of oral and pharyngeal dynamics. However, the videoendoscopic evaluation of swallowing (VEES) does have particular strengths (see Table 10–1) that make it well suited for certain patients with stroke. Due to its portability, videoendoscopy may be advantageous for patients who are critically ill following stroke, that is, patients in the intensive care unit or those who are ventilator dependent. For those patients with significant cognitive impairment and for whom the radiology environment may decrease cooperation and performance, VEES may be a good alternative to VFSS. In addition, VEES is ideal for directly evaluating laryngeal closure and airway protection. Once baseline swallowing biomechanics are identified, VEES may be a valid follow-up assessment to identify change in bolus flow (e.g., aspiration, residue), thus limiting radiation exposure by re-evaluating with VFSS only when change in physiological patterns is suspected.

EXECUTING THE VIDEOENDOSCOPIC EVALUATION OF SWALLOWING

Videoendoscopic Setup

When using VEES, a flexible laryngoscope and light source are required. As with the VFSS, it is ideal to have the evaluation recorded, to have a microphone to capture audio, and to use a counter timer to record time. Hey and colleagues (2015) studied two conditions of interpreting endoscopic images: video-recorded examinations and simulated exams without recording. Intra- and interrater reliability were both significantly improved with recording; use of recording also allowed for more reliable identification of aspiration and penetration. A clinician may piece together a videoendoscopic setup or choose predesigned models. With advances in technology, newer systems are recording video with a wireless system (Sakakura et al., 2017).

Patient and Videoendoscope Positioning

Patients may be evaluated while sitting in bed or seated in a chair or wheelchair. Unlike VFSS, patient positioning is not a critical issue, and likely less time and effort are required to achieve optimal viewing of pharyngeal and laryngeal structures. The clinician should, however, be prepared to reposition the scope as patients with stroke may move, thereby disrupting optimal scope positioning.

The use of topical anesthesia is debated in performing VEES. No difference in patient comfort was identified with or without the use of a topical anesthetic by one research group (Leder, Ross, Briskin, & Sasaki, 1997). Other groups have published conflicting data. O'Dea and colleagues (2015) have identified significantly lower pain scores in the anesthetized condition compared with a decongestant only condition based on a validated scale. This same group found no difference between the groups in Penetration-Aspiration (P-A) Scale scores or pharyngeal residue for standardized boluses. A similar study by Fife et al. (2015) also found no significant change in P-A Scale scores, but the odds of aspirating were 33% higher in the anesthetized condition. Their participants also reported significantly less pain and improved tolerance of the procedure with anesthesia. The need for anesthesia may depend heavily on the patient and the experience of the clinician in handling the endoscope. The confidence of the endoscopist may go a long way to decreasing perceived discomfort and improving tolerance, thus allowing a non-anesthetized study to be completed without negatively affecting swallowing. If anesthesia is considered necessary, topical anesthesia, such as 2% viscous lidocaine, may be used to anesthetize the nares. Aerosol anesthetic should be avoided due to the potential for spread, thereby affecting pharyngeal sensation.

The endoscope is placed transnasally generally alongside or under the inferior turbinate. If a small-bore nasogastric tube (NGT) for feeding is in place, the scope can usually be passed on the same side following the same route. If a large-bore NGT is present, the scope may need to be passed through the other nares. At the entrance to the nasopharynx, if incompetence of velopharyngeal closure is suspected and the patient can produce volitional speech, evaluation of palatal functioning should be completed at this point. Velopharyngeal functioning is determined by having the patient repeatedly contrast oral plosives and nasal resonance sounds, such as "duh-nuh." Following evaluation of velopharyngeal competence, the scope is inserted further until the distal end is placed above the uvula (Figure 12–1). This position should be maintained prior to each swallow, as it allows a view of the epiglottis, base of tongue, hypopharynx, and larynx. After each swallow, the clinician should quickly advance the scope further to determine whether residual material is in the larynx or the trachea. The scope then is retracted to the more superior position before the next swallow.

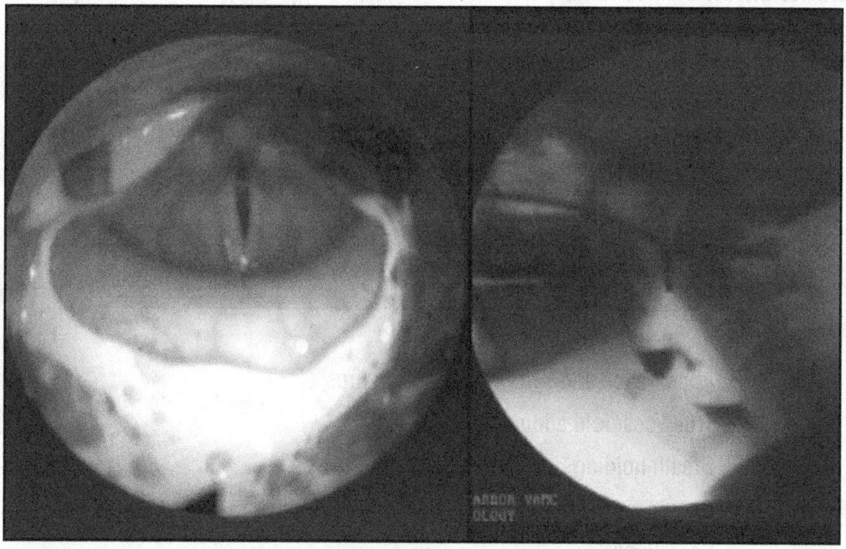

Figure 12–1. Correct placement of the endoscope to view the pharynx and larynx for swallowing. (Figure courtesy of Dr. Joseph Murray)

Pre-Swallow Observations

Numerous observations in addition to the evaluation of velopharyngeal competence should be completed prior to administration of food and liquid (Table 12–1). The appearance and symmetry of structures and recesses (valleculae, pyriform sinuses) should be observed, with any deviations noted. Integrity of true vocal fold (TVF) functioning is completed by having the patient phonate /ee/. The clinician should note the magnitude and symmetry of TVF movement and closure as well as vocal quality. As with velopharyngeal incompetence, unilateral vocal fold paresis frequently may be seen in patients with a lateral medullary stroke.

Breath holding is assessed by having the patient hold his or her breath with notation of: (1) ability to achieve breath holding, (2) duration of breath holding, and (3) adduction of TVF and ventricular vocal fold closure. Cough is evaluated by volitional production. Components of the volitional cough include: inspiration (glottic abduction), supraglottic closure with increased tracheal pressure, and glottic abduction with release of pressure (Murray, 1999). Although volitional cough may not relate to the effectiveness of a reflexive cough, it will provide information on the ability to use volitional cough as part of therapeutic intervention and is a good indicator for poor performance when it is weakly produced.

Evaluation of secretion management is completed by documenting the collection of secretions in the pharyngeal recesses and in the

Table 12–1. Features to Assess with Videoendoscopy Prior to the Administration of Food or Liquid

- Velopharyngeal competence
- Appearance and symmetry of structures
- True vocal fold adduction
- Breath holding
- Cough
- Secretions
- Sensation

laryngeal vestibule. The amount and location of secretions should be noted as well as any response from the patient in an attempt to clear the material. Does the patient spontaneously swallow, throat clear, or cough in an attempt to clear, or is there no response to the accumulation of secretions? Is the patient successful in attempts to clear secretions? Pooling of secretions in the laryngeal vestibule is associated with wet vocal quality and may be evident following stroke. Pooling of secretions in the laryngeal vestibule is strongly associated with aspiration of food and liquid (Murray, Langmore, Ginsberg, & Dostie, 1996).

Sensation initially may be evaluated by noting the patient's response to pooled secretions, post-swallow residual, and aspiration. That is, does the patient repeatedly swallow or cough to clear secretions or residue? Does the patient cough in response to aspiration? Although not a quantitative measure, the patient's response to material in the larynx and pharynx is the most clinically relevant measure of laryngopharyngeal sensation in the context of ingestion.

Bolus Presentation Guidelines

The same guidelines suggested with the clinical swallowing examination or VFSS should be followed for VEES. As with these other evaluations, initiating VEES with small liquid volumes is strongly encouraged with patients following stroke to reduce the amount of aspiration and to prevent contamination of subsequent swallows with significant post-swallow residual. Murray (1999) recommends beginning the examination with ice chips for those patients who demonstrate accumulation of secretions in the laryngeal vestibule or who have been without oral feedings for an extended period. This will prevent a large amount of aspiration in those patients who are at high risk of aspiration and may help "alert" the swallowing system in those patients who have been without oral intake for a period of time.

As VEES does not involve ingestion of barium, the clinician is free to use real food and liquid. At a minimum, the clinician should consider assessing swallowing of liquids, semisolids, and solids, but as with the other evaluation methods, progression to larger volumes and thicker consistencies depends on the patient's response to small liquid volumes. Early in the use of VEES, food coloring was added to material ingested to facilitate visualization of the bolus. One study, however, suggests that nondyed food (milk, pudding) is as reliable as dyed material for completing critical swallowing measures (Leder, Acton, Lisitano, & Murray, 2005). The authors suggest that the ability of a bolus to reflect light is the critical feature for determining the visibility of a bolus in the laryngopharyngeal region. Thus, milk-based products, particularly liquids, are frequently suggested in VEES. A more recent study was in agreement that use of food dye did not influence detection of aspiration significantly among the full cohort; however, when white secretions were present in the pharynx, use of colored dye increased detection of airway invasion (Marvin, Gustafson, & Thibeault, 2016). Additionally, dyed boluses were more likely to be observed with supraglottic penetration of large volumes, and colored liquids were interpreted with better test-retest reliability than undyed boluses. These authors consequently suggest that the use of dyed boluses is indicated for VEES.

By having no time constraints on the length of the VEES, the clinician can extend the assessment to evaluate the effects of fatigue or swallowing behavior over time. The repeated use of compensatory strategies can be evaluated; this is important for the patient with stroke for whom the clinician has concern for continuous employment of a posture without clinician cue. VEES also may be used to provide visual feedback during the initial assessment or in treatment to instruct the patient on the implementation of compensatory strategies such as the super-supraglottic swallow.

INTERPRETING THE VIDEOENDOSCOPIC EVALUATION OF SWALLOWING

Interpreting the VEES can be challenging, as the oral cavity is not viewed and the view is obscured during velar elevation or when the base of tongue contacts the posterior pharyngeal wall, both of which will trap the lens with light from the endoscope reflecting back into the lens. The obscuring of the view is frequently termed "whiteout" and results in loss of view of critical portions of the swallowing event. Thus, judgments of oral and pharyngeal motility must be inferred by viewing observable bolus flow patterns such as pre-swallow pharyngeal pooling and post-swallow residual patterns.

Anatomic Abnormalities

Detailed information concerning pharyngeal and laryngeal anatomy can be obtained with VEES. The superior view of mucosa covering the structures obtained with VEES may provide more detail about anatomic deviations, particularly evidence of a mass, in the pharynx and larynx compared with the lateral view with VFSS. Abnormality in appearance and symmetry should be reported as well as the effects on swallowing, and any suspicious anatomic observations should prompt a referral to otolaryngology for follow-up. The pre-swallow observations on secretions, breath holding, and so forth will provide the clinician with information on glottic function and sensation which are important for swallowing and can assist in forming an impression as to how well the patient may perform during subsequent presentations of food and liquid.

Bolus Flow

Information on bolus timing through the oral cavity and pharynx cannot be obtained with VEES, as the oral cavity is not visualized, and whiteout obscures the actual swallow. Although different from VFSS, information concerning stage transit duration can be determined by observing the entry of the bolus into the pharynx (onset) through the point of whiteout (offset). In this fashion, delay in evocation of the pharyngeal swallow can be determined.

Timing of airway invasion can only be measured if it occurs pre-swallow or post-swallow. Intra-swallow aspiration is determined if material is visualized in the airway after the period of whiteout is over. Unlike VFSS, the clinician will not be able to view intra-swallow airway invasion as it happens. Distinguishing between pre-swallow laryngeal penetration and aspiration may be difficult at times if whiteout occurs before visualization of entry of material into the trachea. Only by inspecting the trachea for residual material once the swallow is completed can intra-swallow aspiration be identified.

Post-swallow residue can be viewed in the pharynx using VEES. Unlike VFSS, which provides a lateral or anterior-posterior view of the depth of residual, the clinician must identify residual material and subjectively determine amount from a superior view. The pyriform sinuses and valleculae are easily viewed with VEES. As with VFSS, it is ideal for clinicians to have a working knowledge of what is normal residue for various consistencies before judging abnormal clearance. Research has suggested that pharyngeal residue is judged to be greater in VEES compared with VFSS (Kelly, Leslie, Beale, Payten, & Drinnan, 2006). Thus, it is critical that clinicians new to the use of VEES internally calibrate their judgment of post-swallow residual with experienced endoscopists and against VFSS findings.

Temporal Coordination and Extent of Structural Movement

Aside from airway protection, any dysfunction in swallowing biomechanics must be inferred using VEES. That is, the clinician must use information gleaned from swallowing function prior to the onset of the whiteout as well as information obtained after the swallow (e.g., post-swallow residual) to determine the area of dysfunction. For example, entry of material into the pharynx before onset of whiteout may be due to pre-swallow pooling or to delayed elicitation of the pharyngeal swallow. Without viewing the oral cavity, this may be very difficult to distinguish. Impaired oral containment or delayed initiation of oral transfer also may be inferred by delayed appearance of the bolus in the pharynx or delayed whiteout. The presence and location of post-swallow residual must be used to judge pharyngeal motility. Vallecular residue may indicate decreased base of tongue retraction and/or reduced epiglottic inversion. Pyriform sinus residue may indicate reduced anterior hyolaryngeal movement and/or decreased upper esophageal sphincter opening.

Rather than inferring oral phase behavior from pharyngeal observation, Farneti, Fattori, and Bastiani (2017) published a novel application of VEES, termed O-FEES, which incorporates specific evaluation of the oral cavity as an accompaniment to a traditional endoscopic evaluation. The protocol requires inversion of the endoscopic tip at the oropharyngeal level to view the oral cavity up to the teeth from the posterior aspects. The researchers reported tolerance of the assessment consistent with tolerance of the endoscopic procedure in general. Additionally, the researchers reported what they considered to be strong validity compared with VFSS, using a very coarse measure of agreement.

Scales for Rating VEES

As with any instrument used in swallowing assessment, attention to the reliability and validity of the technique is of interest. Pilz et al. (2016) evaluated the reliability of two clinicians in rating VEES in 60 patients. The clinicians were trained to four descriptive, ordinal scales: piecemeal deglutition (five levels), post-swallow vallecular retention (three levels), post-swallow pyriform sinus retention (three levels), and laryngeal penetration/tracheal aspiration (three levels). Weighted kappa coefficients identified intrarater agreement between 0.76 and 0.93, with interrater agreement between 0.61 and 0.88. The authors elaborated that etiology of dysphagia did not influence agreement among raters but that liquid bolus swallows were predictive of poorer agreement.

In an effort to provide quantification of VEES, rating scales have been developed to assess a variety of endoscopically observed behaviors. Murray et al. (1996) reported on development of a 4-point secretion severity scale that evaluated presence of secretions at rest, rather than specific residual in response to oral intake. An increased composite severity score was found to be highly predictive of aspiration of food and liquid. This scale was further developed by Pluschinski et al. (2016), who reported very high inter- and intrarater reliability and agreement with a reference standard for interpretation of videorecordings of endoscopic examinations.

The P-A Scale, as reviewed in Chapter 10, was designed for use during VFSS (Rosenbek, Robbins, Roecker, Coyle, & Wood, 1996); however, reliability in scoring has also been demonstrated with VEES (Butler, Markley, Sanders, & Stuart, 2015; Colodny, 2002). Again, the clinician is cautioned that depth of airway invasion in the larynx, one of the measures of the P-A Scale, may be difficult to determine using VEES. Furthermore, and not surprisingly, assignment of higher P-A scores using videoendoscopy compared with VFSS has been identified (Kelly, Drinnan, & Leslie, 2007).

Dziewas, Warnecke, and colleagues completed a series of VEES studies in patients with acute stroke to evaluate the 6-point fiberoptic endoscopic dysphagia severity scale. In their protocol, the following are evaluated in this order: secretion management, puree, liquids, and soft solid food (bread without crust) (Dziewas, Warnecke, Ölenberg, et al., 2008). If airway invasion is evident with secretions, the evaluation is terminated. For food/liquid boluses, three trials are completed at 3 mL volumes for each consistency. The presence of airway invasion with spontaneous elicitation of protective response (e.g., cough, swallow) is evaluated with each swallow. A reflexive response is considered present if evident on one of the three trials. Subsequent consistencies are not provided if airway invasion is evident with any of the three trials at that consistency, regardless of evidence of a protective response. For the solid consistency, residue of more than 50% of the bolus is also determined. Penetration or aspiration of secretions (score 6), puree without a protective reflex (score 5), puree with a protective reflex (score 4), and liquids without a protective reflex (score 4) result in recommendation of no oral intake. Airway invasion of liquids with evidence of a protective response results in recommendation of puree oral intake but no oral liquids (score 3). If greater than 50% residue of the bread bolus is evident (score 2), liquids and purees are recommended. If less than 50% residue with the bread, soft solids and liquids are recommended. The protocol and procedure were determined to be safe (Warnecke, Tiesmann, et al., 2009a) and predictive of functional recovery (Warnecke, Ritter, et al., 2009) and to have sufficient reliability in interpretation (Dziewas, Warnecke, Ölenberg, et al., 2008; Warnecke, Tiesmann, et al., 2009b). The astute clinician, however, will note that this is an extremely conservative protocol with termination of the evaluation with a single instance of airway invasion, which can be normal in healthy, particularly older, adults (see Table 3–1), and no evaluation of compensatory strategies.

Farneti and colleagues (2014) developed a scale not to quantify degree of aspiration but to evaluate endoscopically observed pre-swallow pooling. Intraclass correlation coefficient (ICC) values representing reliability of assessment for pre-swallow site, amount, management, and the composite P-score total were found to be, respectively, 0.999, 0.997, 1.00, and 0.999. Bolus type did not influence reliability.

Post-swallow residual was the focus of evaluation with the development of the Boston Residue and Clearance Scale (Kaneoka et al., 2013). This 11-point ordinal residue rating scale scores three aspects of residue: (1) the amount and location of residue, (2) the presence of spontaneous clearing swallows, and (3) the effectiveness of clearing swallows. Based on the ratings of 63 recorded swallows by four raters, the scale showed high interrater reliability (ICC = 0.81), intrarater reliability (ICC = 0.82–0.92), concurrent validity (Pearson's $r = 0.76$), and internal consistency (Cronbach's $\alpha = 0.86$).

A similar scale, albeit with fewer items, was developed by Neubauer, Rademaker, and Leder (2015). The Yale Pharyngeal Residual Severity Rating Scale was evaluated by 20 raters representing a wide range of skill level. The researchers documented high intra- and interrater reliability and construct validity of the tool for identifying severity and anatomical location of post-swallow pharyngeal residual. However, reliability was based on assessment of still images rather than the moving endoscopic assessment, as would be encountered in clinical routine. A systematic review of scales for endoscopic swallowing assessment was completed by this same research group (Neubauer, Hersey, & Leder, 2016), and not surprisingly, they concluded that their residue scale was the only one with adequate psychometric validation for clinical use.

Response to Compensatory Strategies and Determining the Treatment Plan

The implementation and use of specific management techniques is the same with VEES as it is with VFSS. As time is not an issue with VEES, the clinician may spend more time instructing and having the patient practice various compensatory techniques. Although persistence or resolution of the signs of dysphagia, that is, post-swallow residual or aspiration, is viewed with VEES, the effect on the swallowing biomechanics is not observed. For example, the head-lift exercise may be implemented in a patient with reduced hyolaryngeal movement and post-swallow pyriform sinus residual. Following a course of effective rehabilitation, the clinician would see reduced residual using VEES, whereas with VFSS, the clinician could observe improved hyolaryngeal excursion as well as reduced post-swallow residual.

13 The Instrumental Swallowing Examination

Manometric Evaluation of Swallowing[1]

As discussed in previous chapters, the videofluoroscopic swallowing study (VFSS) provides critical information about swallowing biomechanics through observations of structural and soft tissue movement and bolus flow. The videoendoscopic evaluation of swallowing nicely augments this information by providing optimal visualization of anatomy and airway closure mechanisms. These are undoubtedly very valuable and irreplaceable tools but can be limited by the subjective nature of interpretation of some aspects of swallowing biomechanics, resulting in compromised reliability and questionable validity (Kuhlemeier, Yates, & Palmer, 1998; McCullough, Wertz, Rosenbek, Mills, et al., 2001; Scott, Perry, & Bench, 1998; Stoeckli, Huisman, Seifert, & Martin-Harris, 2003; Wilcox, Liss, & Siegel, 1996).

Manometry provides a measure of pressure and can contribute information about the amplitude and timing of pressure events within the pharyngeal cavity and upper esophageal sphincter (UES) to the diagnostic dysphagia evaluation. Although this technique provides no direct visualization of swallowing events, the issue of subjectivity and subsequent reliability is minimized through the provision of quantitative measures of swallowing biomechanics. Further, this technique can provide clarification and quantification of diagnostic features identified through other techniques. It has been used for more than 20 years to evaluate numerous parameters of swallowing physiology in various populations of individuals with dysphagia, including stroke (Bülow, Olsson, & Ekberg, 1999; Martino, Terrault, Ezerzer, Mikulis, & Diamant, 2001). Manometry can also be utilized as a biofeedback modality

[1]Some content reprinted with permission of Karger Publishers: Huckabee, M. L., Macrae, P., and Lamvik, K. (2015). Expanding instrumental options for dysphagia diagnosis and research: Ultrasound and manometry. *Folia Phoniatrica et Logopaedica*, *67*(6), 269–284.

during rehabilitation, as discussed further in Chapter 22 (Huckabee, Lamvik, & Jones, 2014; Lamvik, Jones, Sauer, Erfmann, & Huckabee, 2015; O'Rourke & Humphries, 2017).

Despite these possible applications, pharyngeal manometry has been slow to emerge into routine clinical practice (Ravich, 1995). In a recent survey of 206 speech pathologists, only 3.5% of respondents reported having access to manometry in their workplace (Jones, Knigge, & McCulloch, 2014). This is compounded by the finding that of those who had access to manometry, only half reported they would pursue a manometric evaluation in a case study of UES dysfunction. This highlights the need for continued education regarding the utility of this technique.

MANOMETRIC APPROACHES

The American Speech-Language-Hearing Association has included pharyngeal manometry as part of the Preferred Practice Patterns for the Profession of Speech-Language Pathology (2004) and as a recommendation for inclusion in the Graduate Curriculum on Swallowing and Swallowing Disorders (2007). The manometric evaluation in clinical settings may be completed jointly by the gastroenterologist and the speech pathologist. Perhaps the best option is joint manometry with a VFSS, termed in the literature "manofluoroscopy." Manofluoroscopy is considered the gold standard in evaluation of swallowing function (Nativ-Zeltzer, Kahrilas, & Logemann, 2012). With visualization of bolus flow time-locked to pressure recordings, the clinician is able to gain greater insights into the relationships between pressure and pharyngeal biomechanics (Bodén, Hallgren, & Witt Hedstrom, 2006; Feinberg, 1993; Kahrilas & Shi, 1998; McConnel, 1988; Salassa, DeVault, & McConnel, 1998). While a typical VFSS is ideally recorded at 30 frames per second, manometry can provide temporal information in the millisecond range (Barbiera et al., 2006). Thus, the clinician is able to quantify the observed pharyngeal events with an objective measure. This provides great advantages over VFSS in isolation. This technique also allows for confirmation of sensor placement through observation. To complete this examination, the manometric catheter can be placed prior to or during the study (radiographically guided) and the recording equipment for both techniques integrated into a single acquisition system.

Another option for completing manometry is to pair this technique with endoscopy, termed "manoendoscopy" by Butler (2006). This option has benefits in flexibility and portability and allows the clinician to visually confirm placement of pharyngeal sensors. Execution of pharyngeal swallowing produces a "white-out" on endoscopy; thus, the period of bolus flow over the manometric sensors is not visualized using this technique. Intrabolus pressure can only be inferred and loses the precision gained from manofluorography. Regardless, in individuals who are unable to transfer to the videofluoroscopy suite and require examinations performed at bedside, the manoendoscopic study will provide valuable information.

Finally, the "bare bones" approach to manometry consists of pharyngeal manometry completed in isolation. This type of assessment would only be appropriate when prior diagnostic studies have been completed and there is a specific differential diagnosis required; manometry in isolation relies on investigation of the timing and amplitude of pharyngeal contact pressure alone. Performing manometry in isolation is contraindicated in individuals with a known or suspected Zenker's diverticulum, as visualization is required to navigate safe placement and reduce the risk of perforation of a diverticulum.

LOW-RESOLUTION MANOMETRY

Low-resolution, solid-state manometry, developed primarily for use in the esophagus, was an advancement on traditional water-perfusion techniques (Dodds, Kahrilas, Dent, & Hogan, 1987). Salassa et al. (1998) present a valuable review of manometric methods that should be requisite reading for any clinicians who wish to include low-resolution manometry in their diagnostic workup. They propose an optimal "standard" catheter design for pharyngeal manometry or manofluoroscopy. The ideal standard pharyngeal manometry catheter is recommended to:

- be 2.1 mm (or smaller) in diameter, ovoid in shape, and 100 cm long

- be marked in cm with anterior to posterior orientation
- have a slightly malleable 3 to 4 cm length of catheter without sensors beyond the most distal sensor
- use solid-state transducers with one sensor each in three or four locations:
  - tongue base
  - hypopharynx
  - UES
  - esophagus (as optional fourth sensor)
- have sensor spacing of 2 cm between tongue base and hypopharynx and 3 cm between the hypopharynx and UES.

Insertion and Analysis

As the procedure requires contact with potentially infectious bodily fluids via intraoral or intranarial catheter placement, adherence to facility-approved infection control procedures is important. After calibrating the catheter to the manufacturer's specifications, the clinician should prepare the catheter by applying a small amount of water-based lubricant to facilitate ease of transfer through the nasal cavity. Topical nasal anesthetic is not necessary with these small-diameter catheters and may adversely affect sensorimotor aspects of pharyngeal swallowing (Guiu Hernandez, Gozdzikowska, Apperley, & Huckabee, 2018). As with all diagnostic procedures, clear instructions should be given prior to initiation of the examination.

With the sensors facing the ceiling, the catheter is passed into and through the nasal cavity, taking care to maintain position below the inferior turbinate. The clinician will feel slight resistance as the catheter abuts the posterior pharyngeal wall. If the catheter does not easily pass from the horizontally oriented nasal cavity into the more vertically oriented pharyngeal cavity, asking the individual to look up to the ceiling will reduce the angle at the nasopharyngeal junction and allow transfer. As the catheter enters the pharynx, the sensors will now be oriented toward the posterior pharyngeal wall. During blind placement, care must be taken to avoid laryngeal irritation or invasion with the tip of the catheter. To accomplish this, it is best to let the individual control placement by executing either dry or, if tolerated, water swallows. In this case, the individual "swallows" the catheter into the esophagus, thus protecting the airway as the tip of the catheter moves through the hypopharynx. If resistance is encountered in passing the catheter through the UES, a slight quarter-turn rotation of the catheter may facilitate guidance through the lateral channels and into the esophagus.

After the uppermost sensor is placed within the esophagus, up to 40 cm from the tip of the nose, the clinician must correctly position the catheter. This is accomplished using a "pull through" technique. With the waveform display running, the catheter is slowly withdrawn. As the uppermost sensor passes through the high-pressure zone of the UES, pressure recordings in this channel will increase and then subsequently decrease as the sensor exits into the hypopharynx. Similarly, the mid-pharyngeal sensor will produce a waxing and waning amplitude as it passes through the cricopharyngeus and into the pharynx. As the lowermost sensor passes through the UES, the clinician will pull through the pressure zone and then push the catheter very slightly back into the zone of high pressure; approximately 1 cm after peak pressure is achieved. In so doing, the lowermost sensor is resting near the top of the cricopharyngeus. During swallowing, if the catheter is appropriately positioned, the clinician will observe a typical "M-wave" (Castell, Dalton, & Castell, 1990; Richter & Castell, 1989), as displayed in Figure 13–1. Baseline pressure, although not maximal resting pressure, is evident at rest. As hyolaryngeal excursion is initiated, the cricopharyngeus is pulled fully over the lowermost sensor, resulting in peak amplitude, or the first peak in the "M." Cricopharyngeal relaxation then produces a substantive drop in pressure as the UES is maximally opened; this produces the middle drop in the "M-wave." The cricopharyngeus then contracts after bolus transfer with again a maximal rise in pressure, then subsequently returns to a lower resting average as passive return of hyolaryngeal excursion drops the cricopharyngeus back to the inferior aspect of the lowermost sensor.

When the catheter is appropriately positioned, the clinician should ensure that the guide numbers on the catheter are facing up at the nose, indicating that the sensors within the pharynx are posteriorly oriented. The catheter then should be secured to the nose with standard medical tape, and the individual is allowed time to adjust to the catheter in vivo. Figure 13–2A displays a catheter in vivo at rest; Figure 13–2B displays a manometry catheter in vivo during pharyngeal swallowing with the pharynx fully closed around the catheter.

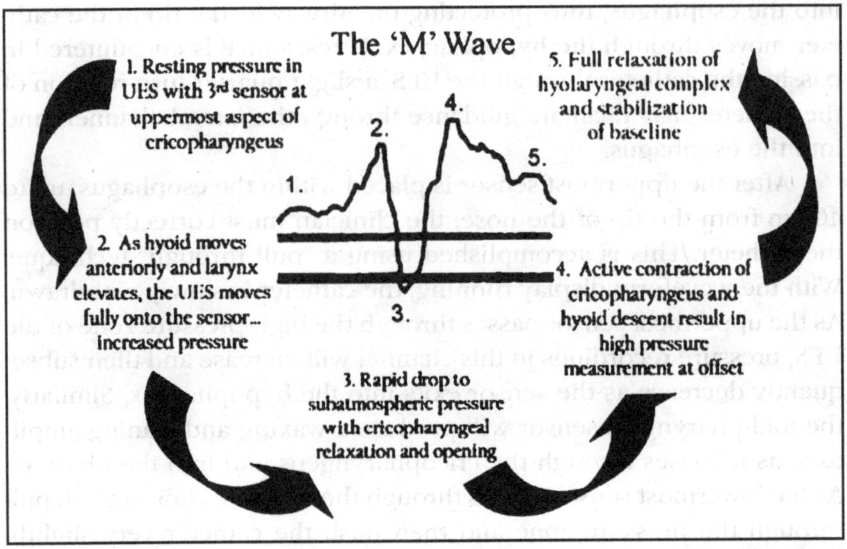

Figure 13–1. The characteristic "M-wave." UES = upper esophageal sphincter.

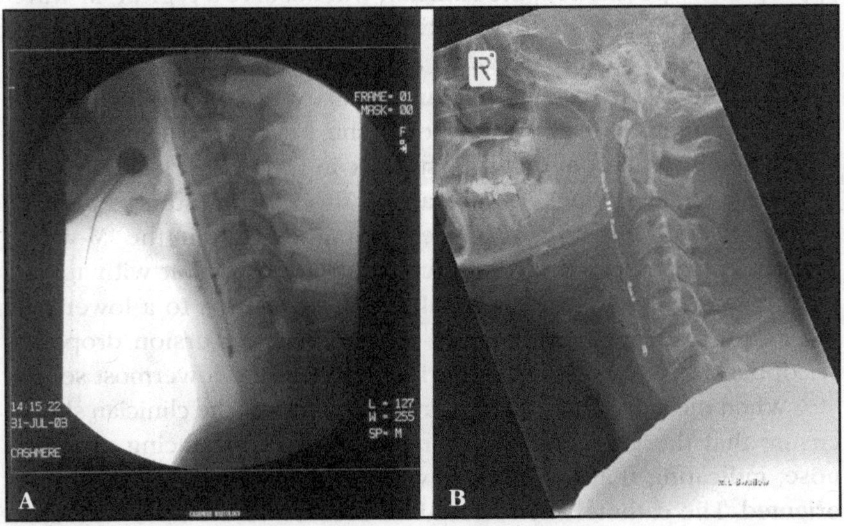

Figure 13–2. Pharyngeal manometric catheter in vivo at rest (**A**) and during swallowing (**B**).

Interpretation of Low-Resolution Manometry

As a measurement of pressure, low-resolution manometry provides quantitative information about the amplitude and duration of pressure events within the pharyngeal cavity and UES. Perhaps more importantly, valuable information can be gained about the sequencing of pharyngeal events. Figure 13–3 represents three low-resolution manometry waveforms from saliva swallowing in a healthy individual.

The uppermost waveform represents pressure generation in the proximal pharynx, at about the level of the base of tongue to the posterior pharyngeal wall approximation. The middle waveform represents pressure generation in the mid-pharynx, at approximately the level of the laryngeal aditus. For both waveforms, at rest there is a flat baseline at approximately atmospheric pressure. During swallowing, a short peak is visualized. The point of a sharp increase in pressure is subtracted from the return to baseline post-swallow for calculation of duration of pharyngeal pressure. Peak pressure is identified as the nadir amplitude during swallowing. The lowermost sensor rests at the upper margin of the UES. At rest the baseline is measured with positive pressure. As the hyoid elevates and pulls the UES over the sensor, there is a peak in amplitude that represents peak pressure within the cricopharyngeus before relaxation. The waveform then drops dramatically to atmospheric or sub-atmospheric pressure levels as the UES is pulled open. Peak negative pressure is termed "nadir pressure" during this drop. As the cricopharyngeus contracts at the conclusion of swallowing, there is again a sharp rise in pressure that represents peak offset. Subtracting onset time from offset time derives duration of UES opening.

In addition to peak and durational measures, it is of interest to evaluate sequencing of pressure generation. This is easily visualized by using overlapping waveforms as shown in Figure 13–4. Onset of pressure in the upper pharynx should precede onset of pressure in the lower pharynx. The onset of UES opening should occur prior to peak pressure in the upper pharynx, and the offset of UES opening should occur after peak pressure in the mid-pharynx.

The waveform in Figure 13–4 is an example of contact pressure. It is important that the clinician differentiate contact pressure from intrabolus pressure. Intrabolus pressure is defined as brief, moderate pressure increase elicited by the bolus passing the pharyngeal sensors (Cerenko, McConnel, & Jackson, 1989; Kahrilas, Logemannn, Lin,

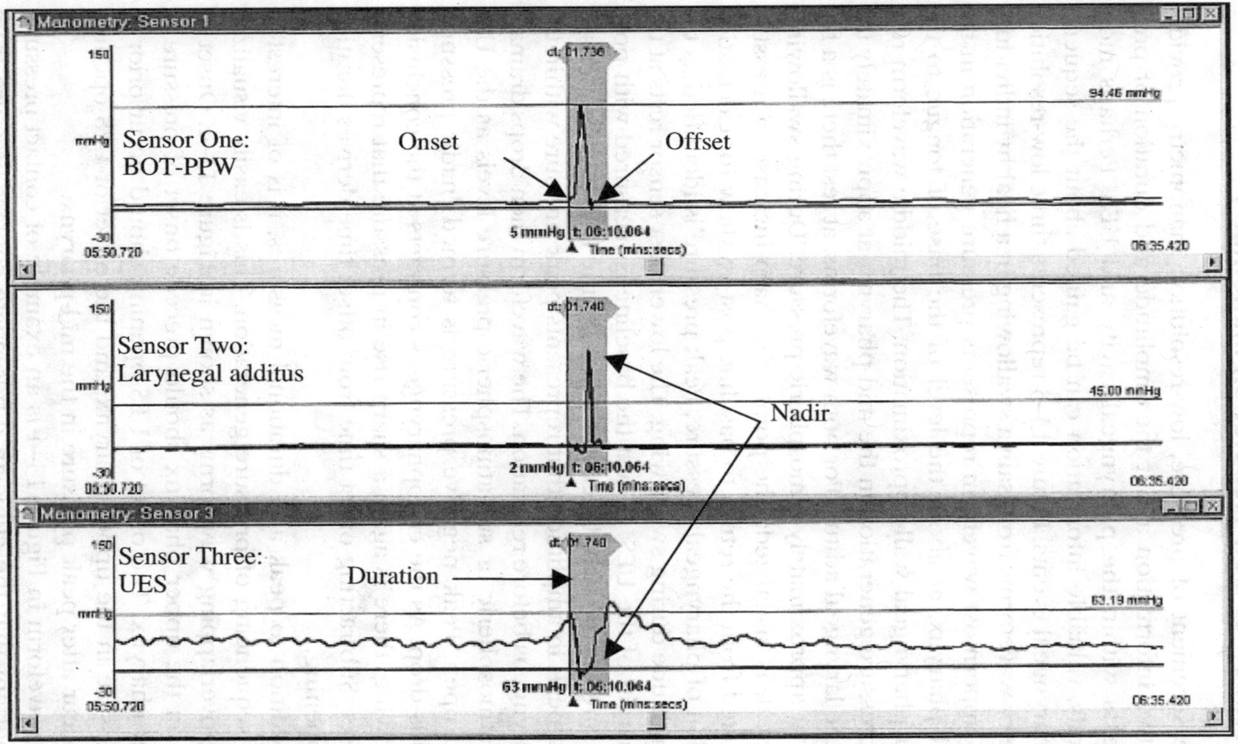

Figure 13–3. Interpretation of the pharyngeal manometry waveform includes measurement of amplitude at nadir, as well as time of onset and offset, which allows calculation of duration. BOT = base of tongue; PPW = posterior pharyngeal wall; UES = upper esophageal sphincter.

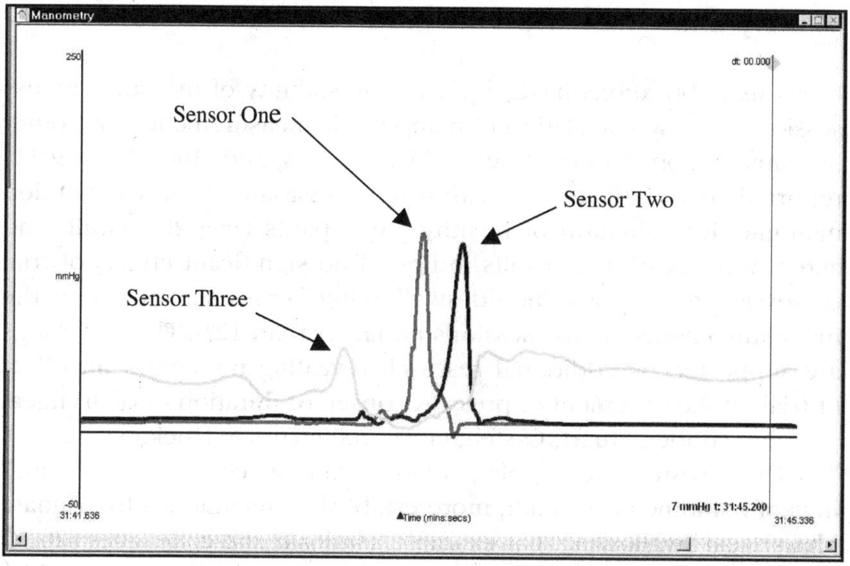

Figure 13–4. Overlapping waveforms acquired through pharyngeal manometric evaluation allow for clear visualization of sequencing of pharyngeal pressure generation.

& Ergun, 1992; McConnel, 1988). This is a measure of the pressure exerted *by* the bolus. This measure is reliably identified only with manofluoroscopy, as visualization of the bolus relative to sensors is a prerequisite to determining whether pressure is indeed exerted from the passing bolus. This is contrasted with pharyngeal contact pressure, which is the pressure exerted by approximation of pharyngeal structures after the bolus passes.

Normative data exist regarding the amplitude and duration of pharyngeal pressure, degree of UES relaxation, and the coordination of timing of UES relaxation relative to pharyngeal pressures (Butler, Stuart, Castell, et al., 2009; Lamvik, Macrae, Doeltgen, Collings, & Huckabee, 2014). Studies have revealed differences based on sex and age (Butler, Stuart, Castell, et al., 2009; Meier-Ewert et al., 2001; van Herwaarden et al., 2003). Further research indicates low-resolution manometry to be sensitive to differences in swallowing conditions, such as spontaneous versus reflexive swallowing and variable bolus sizes (Al-Toubi, Doeltgen, Daniels, Corey, & Huckabee, 2015).

Validity and Reliability

Previous publications have explored the stability of measures across sessions and the correlation of manometric measurements with other instrumentation devices. Macrae, Myall, Jones, and Huckabee (2011) reported an investigation of within-subject variance in low-resolution manometric evaluation of healthy participants (n = 20) within and across three sessions. Results indicated no significant effects of trial or session for dry and liquid swallowing across sensors, with the maximum change across sessions no larger than 12%. These findings are supported by additional research revealing no significant effect of trial on measurement of pressure, onset, or duration of pharyngeal pressure (Butler, Stuart, Castell, et al., 2009; Hiss & Huckabee, 2005).

These results are supplemented by studies correlating the findings of manometry to other, more established techniques to evaluate pharyngeal swallowing. For example, Pauloski and colleagues (2009) evaluated the relationship between VFSS and manometry in healthy adults (n = 7) and patients with dysphagia (n = 11). Results indicated that increases in amplitude of pharyngeal pressure correlate with duration of tongue base to posterior pharyngeal wall approximation. These findings are mirrored in a more recent study by Leonard, Rees, Belafsky, and Allen (2011), who evaluated the relationship between pharyngeal manometry and a measure of pharyngeal constriction on VFSS in patients with dysphagia (n = 25). A significant inverse correlation ($r = -0.72$) was identified between manometric pressure and pharyngeal constriction ratio, indicating that greater manometric pressure is related to a functional pharyngeal constriction (e.g., obliteration of the intraluminal pharyngeal airspace during swallowing).

Limitations

Despite the diagnostic value offered by low-resolution manometry, there are considerable limitations that have hindered its widespread acceptance. The primary limitation of low-resolution manometry is sensor positioning arising from fixed sensor placement along the catheter. Placement of the catheter requires the clinician to be meticulous in monitoring placement throughout the study. Research indicates a typical pharynx can range between 7 cm and 13 cm in healthy individuals (Ergun, Kahrilas, & Logemann, 1993). With fixed sensor positions along the catheter, measurement accuracy may be reduced across individuals of varying height. Further, users of low-resolution pharyngeal manometry must be cautious of intra-swallow catheter movement altering recording location of each sensor area, especially in blind manometric studies where catheter placement is not visually monitored with VFSS. Intra-swallow catheter movement is thought to arise from early movement resulting from velopharyngeal closure, followed by a non-synchronous change in the length of the pharynx and position of the UES (Ravich, 1995).

Another limitation is the use of the "M-wave" for catheter positioning. Although use of the "M-wave" for catheter positioning and placement is published routinely (Al-Toubi et al., 2015; Balou et al., 2014; Huckabee & Steele, 2006; Lamvik et al., 2014; Witte, Huckabee, Doeltgen, Gumbley, & Robb, 2008), the validity and reliability of this positioning technique warrants further investigation. Of note, original publications describing use of the "M-wave" did not validate against other techniques, such as VFSS (Castell & Castell, 1993). This is concerning, as incorrect positioning based on the M-wave can misdiagnose impaired UES functioning. If an individual has sufficient hyolaryngeal excursion, it is possible that inappropriate placement can lead to the sensor measuring pressure from the cervical esophagus, a negative pressure zone, artificially reducing the nadir pressure measured in the UES sensor. The advent of high-resolution manometry (HRM) has highlighted this limitation of low-resolution manometry further, as the UES region has been found to readily span three to five HRM pressure sensors (Jones, Ciucci, Hammer, & McCulloch, 2015). As discussed below, HRM may be superior in specific assessment of UES function to low-resolution manometry, unless adjunct imaging, such as VFSS, is concurrently utilized to overcome placement limitations.

Additionally, low-resolution manometry uses primarily unidirectional sensors that face the posterior pharyngeal wall, and thus complex pressure patterns generated within the irregularly shaped pharyngeal lumen are inferred based on information from unidirectional measures. Doeltgen and colleagues (2007) evaluated the placement of a catheter following insertion in either the right or left nares in healthy participants ($n = 10$). Based on analysis of still radiographic images, the catheter was positioned in the pharyngeal midline for only 20% of trials, with a deviation from 1.7 to 14.7 mm from midline. Previous publications have reported that radial asymmetry in pressure measurement can vary as high as 86 ± 13 mm Hg to 365 ± 29 mm Hg in lateral and posterior directions, respectively (Castell & Castell, 1993). This is compounded by inability to confirm specific intraluminal catheter placement when performing manometry without adjunct visualization techniques.

Despite these limitations, low-resolution manometry is a highly useful adjunct to clinical evaluations, providing robust, quantitative data regarding oropharyngeal swallowing function with high temporal resolutions. Although HRM advances this technology, as discussed in the subsequent section, fewer clinicians have access to this sophisticated equipment. Low-resolution manometry remains readily available, and therefore, still clinically relevant to research and clinical practice.

HIGH-RESOLUTION MANOMETRY

HRM has grown in popularity in the evaluation of pharyngeal swallowing. Considered the gold standard in the assessment of esophageal function by gastroenterologists, this tool has emerged as valuable in evaluating pharyngeal swallowing biomechanics (Rice & Shay, 2011; Takasaki et al., 2008). By increasing the number of recording sensors from 3 to 36, HRM enables continuous evaluation of intraluminal pressure along the aerodigestive tract. Each of the 36 pressure sensors comprises up to 16 measurement segments, creating an averaged, circumferential pressure reading within each sensor. Pharyngeal HRM has been used to evaluate normal swallowing (Takasaki et al., 2008), dysphagia following stroke (Lan et al., 2015), and swallowing using various maneuvers, including tongue-hold (Hammer, Jones, Mielens, Kim, & McCulloch, 2014), effortful swallowing (Hoffman et al., 2012; Takasaki, Umeki, Hara, Kumagami, & Takahashi, 2011), Mendelsohn maneuver (Hoffman et al., 2012), head turn (Balou et al., 2014; McCulloch, Hoffman, & Ciucci, 2010), and chin tuck (Balou et al., 2014; McCulloch et al., 2010). With robust spatial resolution paired with high temporal resolution, pharyngeal HRM has become increasingly common in research (Hoffman, Ciucci, Mielens, Jiang, & McCulloch, 2010; Hoffman et al., 2013; Mielens, Hoffman, Ciucci, McCulloch, & Jiang,

2012; Pandolfino, Fox, Bredenoord, & Kahrilas, 2009; Takasaki et al., 2008) and clinical practice (Knigge, Thibeault, & McCulloch, 2014).

Insertion and Analysis

As with low-resolution manometry, adherence to facility-approved infection control procedures is critical for this invasive technique. After calibrating the catheter to the manufacturer's specifications, the clinician should prepare the catheter by applying a small amount of water-based lubricant to facilitate ease of transfer through the nasal cavity. Though previous publications recommend use of topical nasal anesthetic (Knigge et al., 2014), a double-blind study investigated whether topical nasal anesthetic improves procedure tolerability or affects pharyngeal pressure ($n = 20$) when using a 2.75-mm HRM catheter (Guiu Hernandez et al., 2018). Results indicated that use of even a small dose (0.4 mL of 2% viscous lidocaine hydrochloride) affected sensorimotor aspects of pharyngeal swallowing, without offering any significant improvement in self-rated procedure comfort. Once the water-based lubricant has been applied, the individual "swallows" the catheter into the esophagus, thus protecting the airway as the tip of the catheter moves through the hypopharynx to esophageal entry, similar to low-resolution manometry. As pharyngeal pressure is measured continuously along the length of the pharynx, and the sensors are circumferential, precise placement of the catheter is less critical; once the clinician has inserted the sensor portion of the catheter in its entirety, the process is complete. The catheter then should be secured to the nose with standard medical tape, and the individual is allowed time to adjust to the catheter in vivo.

Interpretation of High-Resolution Manometry

HRM pressures can be displayed as waveforms, similar to low-resolution manometry, and as a topographical contour plot, as seen on the PluralPlus companion website. This allows a display of a continuous pressure spectrum with pharyngeal position on the vertical axis and time on the horizontal access. Pressure is represented by a color gradient, with warmer colors (e.g., reds) representing higher pressure and cooler colors (e.g., blues) representing lower pressure.

HRM was designed for evaluation of the esophagus; this is reflected in the existing analysis software available on HRM systems, which are not designed for use in the pharynx. Although ongoing work is exploring classification models of pharyngeal swallowing and developing analysis tools, there is no consensus on optimal measurements of pharyngeal HRM at present. Thus, most publications rely on exporting the results of an HRM study to external programs such as MATLAB to analyze pharyngeal swallowing with custom-made algorithms, which are not clinically available (Hammer et al., 2014; Hoffman et al., 2010, 2012; Jones, Hammer, Hoffman, & McCulloch, 2014; Ryu, Park, & Kang, 2015). Currently, there is only one freely available integrated platform available for analysis of pharyngeal swallowing, called Swallow Gateway (https://www.swallowgateway.com/). This online tool uses measurements that have been validated against tools including VFSS and has demonstrated robust reliability (Omari, Papathanasopoulos, et al., 2011; Omari et al., 2016). For an overview of existing measures, readers are encouraged to review Cock and Omari (2017). The Swallow Gateway enables analysis of pressure-only and combined pressure-impedance recordings and allows collaboration in analysis between clinicians through the ability to securely share studies online. To utilize this software, clinicians need to export data from an HRM study to a *text file* and then reimport to the online Swallow Gateway. Users are then able to locate anatomic areas of interest and analyze specific pressure and bolus flow parameters. This reflects the currently cumbersome nature of HRM analysis of pharyngeal swallowing. However, thanks to efforts of numerous working groups, improved analysis software and development of consensus of measurement may be increasingly available in the coming years.

Validity and Reliability

In the first publication investigating pharyngeal HRM, Takasaki et al. (2008) performed a feasibility study to assess the potential for application of HRM in oropharyngeal swallowing. The authors selected three anatomic regions for measurement and averaged pressure across the selected sensors in each region: the velopharynx, meso-hypopharynx, and UES. They argued that these measurement locations were optimal due to ease in accurate identification of each region: the UES has a clear band of pressure at rest and the velopharynx can be identified by non-swallow speech tasks, such as production of /kaka/. These anatomic definitions have been used for measurement in numerous subsequent research activities (Hoffman et al., 2010; Knigge et al., 2014; Lin et al., 2014; McCulloch, 2010; Takasaki et al., 2011) and this framework has been adapted in automated analysis programs described in the literature (Jones, Hoffman, et al., 2014).

Importantly, however, the authors did not validate the accuracy of this measurement technique against gold-standard instrumental techniques, such as VFSS. This is critical, as recent research has revealed that intra-swallow catheter movement contributes to poor identification of anatomic landmarks compared with VFSS (Jones et al., 2015). Movement associated with UES elevation occurs independently of additional intra-swallow catheter movement related to velopharyngeal closure. Further, the authors posit that the optimal location for measurement of nadir UES pressure based on waveforms or topographical plots is unknown. This is mirrored in a study investigating the reliability of an automated analysis of UES pressure compared with visual analysis by trained clinicians (Lee et al., 2014). Lee and colleagues stated that automated analysis of UES relaxation with HRM is similarly not accurate and called for development of novel analysis techniques. While HRM is the optimal technique for evaluating UES function and overcoming limitations in sensor placement that plague low-resolution manometry, poor reliability in existing analysis techniques limits the utility of this technique.

Difficulties with reliable selection of anatomic areas of interest may be compounded by questionable validity. By measuring only three anatomic areas (Knigge et al., 2014), namely, the velopharynx, hypopharynx, and UES, the user reduces the high-resolution information garnered from closely spaced sensors to three points of interest. The results become roughly comparable to output of low-resolution manometric systems, which report pressure and temporal data from three similar anatomic areas, namely superior pharynx, inferior pharynx, and UES. By averaging across sensors and over time, the numerous publications implementing this method may reduce the specificity of measurement and minimize the advantages of HRM itself (Knigge et al., 2014). This is critical to consider, especially with ongoing development of pharyngeal HRM automated measurement algorithms. At present, further research is needed to continue development of reliable and valid analysis methods suitable for clinical practice.

Limitations

While it is evident that the advent of high-resolution manometry has overcome many of the limitations of low-resolution pharyngeal manometry, HRM systems have important limitations which should be discussed, in addition to the abovementioned difficulties in analysis. Primarily, HRM is limited by catheter diameter; the use of adult circumferential sensors mandates an increase in catheter diameter up to 4.2 mm in HRM systems (compared with 2.1 mm in low-resolution manometry). While this may affect comfort and tolerance of the procedure, this increased diameter may also affect timing and amplitude of pharyngeal pressure.

Additionally, a measurement error has been reported in the ManoScan™ system, which is the most commonly used HRM system in clinical practice (Babaei, Lin, Szabo, & Massey, 2015; Babaei, Szabo, Yorio, & Massey, 2018; Lamvik, Guiu Hernandez, Jones, & Huckabee, 2016; Robertson et al., 2012). Previous reports have revealed this measurement error can be as substantial as 11.1 mm Hg (interquartile range, 9.9 mm Hg) for an average duration study (Robertson et al., 2012). While the manufacturer recommends applying a correction to all studies prior to analysis, use of this correction is rarely reported in published manuscripts, and the measurement error and use of standard correction methods were not mentioned in the clinical protocols of pharyngeal HRM (Knigge et al., 2014). At present, users of HRM are advised to interpret existing normative HRM data with caution until further studies can replicate data after correcting for measurement error. Long-term, however, HRM will likely serve an important role in the assessment of pharyngeal swallowing biomechanics and providing outcome measures for rehabilitation effectiveness.

IMPEDANCE

The basic technique of high-resolution manometry has been expanded to include measurements of pharyngeal impedance to detect intraluminal bolus flow (Omari et al., 2006). Similar to manometry, intraluminal electrical impedance is commonly used in the field of gastroenterology in functional evaluations of esophageal motility. In recent years, it has similarly been applied to evaluation of bolus flow in pharyngeal swallowing (Kuo, Holloway, & Nguyen, 2012). The aim of impedance is to monitor both antegrade and retrograde bolus flow in attempts to overcome this limitation of pharyngeal manometry (Kahrilas & Sifrim, 2008).

Impedance is based on the communication (e.g., current loop) between adjacent electrodes. These electrodes respond to alterations in conductivity based on the intraluminal environment, such as air, mucosa, and bolus (Kahrilas & Sifrim, 2008). A highly conductive ionic bolus (e.g., saline) has low resistance to current flow and can be easily recorded to investigate bolus transfer and any residual (Pandolfino et al., 2009), thus, "impedance allows for inferences to be made about the relationship between abnormalities of motility seen on manometry with the abnormalities in bolus transit seen on impedance" (Kuo et al., 2012, p. 27). The impedance sensors are typically distributed between the manometric pressure sensors in combined systems. For example, there are a total of 18 channels at 20-mm intervals in the ManoScan System. These high-resolution impedance systems enable continuous visualization of the bolus when in contact with adjacent electrodes during transit or at rest (Pandolfino et al., 2009).

Much of the research in impedance is conducted in reference to esophageal swallowing. However, select research groups have investigated application of this method to pharyngeal swallowing. Omari, Dejaeger, Tack, Vanbeckevoort, and Rommel (2012) investigated analysis methods of impedance-manometry data by comparing the relationship between impedance (bolus flow) and pressure. This enables computation of a gestalt "pressure flow" related measure, termed swallow risk index (SRI). The SRI compares four pressure and flow variables to compute an overall risk index (Omari, Dejaeger, et al., 2011). Two studies investigating adult and pediatric patients with dysphagia (n = 43) and healthy controls (n = 10) determined that an SRI cutoff of 9 could predict pharyngeal residue with moderate sensitivity (75%) and specificity (80%) (Omari, Dejaeger, 2011; Omari et al., 2012). Further, they reported that an SRI cutoff score of 15 correlated well with aspiration observed on VFSS.

Omari, Dejaeger, Tack, Van Beckevoort, and Rommel (2013) posit that impedance-based measure may be used in place of VFSS in clinics with limited access or in patients who are difficult to evaluate due to mobility or cognitive deficits. However, it is critical to note that analysis of bolus flow is not the sole purpose of completing a VFSS. With a thorough VFSS, the clinician can not only diagnosis impairments in functional biomechanics and airway protection, but also generate compensatory and rehabilitation targets. This far surpasses the capabilities of impedance technology. Nevertheless, impedance may serve as an adjunct tool for follow-up and outcome assessments, limiting exposure to radiation.

Although these advances have aided in the translation of research of impedance to clinical practice, it should be noted that impedance is an estimate of bolus flow based on conduction. Therefore, there are important limitations. For example, residual bolus material spanning just one sensor, unable to fulfill the circuit loop of two adjacent sensors, will not be visualized in impedance measures. Further, impedance has reduced ability to detect small liquid quantities and is sensitive to catheter movement, similar to manometry (van Wijk et al., 2009). It is also difficult to quantify the percent or quantity of bolus material ingested with impedance flow, comparable to the limitations of bolus residual estimations in two-dimensional VFSS. An impedance signal depicts presence of residual, without capability to quantify specific amount. With further knowledge of benchmark normative data and standardized analysis methods relevant to pharyngeal swallowing, this technique may prove beneficial as an adjunct screening method for impairments in bolus transit during deglutition, especially when paired with pharyngeal manometry.

WHAT CAN MANOMETRY OFFER TO CLINICAL PRACTICE?

Case Examples

Pharyngeal manometry offers quantification of observed biomechanics that have been documented from other diagnostic tests. This will aid the clinician in differential diagnosis of pharyngeal motility disorders by providing objective measures of pharyngeal events. Unfortunately, data have not yet emerged that quantify pharyngeal motility disorders in stroke. Several clinical cases are presented below that highlight the clinical utility of this technique; however, until a thorough normative data set is established, application in clinical practice will be limited.

Mr. N is a 72-year-old male admitted to the acute hospital with a pontine stroke. He was evaluated clinically for dysphagia secondary to intermittent coughing during meals during his brief four-day hospitalization. VFSS revealed significant post-swallow pharyngeal residual with intermittent aspiration that was cleared with a reflexive cough. The treating clinician was unsure from the examination whether the residual was secondary to overall poor pharyngeal motility or represented a specific impairment of bolus transport through the UES. Mr. N was being considered by the head and neck surgery service for a cricopharyngeal myotomy. A manoendoscopic study was completed with three primary findings (Figure 13–5). First, although resting pressure in the cricopharyngeus was variable, impaired opening of the UES was ruled out. The lowermost cricopharyngeal sensor documented appropriate relaxation to negative pressure during swallowing.

Second, the uppermost and middle pharyngeal sensors documented overall reduced pharyngeal contact pressure generation during swallowing. Average pressures of 17.2 mm Hg (standard deviation [SD] = 8.1) in the upper pharynx and 32.3 mm Hg (SD = 21) in the lower pharynx were compared with local normative values taken from 40 healthy individuals of 99.44 mm Hg (SD = 41.0) at the upper pharyngeal sensor and 116.32 mm Hg (SD = 48.06) at the lower

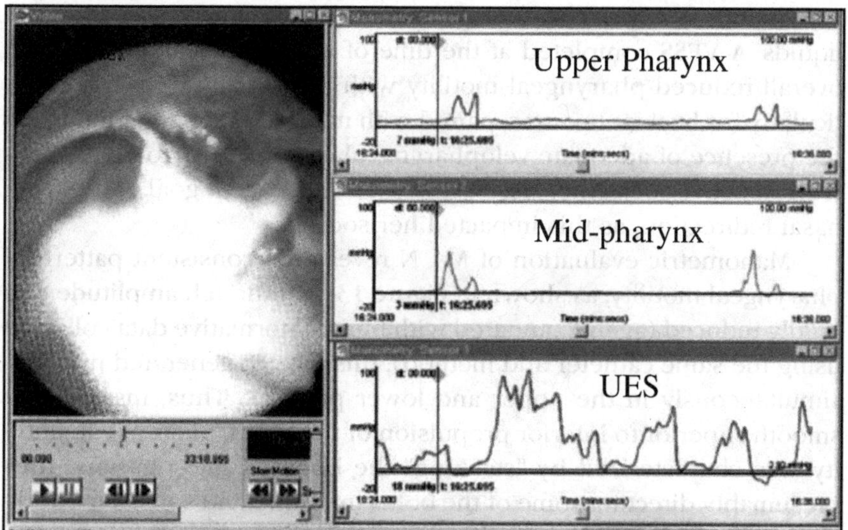

Figure 13–5. Case Study #1. Results of manoendoscopic evaluation reveal very low pressure generation, paired with mis-sequencing of pharyngeal pressure within the pharynx.

sensor using the same methods and catheter. Finally, and perhaps most interestingly, Mr. N presented with an inconsistent mis-sequencing of pharyngeal events. On 67% of swallows, pressure generation was initiated in the lower pharynx an average of 123 msec *before* pressure in the upper pharynx. Based on local normative values, unimpaired individuals will consistently generate pressure in the upper pharynx on average 201 msec before pressure in the lower pharynx. Given this pattern of pharyngeal pressure generation, cricopharyngeal myotomy was determined not to be the appropriate treatment course. Additionally, effortful swallowing was decided to be inappropriate given the improper sequencing of pharyngeal pressure. Fortunately for this patient, the dysphagic presentation resolved within 2 weeks, and he returned to a normal diet.

This individual can be contrasted with Ms. N, who is a 40-year-old female referred for swallowing rehabilitation with a four-year history of chronic pharyngeal phase dysphagia subsequent to brainstem stroke. Shortly post-onset, she underwent surgical true vocal fold medialization secondary to asymmetry in vocal fold closure. She was initially fed via gastrostomy tube, but this was discontinued at approximately three years post-onset. At the time of referral, Ms. N was ambulatory and independent with significant left-sided weakness and gait disturbance. She was consuming a soft, moist, or minced diet with thin liquids. A VFSS completed at the time of referral revealed presumed overall reduced pharyngeal motility with post-swallow residual, particularly for heavier textures, paired with nasal redirection of liquids in the presence of adequate velopharyngeal closure. As a young woman with an active social life, Ms. N expressed a treatment goal of reducing nasal redirection, as this impacted her socially.

Manometric evaluation of Ms. N revealed a consistent pattern of pharyngeal motility, as shown in Figure 13–6. Although amplitude was mildly reduced (again compared with limited normative data collected using the same catheter and method), this patient generated pressure simultaneously in the upper and lower pharynx. Thus, instead of a smooth superior to inferior propulsion of the bolus, pharyngeal motility was characterized by "stacking" the bolus at mid-pharynx, thus presumably directing some of the bolus inferiorly and some superiorly into the nasal cavity. This finding explains her radiographic presentation of pharyngeal residual and nasal redirection. Unfortunately for Ms. N, rehabilitation efforts were only partly effective. She was able to increase diet level tolerance, but therapy did not positively affect

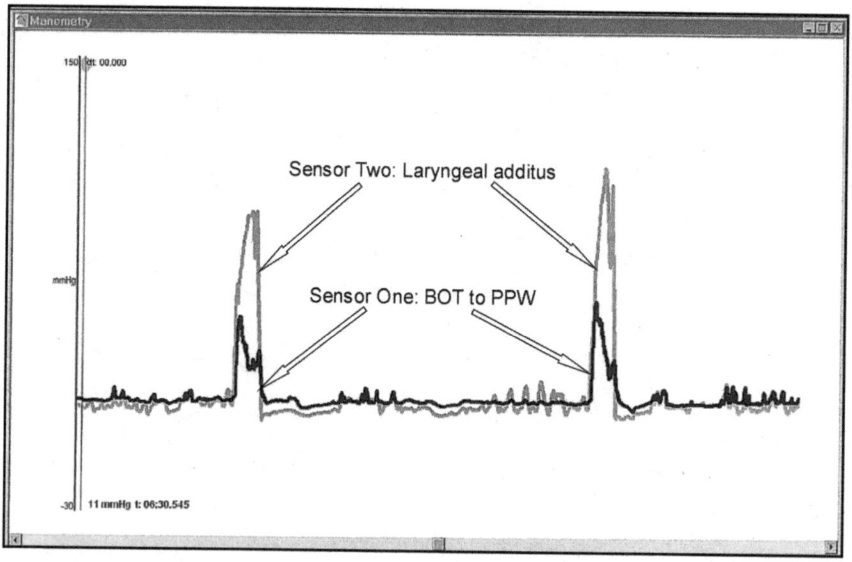

Figure 13–6. Case Study #2. An atypical pattern characterized by the absence of superior to inferior pressure distribution. Clinically, this correlated with nasal redirection and post-swallow residual.

nasal redirection. As discussed in Chapter 22, only limited rehabilitation techniques have been developed to address the phenomenon of "pharyngeal mis-sequencing," perhaps in large part because our diagnostic tools have not allowed for identification of this pathophysiologic feature.

Considerable work remains before low- and high-resolution pharyngeal manometry, with and without impedance, can emerge as a standard diagnostic tool. More specific and objective measurement of pharyngeal biomechanics will help us identify pathophysiologic features of swallowing that are poorly defined based on existing diagnostic techniques. Identification of these features consequently will increase the demand for availability and incorporation of these techniques into routine clinical practice.

14 The Instrumental Swallowing Examination

Ultrasound Evaluation of Swallowing[1]

THE NEED FOR DIAGNOSTIC SPECIFICITY

Throughout this text, we have emphasized that assessment of swallowing physiology—whether for diagnosis or research—depends on instrumentation. This complex mechanism generates too few auditory, visual, or tactile hints of the underlying process to validly define what transpires within the oropharynx by external observation of biomechanical movements alone. Screening protocols produce variable and questionable sensitivity and specificity for identifying the presence or absence of dysphagia (Daniels, Anderson, & Willson, 2012; O'Horo, Rogus-Pulia, Garcia-Arguello, Robbins, & Safdar, 2015; Park, Bang, Han, & Chang, 2015). However, understanding the unique characteristics of that impairment to develop appropriate and specific treatment plans requires observation or measurement of internal biomechanics.

Despite the sophistication of radiographic instrumentation, interpretation of the videofluoroscopic swallowing study (VFSS) has historically relied on comparatively unsophisticated, subjective interpretation by clinicians. Consequently, the VFSS has struggled with poor interrater reliability. Studies have documented insufficient interrater reliability for routine clinical practice (McCullough et al., 2001; Wilcox, Liss, & Siegel, 1996) with higher interrater reliability reported for discrete measures in clinical research (Leonard, Kendall, McKenzie, Gonçalves, & Walker, 2000; Sia, Carvajal, Carnaby-Mann, & Crary, 2012). Martin-

[1]Significant portions of this chapter have been reprinted with permission of Karger Publishers: Huckabee, M. L., Macrae, P., and Lamvik, K. (2015). Expanding instrumental options for dysphagia diagnosis and research: Ultrasound and manometry. *Folia Phoniatrica et Logopaedica*, 67(6), 269–284.

Harris and colleagues (2008) derived a descriptive scale to develop a "common language" for describing impairment at progressive severity levels. Reliability of interpretation is controlled by certifying only those who achieve a targeted degree of agreement. There are specific biomechanical measurements that have been reported in the literature and used in research with reported high interrater reliability (Leonard et al., 2000; Martin-Harris et al., 2008; Sia et al., 2012). These require additional software installation, and perhaps more critically for clinical practice, considerable time, thus again potentially limiting translation to the broad clinical community. Another limitation of VFSS is the need to balance the radiation safety issues inherent in increased exposure with the need to collect adequate information for treatment planning, and re-evaluation to assess recovery.

VFSS and videoendoscopic evaluation of swallowing, the other routine diagnostic approach, provide dynamic, integrated imaging of swallowing biomechanics, and will justifiably remain the foundation of diagnostic assessment. However, as our understanding of swallowing impairment increases, so does our recognition of limitations of these two tests. This highlights the need for integration of adjunctive, and preferably quantitative, methods for evaluation of swallowing to supplement currently used imaging techniques.

The use of ultrasound imaging for swallowing was initially described in the 1970s (Skolnick, Zagzebski, & Watkin, 1975; Stevens, 1978) but has not transitioned to routine clinical practice. Newer data on this technique suggest that it may provide valuable, quantifiable, and importantly, non-invasive insights into swallowing biomechanics.

ULTRASOUND IMAGING: THE METHOD

Diagnostic ultrasound imaging is generated by presentation of cyclic sound pressure waves in the range of 2.5 to 10 MHz into biologic tissue using a surface transducer. These sound waves travel through the tissues and are reflected back when there is an acoustic boundary between tissue surfaces, such as that encountered between fluid and soft tissue or soft tissue and bone. The reflected waves are detected by the transducer and converted into an electrical signal. Information on the conductive properties of the tissues, and their relative distance from the transduceris used to produce the ultrasound image, similar to the process of echo-location used by dolphins and bats. Higher frequency sound waves are used to image superficial structures, as they are characterized by a shorter wavelength with reduced tissue penetration and increased resolution. Lower frequency waves are longer and provide better penetration into deep structures, but with poorer resolution, thus are preferable for imaging deep structures. Applications for swallowing diagnostics can be classified into two primary areas: evaluation of muscle morphometry and kinematics of oral, pharyngeal, and laryngeal structures.

MUSCLE MORPHOMETRY

The correlation between muscle fiber enlargement (hypertrophy) and an increase in muscle strength is well recognized (Esposito, Cè, Gobbo, Veicsteinas, & Orizio, 2005; Folland & Williams, 2007; Kanehisa et al., 2002). This adaptation of muscle morphometry following exercise has been well documented in limb muscles (Abernethy, Jürimäe, Logan, Taylor, & Thayer, 1994; Jones, Rutherford, & Parker, 1989) but has scarcely been investigated for muscles innervated by cranial nerves, despite the fact that most dysphagia treatments aim to increase muscle strength (Burkhead, Sapienza, & Rosenbek, 2007). The lingual and submental muscle groups are the target of many swallowing rehabilitation techniques and may consequently demonstrate hypertrophic change in response to strengthening exercise as in the case of limb exercise. However, given the differences in functional, compositional, and neural control between muscles controlled by the spinal nerves and those controlled by cranial nerves (Chhabra & Sapienza, 2007; Kent, 2004), hypertrophic modification in these muscles requires further investigation. Anecdotally, documentation of muscle hypertrophy following exercise may provide valuable information for treatment plan adjustments. A recent patient in our clinic showed significant submental hypertrophy following strengthening exercise; however, no functional change was seen in swallowing. This suggests that while the exercise was having the desired effect on the muscle, isolated muscle weakness was unlikely to be the primary cause of the dysphagic presentation. By altering the treatment approach to address skill in swallowing, rather than strength, the patient was able to achieve functional improvement and return to oral intake.

Muscle morphometry has been assessed using a variety of imaging techniques, including magnetic resonance imaging (MRI) (Aagaard et al., 2001; Robbins et al., 2005; Robbins et al., 2007), computed tomography (Engstrom, Loeb, Reid, Forrest, & Avruch, 1991; Hudash, Albright, McAuley, Martin, & Fulton, 1985), and ultrasonography (Hodges, Pengel, Herbert, & Gandevia, 2003; Maganaris, Baltzopoulos, & Sargeant, 2002; Reimers, Harder, & Saxe, 1998; Watkin et al., 2001). The few investigations documenting muscle morphometry of the corticobulbar muscles involved in swallowing have been based primarily on MRI. These studies have revealed hypertrophy following exercise in the collective tongue muscles (Robbins et al., 2005, 2007) and increased muscle thickness of pharyngeal constrictors following radiotherapy (Popovtzer, Cao, Feng, & Eisbruch, 2009). Corticobulbar muscles were found to behave similarly in this regard to corticospinal muscles; however, MRI is an expensive technique that limits application in both research and clinical practice.

Most typically muscle morphometry has evaluated the floor-of-mouth muscle group with the transducer placed in the coronal plane underneath the chin at midpoint. As seen in Figure 14–1, using this placement, the anterior belly of digastric muscles are observed at the top of the image, one to either side. The mylohoid muscles may be viewed as a thin band inferior to the anterior digastric muscles; however, these are often difficult to visualize in their entirety. Finally, the geniohyoid muscles are observed as one central muscle, as they approximate at midline.

Validation of ultrasound imaging for submental muscle measurement has been the subject of several studies. An early study documented construct validity by identifying greater cross-sectional area (CSA) of the geniohyoid muscles in four patients post-radiotherapy compared with healthy controls (Watkin et al., 2001). This study also reported that tissue composition (proportion of muscle to fat) was greater in patients and older controls than young controls, a second measure of construct validity. While the authors proposed a measure of convergent validity for their ultrasound measures, they did not make the necessary comparisons to achieve this.

Ultrasound imaging of submental muscle morphometry has recently been validated against MRI (Macrae, Jones, Myall, Melzer, & Huckabee, 2013). As a measure of convergent validity, comparisons were made between coronal ultrasound and MR images derived from the submental muscles in 11 healthy participants. Of the three targeted

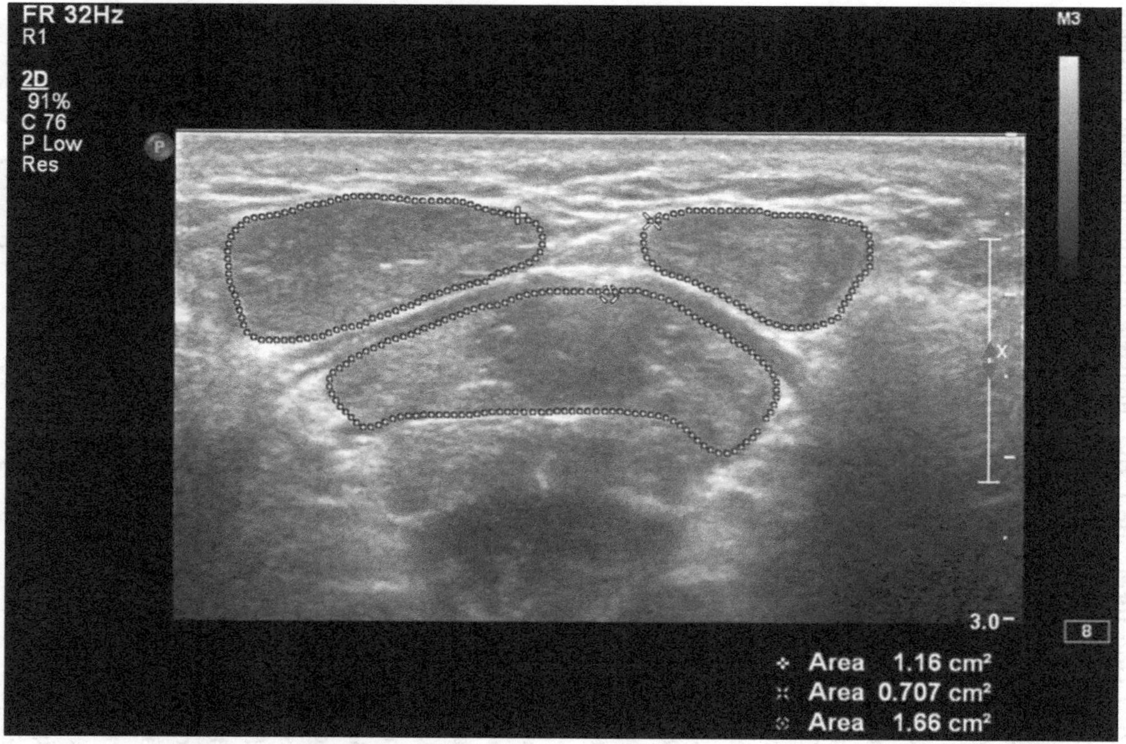

Figure 14–1. Measurement of CSA of submental muscles. The anterior belly of digastric muscles are represented as two circles at the top lateral of the image and the paired geniohyoid muscles are measured together as the outlined image in the center of the screen.

muscles—anterior belly of digastric, mylohyoid, and geniohyoid—only the digastric could be visualized adequately for measurement of CSA using MRI. Using ultrasound, the digastric and geniohyoid muscles could be visualized but not the lateral borders of the mylohyoid; thus, final comparison methods were limited to the anterior belly of the digastric muscles. In summary, CSA measures from the two methods were significantly and fairly highly correlated (left: $r = 0.909$, $p < 0.01$; right: $r = 0.77$, $p < 0.01$), indicating that ultrasound provides measures of submental muscle morphometry that are consistent with those obtained from MRI. Interestingly, ultrasound CSA measurements were smaller than MRI measurements ($p = 0.01$) by 10% (95% CI = −18 to −2). The authors attribute this difference, in part, to positional differences. Muscles were measured approximately mid-point between origin and insertion of the muscle. As MRI is conducted in the supine position, this mid-point may be biased past mid-point and toward the hyoid due to gravitational forces in this position. This potential measurement error, when paired with the capability of ultrasound to image the anterior belly of the digastric and the geniohyoid muscles, suggests that ultrasound may indeed have advantages over MRI quantification. The significantly lower cost of ultrasound imaging and the ease of use make this a clinically assessable instrument for evaluation.

Reliability of ultrasound muscle measurement has also been assessed. An early study evaluated test-retest reliability in 46 patients with temporomandibular joint disorders (Emshoff, Bertram, & Strobl, 1999). Bilateral CSA measurements were derived from most of the masticatory muscles across two sessions. For the anterior belly of the digastric muscles, reliability was high, with an intraclass correlation coefficient (ICC) of 0.91 and a repeatability coefficient (defined as two times the standard deviation of the mean of both measures) of 0.58 mm. A more recent open access thesis that employed ultrasound measures in a treatment study documented strong inter- and intrarater reliability of morphometric measures of submental muscles (Macrae, P., http://hdl.handle.net/10092/6261). For the anterior belly of the digastric muscles, ICCs for inter- and intrarater reliability were calculated at 0.86 and 0.98, respectively. For the geniohyoid muscles, interrater reliability was calculated at 0.80 with intrarater reliability documented at 0.96.

The prior studies have documented validation to other measurement methods and reliability, but what of functional validation? Kajisa and colleagues (2018) examined the relationship between jaw-opening force and CSA of the geniohyoid and mylohyoid muscles in healthy participants. Their data suggest that jaw-opening force was positively associated with CSA of the geniohyoid muscle but not with the anterior belly of the digastric. Further research in patients with stroke may provide valuable insights into the appropriateness of therapeutic approaches on a patient-by-patient basis.

Finally, an interesting study documented the construct validity and rater reliability of tongue thickness, rather than submental muscles (Hsiao, Chang, Chen, Chang, & Wang, 2012). Data were collected from 30 healthy individuals, 30 patients with stroke-related dysphagia, and 30 patients with stroke but no dysphagia. Captured from a coronal image of the tongue, thickness was defined as the height in centimeters between the hyoid shadow inferiorly, the tongue surface superiorly, and midpoint between the acoustic shadows of the right and left mandible. This measure was found to differentiate the three groups. Tongue thickness measures were significantly less in patients with stroke-related dysphagia (0.9 cm) than the healthy participants (1.1 cm) or the patients with stroke but no dysphagia (1.0 cm). A tongue thickness of less than 1.0 cm differentiated tube-fed patients from others, with a sensitivity and specificity of 70.0% and 66.7%, respectively. Intra- and interrater reliability could be considered moderate, with ICC values at 0.71 and 0.68, respectively.

A very recent study evaluated validity of geniohyoid and lingual measures for detection of "sarcopenic" dysphagia (Ogawa et al., 2017). Patients with dysphagia were divided into three groups: those considered to represent sarcopenia, those with likely sarcopenia, and those without sarcopenia. Results from this study suggested that "the area of the tongue muscle and its area of brightness were independent risk factors for sarcopenic dysphagia. However, geniohyoid sagittal muscle area and area of brightness showed no significant independent association with sarcopenic dysphagia" (p. 516).

SWALLOWING KINEMATICS

Ultrasound offers a relatively inexpensive and non-invasive method of investigating several aspects of swallowing kinematics that would otherwise require the more invasive technique of VFSS. Perhaps its greatest application lies in the ability to repeat assessments to quantify the influence of intervention without great cost or radiation exposure. Despite this, the method has resisted integration into the clinical diagnostic armamentarium. While the bony structures of the oral and pharyngeal cavities, such as the hyoid, cannot be visualized directly with ultrasound (Chi-Fishman, 2005), indirect measures of displacement can be made from visualizing the muscular end-points and the acoustic shadow created by bone. Real-time ultrasound provides a simple method by which to quantify temporal measures associated with biomechanical movement (Dejaeger & Pelemans, 1996). When quantifying spatial measures, studies of hyoid displacement utilizing ultrasound have historically required similar complex calibration and transformation processes to those required for VFSS measures (Leonard et al., 2000; Sia et al., 2012). However, other measures that are less sensitive to postural change may avoid these complex analysis procedures. Two primary applications have surfaced for measuring swallowing kinematics: superior-anterior hyoid displacement and thyrohyoid approximation.

Hyolaryngeal movement is a key feature of pharyngeal swallowing. A reduction of movement in either the superior or anterior trajectories can have substantial ramifications for the safety of ingestive swallowing. To measure hyolaryngeal movement, a curvilinear transducer is placed in the sagittal plane such that the shadow cast by the mandible is viewed at one edge of the screen and the shadow cast by the hyoid is viewed at the opposite edge, as seen in Figure 14–2. During swallowing, the shadow cast by the hyoid is observed to move toward the mandibular shadow.

Early validation of hyolaryngeal movement with ultrasound used a relatively complex process of "tracking" hyoid position (as defined by the shadow cast by this structure) on digitized images downloaded into a separate software program, with maximal excursion measured in centimeters from the resting point reference (Chi-Fishman & Sonies, 2002a, 2002b). Using this technique, measurement of hyoid displacement is not referenced to a fixed anatomic point, but rather to the mobile hyoid itself. Quantifiable data validate the capacity of this technique to differentiate hyolaryngeal movements between some aspects of bolus size and viscosity (Chi-Fishman & Sonies, 2002a), as well as the conditions of single versus continuous swallowing (Chi-Fishman & Sonies, 2002b) in healthy individuals. Interrater reliability was documented in the form of a high Pearson correlation coefficient of 0.81. More recently, construct validity of hyolaryngeal movement

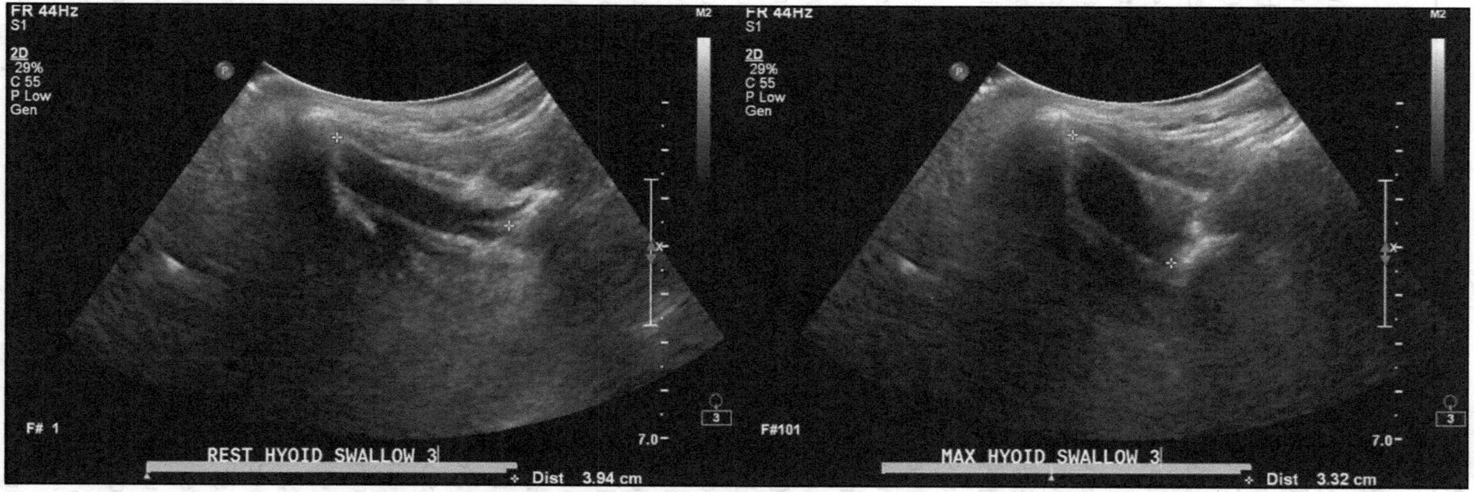

Figure 14–2. Measurement of hyolaryngeal movement at baseline. Ultrasound images are represented, with floor of mouth at the top of the image and tongue at the bottom. The left-sided figure represents rest position of muscles and structures, with the distance between mandibular symphysis and hyoid at the bottom of the screen and white stars denoting points of measurement. The right-sided figure represents the ultrasound frame at peak of hyolaryngeal excursion.

was assessed through ultrasound evaluation of 30 healthy controls, 30 patients with stroke-related dysphagia, and 30 patients with stroke and no dysphagia (Hsiao et al., 2012). Ultrasound measures from patients with dysphagia (1.3 cm) were significantly less than both healthy controls (1.7 cm) and patients without dysphagia (1.6 cm). Hyolaryngeal movement below 1.5 cm was determined to be the cut-off point for dysphagia dependent on tube feeding, with a calculated sensitivity and specificity of 73.3% and 66.7%, respectively. Intra- and interrater reliabilities were reported with ICC values at 0.88 and 0.81, respectively. Of note, measurement of hyoid movement was represented in centimeters as a difference value, with hyoid position at rest and during swallowing compared with the reference point of the mandibular symphysis.

Further research expanded on the approach of using the mandible as an anatomic reference point for measuring hyolaryngeal movement (Macrae, Doeltgen, Jones, & Huckabee, 2012). For this method, electronic calipers were used to measure the distance between the hyoid and the mandible during both a "rest" frame prior to the swallow and a "maximal displacement" frame, at which the hyoid bone was at maximal anterior displacement. The percentage change from rest to maximal excursion was then calculated to represent hyolaryngeal movement. Three raters reviewed the sonographic video sweeps of five discrete swallows from each of five participants for interrater reliability. The primary investigator measured each swallow on two occasions for intrarater reliability. Single-measure ICC was high for interrater agreement at 0.86 for rest measures and 0.86 for maximal displacement. Intrarater reliability was even higher at 0.95 for rest and 0.98 for maximal displacement. These data suggest that this analysis approach involving an anatomic reference point can result in high reliability, and importantly, calculations can be made on the ultrasound instrumentation, where calibration is intrinsically relative to the settings of the image acquisition. Using an approach that expresses displacement as a percent change from rest is crucial for across-participant comparisons.

A recent study evaluated hyoid displacement with the mandible as reference point during 5 mL water swallowing in patients with dysphagia and validated this to Penetration-Aspiration (P-A) Scale scores from VFSS (Lee, Lee, Kang, Yi, & Kim, 2016). They were grouped based on P-A Scale scores as non-aspirators (P-A Score 1), penetrators (P-A Scores 2–5), or aspirators (P-A Scores 6–8). Hyoid displacement was significantly greater in patients who did not aspirate than in those who penetrated or aspirated. Sensitivity and specificity for identifying those with airway compromise (penetration or aspiration) were 83.9% and 81%, respectively, using a cutoff of 13.5 mm.

Thyrohyoid approximation is another biomechanical feature of swallowing that has been investigated using ultrasound. This feature of swallowing plays a critical role in supraglottic airway compression. A non-invasive method to document this movement would potentially be of great clinical value. Given the close proximity of the thyroid and hyoid cartilages and the relatively clear boundaries, direct measurement in centimeters is possible, without complex manipulation of the data. An initial study of 44 healthy controls and 18 patients with dysphagia provided the first documentation of construct validity (Hsiao et al., 2012). Of note, the classification of dysphagia was based solely on a water swallowing test and was not confirmed with other instrumental assessment. The two groups demonstrated similar distance between the thyroid and hyoid at rest. However, the patient group demonstrated significantly less thyrohyoid approximation during water swallowing. Limitations of this study include the lack of a suitable "gold standard" and the absence of reported reliability; however, it addresses an important metric of swallowing that requires further evaluation.

A consequent study (Huang, Hsieh, Chang, Chen, & Wang, 2009) addressed these weaknesses in design. Ten patients with stroke and 15 healthy controls were evaluated with both ultrasound and VFSS. As a measure of convergent validity, measures of thyrohyoid approximation in patients with stroke were very similar between ultrasound (40.4 ± 7.1%) and VFSS (42 ±16.1%). Construct validity was provided by documenting greater thyrohyoid approximation in healthy individuals (47.2 ± 4.9%) than in patients with normal swallowing (42.6 ± 8.3%, $p = 0.02$) and patients with dysphagia (34.0 ± 10.9%, $p = 0.02$). These measures produced a sensitivity of 0.75, and specificity of 0.77 to detect dysphagia. Finally, interrater reliability assessment produced an ICC >0.97 for measures in each of the groups.

EMERGING APPLICATIONS

The use of ultrasound in swallowing assessment appears to be gaining some traction. Additional work has started to emerge on the use of this technology for measuring lateral pharyngeal wall placement (Kim

& Kim, 2012), upper esophageal sphincter opening (Morinière et al., 2013), and observed aspiration (Miura et al., 2014). Of particular interest is the potential for observation of aspiration using non-invasive methods; however, sensitivity is not promising at 0.64, and interrater reliability has not been documented.

Translating ultrasound imaging into clinical practice will require attention to several measurement details. Maintaining the position of the transducer relative to the position of the head is crucial to control for movement artefact and to ensure that accurate measures of true hyoid displacement are obtained (Chi-Fishman, 2005). Studies have employed head and neck stabilization by securing participants' heads to the head rest of a dental chair with a soft headband (Chi-Fishman & Sonies, 2002a, 2002b). These same studies also secured the transducer with an adjustable assembly allowing movements in three dimensions. While more stringent methods are available for head and transducer stabilization, these units are often cumbersome and not portable, and have historically been utilized for analysis of tongue motion. A review of these methods has been previously published (Stone, 2005). Utilizing an anatomical reference point by which to compare hyoid position eliminates some of the issues with head movement. However, the effect of differential posturing on hyoid measures across sessions may warrant some form of movement restriction. A recent study compared hand-held transducer placement to stabilized head and transducer placement with data taken from healthy individuals (Perry, Winkelman, & Huckabee, 2017). No main effect of scanning method was detected in this research. There was up to 47% greater variability in measures of hyoid excursion when using the fixed transducer compared with hand-held. For submental muscle measurement, slightly greater within-session variability was calculated for hand-held transducer measurements, but slightly greater across-session variability was seen for fixed transducer measurements. These data suggest that stabilization may not provide superior measurement to a simple, hand-held transducer. If this is confirmed with further research, it may facilitate clinical translation.

Importantly, ultrasound technology is improving remarkably, allowing for refined resolution in small instrumentation. Unlike VFSS, measurements can be made on the recording system quickly and efficiently, thus allowing greater access to quantitative measures. With the development of portable devices that record into a table or a smartphone, the cost of ultrasound technology is quickly moving into the affordable range for clinical speech pathology. With quite high sensitivity and specificity for detection of those at risk of aspiration and a cost less than $10,000 USD in some cases, ultrasound has the potential to be a viable advanced screening tool for those working in community settings or rural regions where other instrumentation is not readily available.

In summary, ultrasound offers a non-invasive and less expensive method of assessment and reassessment, allowing more direct quantification of several aspects of swallowing. Emerging data are suggesting quite reasonable validity and reliability of measurement. This technique is not proposed as a replacement for VFSS; however, incorporation of ultrasound into clinical practice will allow the luxury of intermittent and quantifiable assessment of change, comparison of patient behavior to a healthy normative database, and access to instrumental assessment in regions where instrumentation is not readily available.

15 Professional Responsibilities

Dysphagia Diagnosis in Stroke

A medical diagnosis, although hypothesized through careful history, observation, and non-instrumental assessment by a health care provider, requires instrumental or laboratory assessment for confirmation. Dysphagia is a medical diagnosis, and as such, instrumental assessment is presumed to follow a clinical swallowing examination (CSE) in patients with suspected dysphagia following stroke. Indeed, more than one assessment may be required to explicitly define the nature of pathophysiology and develop efficacious and cost-efficient treatment. Failure to do so carries serious consequences for patient outcomes and consequent professional integrity. However, this standard of practice does not always appear to be accepted or acted on in many clinical settings. So what impedes best practice? Based on our earlier model, rather than accepting a sign of clinical impairment as the final step in assessment, an exploration of the underlying pathophysiology is appropriate. In this medical arena of clinical practice, we appear to be plagued by either underconfidence or overconfidence, both of which are complicated by resource issues and both of which can hinder our work.

For the speech pathologist who is comfortable and confident in the health care arena, the medical model of diagnosis and the implications of this are apparent. However, as a profession, our uneasiness in this setting sometimes becomes noticeable when approaching diagnosis of swallowing impairment. Speech-language pathology is a profession that historically has provided diagnoses based on a careful history, astute observation, and critical listening. Additionally, early on, speech pathologists were lacking appropriate instrumental techniques and a detailed recognition of the complexities of swallowing pathophysiology. Times have changed and clinical practice must change with it. Instrumentation for swallowing is an accepted and necessary component of practice (American Speech-Language-Hearing Association, 1992). However, it appears that as professionals, speech pathologists have become accustomed to practicing with limited resources without insisting on what is required for optimal patient management. Timidity in requiring orders for instrumental assessment does not benefit anyone. It fails the patient through inadequate diagnosis and inappropriate rehabilitation plans. It fails the profession by perpetuating the myth that clinicians can gather the necessary information through observation. The provision of optimal assessment and care of the client with dysphagia is the responsibility of the clinician. All clinicians will require confidence in their professional problem-solving and negotiation skills to ensure that this responsibility is met. Anything less is unacceptable and unethical. Speech pathologists have earned a place in the health care system and should maintain that place as confident and contributing members of the health care team.

Equally hindering the management of the client with dysphagia is overconfidence in our clinical skills and techniques. Many of the wisest clinicians have learned the hard way that overestimation of our clinical abilities or overconfidence in clinical assessment procedures can have adverse effects. Our data and clinical evidence support this. Certainly every single referral cannot have an instrumental assessment. There will be some who are culled for very justifiable reasons; they may not be appropriate for oral intake regardless of what the instrumental assessment reveals. But caution should be exercised in exaggerating clinical accuracy under the guise of "judicious use of clinical resources," particularly in patients with stroke who, because of potential sensory deficit and cognitive impairment, cannot assist with detection of dysphagia. Sparing resources by deferring diagnostic examination may ultimately cost the health care system more in the long term. In an analysis of almost 184,000 stroke hospitalizations, Wilson (2012) identified that the average cost per hospitalization for stroke with pneumonia was almost three times greater than the average cost per hospitalization without concomitant pneumonia ($34,706 vs. $11,604, respectively). In that same year, Wilson and Howe (2012) documented the cost-effectiveness of first-time videofluoroscopic swallowing studies (VFSS), based on an average cost of $337 as reported in Medicare fee schedules. Although health care funding models are complex, $337 compared with the blowout costs associated with pneumonia seems quite a justifiable expense. Additionally, underreferral for instrumental assessment has professional implications. If clinicians propose that they can infer a diagnosis for one patient with stroke without instrumental assessment, then they weaken the argument for instrumental assessment in the next. The bottom line is that one cannot see what cannot be seen. This does not reflect on the clinician, rather it reflects on the nature of the disorder and limitations of observational assessment.

Although this text presents a "hard line" on the use of instrumentation, it is acknowledged that resourcing issues are ever-present in health care settings. The current reality is that the VFSS or other diagnostic techniques may not be currently and readily available in some rural regions or specific settings. In this case, the following are recommended:

1. In the short term:
   a. Maximize the accuracy of the clinical assessment through a thorough investigation rather than a cursory observation of oral intake. Pay close attention to history and cranial nerve findings in the stroke population to provide guidance of the underlying pathophysiology. Use less invasive and less expensive instrumental adjuncts to the clinical assessment such as cough reflex testing, pulse oximetry, and auscultation when they are appropriate and interpreted with caution.
   b. Document the need for diagnostic assessment and the limitations of clinical assessment.
   c. Make it clear in notes to the health care team and to the patient that clinical impressions are not diagnostic in nature but are speculations based on observable behavior.
   d. Make it clear in notes to the health care team and to the patient that any recommended management approach has the potential for a positive effect, a neutral effect, or even an adverse effect without the benefit of diagnostic examination for clarity.
2. In the long term:
   a. Advocate for patients. No one will provide resources if clinicians do not argue strongly for their necessity. Prepare proposals for resources that are strongly substantiated by the literature.
   b. Once again, the clinician must document. In order to effect a change in practice, it may be necessary to perpetually document what is needed to do the job well. Accepting less will not change practice, attitudes, or resources.

c. Investigate all diagnostic options. If VFSS is clearly not available, then look into alternatives such as the mobile VFSS and videoendoscopic swallowing study units. Budgeting for this service may not be prohibitive for your system.

d. As well, if VFSS is not available, enhance collaborations with colleagues in gastroenterology and otolaryngology. Pooled financial and skill resources may facilitate the establishment of pharyngeal manometry or endoscopy clinics. Although in the stroke population these may be considered adjunctive instrumental examinations, something is better than nothing to support the CSE.

CASE EXAMPLE

MF, a 76-year-old female, was admitted from her internist's office to the hospital with a right parietal stroke. Neurologic impairments documented in her admission notes included mild left-sided weakness, decreased left sensation, left visual and sensory neglect, impaired balance, mild oropharyngeal dysphagia, and mild dysarthria. Her past medical history was significant for mitral valve repair, type II non-insulin-dependent diabetes, atrial fibrillation, and osteoporosis. Although the patient reported to the health care team an acute onset of dysphagia for solids, no formal clinical or diagnostic swallowing evaluation was initiated. She completed her acute hospitalization with no indication of nutritional or pulmonary compromise.

Not long after admission, the patient was transferred to an acute inpatient rehabilitation setting. Again, no swallowing evaluation was included as part of her admission workup. Two weeks following rehab admission, the speech pathologist was consulted to evaluate the patient for dysphagia. After clinical assessment and observation of a meal, the clinician concluded: "MF finished her meal without difficulties. No oral or pharyngeal phase swallowing problems were apparent. The patient is apprehensive about eating solids. Recommend: soft diet, thin liquids." Ten days later, nursing notes included the following comment: "The patient is apprehensive about eating lunch yet appeared to manage a soft diet." Two weeks later: "The patient choked on solids at lunch; plan to supervise meals." At this point her albumin levels suggested potential undernutrition. However, speech pathology was not re-consulted for a follow-up evaluation. She demonstrated no evidence of pulmonary compromise.

Approximately 2 months post-stroke, the patient was transferred to a nursing home. One month later, she was visited by a dietician through a home health care agency, who documented: "The patient prefers minced, pureed food. She has self-selected a pureed diet due to difficulty swallowing solids." Again, no further evaluation was recommended.

A referral for outpatient swallowing evaluation was sought by the patient's family one year later due to increasing dysphagic symptoms. On evaluation, she continued to complain of increasing dysphagia for solids, with more recent difficulty managing liquids. Rigorous coughing during meals was frequent and discomforting. She experienced a substantial weight loss since her onset admission. No strongly lateralizing cranial nerve findings were present. However, vocal quality was weak and wet. Speech was mildly dysarthric of the flaccid type. VFSS revealed a moderate pharyngeal phase dysphagia with overall poor pharyngeal motility and diffuse residual. Of note was the presence of a pronounced filling Zenker's diverticulum with backflow of contents into the pharynx on completion of swallowing and post-swallow aspiration.

The patient was referred for surgical evaluation of diverticulum excision but was deemed an unsuitable candidate due to complicating cardiac factors. Rehabilitation of dysphagia at this point was unlikely to be effective due to the size of the pouch; thus, conservative compensatory management was implemented to decrease risks. Despite this, the patient developed pulmonary infection and expired within 8 months.

There are several possibilities with this patient. It is possible that she had a long-standing dysphagia that was not recognized until the onset of her stroke, although the patient reported acute onset. It is possible that the diverticulum would have developed regardless of her stroke; that is, it represented a coincidental occurrence. From her history, however, the most likely scenario is that her neurologic impairment led to specific dysfunction of the cricopharyngeus muscle with an acute-onset dysphagia for solids secondary to impaired upper esophageal sphincter opening. This was not diagnosed acutely or subacutely and within the ensuing year resulted in the development of the pouch. Unfortunately for this patient, there are many options for rehabilitation of cricopharyngeal abnormalities that were not made available to her because of a failure to diagnose. Whether the responsibility for this failure is on the shoulders of the clinician, the physician, or the health care system is irrelevant to the patient and her family. By treating without optimal information, the clinician may undermine not only positive outcomes for the patient but also the advancement of clinical practice. It is acknowledged that sometimes restraints of resources and support may inhibit optimal practice. However, if the clinician proceeds down this route, the potential consequences must be recognized.

16 Diagnosis of Dysphagia in Stroke

Establishing an accurate diagnosis of dysphagia is a process of problem solving through what is inferred from the clinical assessment and what is visualized on the instrumental evaluation. Only after this careful problem solving is completed can the clinician translate that knowledge to the variety of scales used to quantify findings (as discussed in Chapter 10) and compare the patient data with both normative values and the limited etiology-specific data that are available. The diagnosis of dysphagia frequently is initiated from a consideration of the signs presented—for example, post-swallow residue. However, the thorough examination is incomplete if the clinician fails to identify the underlying physiologic basis of the dysfunction. Both components are of substantial importance. Signs of dysphagia more often are addressed through compensatory management, whereas the physiologic abnormality is targeted by direct rehabilitative approaches. Elucidation of one without the other leaves the patient with dysphagia with an incomplete treatment plan and reduced potential for positive outcome. Unfortunately, our currently available diagnostic tools allow us to only view biomechanics, rather than elucidate the lower-level underlying physiology (such as weakness, discoordination, spasticity) that causes those biomechanical changes. Until our techniques become more refined, we report a biomechanical level of specificity. Table 16–1 provides a list of dysphagic signs and biomechanical etiologies.

In this chapter, we present a format for diagnosis of oropharyngeal dysphagia by identifying signs and then determining the underlying basis of each sign through an understanding of specific biomechanics. This methodical approach suits the nature of data available from many of our instrumental examinations. The signs of dysphagia (e.g., pre-swallow pooling, post-swallow residual) are more often static and thus frequently easier to visualize. The clinician can observe these features over a longer period of time. In comparison, underlying biomechanics (e.g., hyoid movement, epiglottic deflection) are frequently dynamic and require a "quick eye" to visualize. Thus, direct observation can be more challenging.

Table 16–1. Differentiation Between Signs and Biomechanical Abnormalities Underlying Dysphagia

Signs	***Biomechanical Abnormalities***
• Inadequate bolus preparation	• Oral motor impairment
• Anterior leakage	• Delayed pharyngeal swallow
• Post-swallow oral residual	• Inadequate BOT to PPW approximation
• Pre-swallow pharyngeal pooling to the level of the ___	• Weakened pharyngeal contraction/poor stripping
• Inadequate epiglottic deflection*	• Inadequate epiglottic to arytenoid deflection*
• Inadequate opening of the UES*	• Inadequate hyolaryngeal excursion
• Post-swallow vallecular residual	• Incomplete velopharyngeal closure
• Post-swallow pyriform sinus residual	• Impaired opening of the UES
• Aspiration	
• Penetration	

Note. UES = upper esophageal sphincter; BOT = base of tongue; PPW = posterior pharyngeal wall.
*May be both sign and biomechanical abnormality.

A structured approach to problem solving will focus the clinician toward an accurate diagnosis without distraction from the dynamic array of diagnostic data. At the conclusion of the examination and based on the identified sign, the clinician should be able to present a diagnostic summary that reflects the sequence of problem solving in the following format:

> "The patient presents with *[which phase]* dysphagia characterized by *[signs]* secondary to *[biomechanical abnormality]*."

Frequently, a single biomechanical abnormality can result in a number of observed signs and symptoms. Thus, written presentation of data may be facilitated by structuring the diagnostic summary with the biomechanical abnormality first.

> "The patient presents with *[which phase]* dysphagia characterized by *[biomechanical abnormality]* resulting in *[signs]*."

To facilitate understanding and clinical carryover, two table formats are presented. The first, Table 16–2, supports the approach that clinical problem solving starts at the signs and works its way into the biomechanical abnormality. The second, Table 16–3, may aid the clinician in clear documentation by presenting biomechanical abnormalities followed by their consequent signs.

ORAL PHASE

Within the oral phase of swallowing, an array of signs can be visualized on both clinical and diagnostic examination. These are summarized in Table 16–3, and all are a consequence of the primary biomechanical abnormality of poor orolingual control. Unfortunately, as discussed, a more specific and objective physiologic definition of this biomechanical abnormality is difficult with our current instrumentation and, thus, requires more subjective speculation. Poor orolingual control may feasibly be secondary to bilateral or hemi-weakness, spasticity, or a discoordinated quality characteristic of apraxia. The term "apraxia of swallowing" has been applied to patients with "the inability to organize the front-to-back lingual and bolus movement normally characteristic of a swallow or . . . simply holding the bolus without initiating any oral activity" (Logemann, 1998, p. 83). Describing this disorder as "apraxia," however, implicates specific principles in the act of swallowing. It suggests that swallowing is a learned, skilled movement and that the abnormal movement pattern is not attributable to sensory or elemental motor deficits. The similarities and differences of apraxia of swallowing with more traditional disturbances of the praxis system (limb apraxia, buccofacial apraxia, apraxia of speech) have previously been reviewed (Daniels, 2000) and deserves yet considerable further investigation.

Regardless of the semantic or theoretical issues, however, there *is* an oral dysmotility disturbance that is characterized by repetitive, disorganized anterior-posterior bolus movement in the oral cavity, which prolongs oral transfer and is evident in patients with stroke (Daniels, Brailey, & Foundas, 1999; Robbins & Levine, 1988; Robbins, Levine, Maser, Rosenbek, & Kempster, 1993).

Table 16–2. Swallowing Signs Associated with Specific Biomechanical Abnormalities

Occurring	*The Signs Of*	*Can Be Secondary To*	*In Which Phase*
Pre-swallow	Anterior leakage	Poor orolingual control	Oral
	Inadequate bolus preparation		
	Inadequate bolus formation		
Post-swallow	Oral residual		
Pre-swallow	Pharyngeal pooling to the level of ____	Delayed pharyngeal swallow	Pharyngeal
During the swallow	Nasal regurgitation	Discoordinated/impaired pharyngeal motility	
	Inadequate epiglottic deflection*	Intrinsic structural changes in supportive tissue	
		Decreased anterior hyoid movement	
	Inadequate opening of the UES*	Intrinsic structural functional changes in cricopharyngeus noncompliance	
Post-swallow	Vallecular residual	Decreased base of tongue to posterior pharyngeal wall approximation	
		Inadequate epiglottic deflection*	
	Pyriform sinus residual	Decreased anterior hyoid movement*	
		Inadequate opening of the UES*	

Table 16–2. *continued*

Occurring	*The Signs Of*	*Can Be Secondary To*	*In Which Phase*
Pre-swallow	Penetration/ Aspiration	Pharyngeal pooling*	Oral
			Pharyngeal
During the swallow	Penetration	Inadequate epiglottic deflection*	Pharyngeal
	Aspiration	Inadequate supraglottic shortening/laryngeal elevation*	
		Impaired or delayed vocal fold closure	
Post-swallow	Penetration/ Aspiration	Oral residual*	Oral
		Pharyngeal residual*	Pharyngeal

Note. UES = upper esophageal sphincter.
*Occasionally a sign will be caused by another sign, which requires the clinician to problem solve through to the initial presenting biomechanical abnormality.

Oral biomechanical abnormalities may also be disguised as, or exacerbated by, decreased attention. In these cases, the prolonged and inefficient oral phase of swallowing is not solely biomechanically based but is complicated by cognitive factors. Augmentative instrumental assessments, such as oral manometry (e.g., Iowa Oral Pressure Instrument [IOPI]), or the more invasive intramuscular electromyography (EMG) may provide valuable information. While the IOPI is being used more often in clinical practice and normative data are available, the equipment is still quite expensive, thus may not be readily available to many clinicians. Intramuscular EMG is rarely incorporated into clinical practice, and specific expertise is required. This limitation on availability discourages clinical application. Integration of cranial nerve findings will assist in differential diagnosis of oral inefficiency. A patient with no evidence of hypoglossal nerve damage on assessment but who demonstrates oral inefficiency during ingestion more likely may present with cognitive inattention as the primary etiology.

Table 16–3. Biomechanical Abnormalities with Their Consequent Signs

	The patient presents with oral phase dysphagia characterized by poor oral lingual control resulting in:
Pre-swallow	• Anterior leakage • Inadequate bolus preparation • Pharyngeal pooling to the level of _____ • Inadequate mastication • Supraglottic penetration of pre-swallow pooling • Aspiration of pre-swallow pooling
During the swallow	• Supraglottic penetration of pooled material • Aspiration of pooled material
Post-swallow	• Anterior leakage of post-swallow oral residual • Post-swallow oral residual • Post-swallow pharyngeal pooling of oral residuals to the level of ____ • Supraglottic penetration of post-swallow oral residual that pools into pharynx • Aspiration of post-swallow oral residual that pools into pharynx
	The patient presents with pharyngeal dysphagia characterized by delayed pharyngeal swallow resulting in:
Pre-swallow	• Pharyngeal pooling to the level of _____ • Supraglottic penetration of pre-swallow pooling • Aspiration of pre-swallow pooling
During the swallow	• Supraglottic penetration of pooled material • Aspiration of pooled material
Post-swallow	• None
	The patient presents with pharyngeal dysphagia characterized by inadequate anterior hyoid movement resulting in:
Pre-swallow	• None
During the swallow	• Decreased epiglottic deflection[1] • Decreased traction force for UES opening[2] • Supraglottic penetration

Table 16–3. *continued*

Post-swallow	• Vallecular residual >pyriform sinus as a secondary effect[1] • Pyriform sinus residual >vallecular as a secondary effect[2] • Supraglottic residual • Aspiration of supraglottic or pharyngeal residual
The patient presents with pharyngeal dysphagia characterized by inadequate base of tongue to posterior pharyngeal wall resulting in:	
Pre-swallow	• None
During the swallow	• Impaired bolus transport through proximal pharynx
Post-swallow	• Post-swallow vallecular residual (>pyriform sinus residual) • Supraglottic penetration of residual • Aspiration of supraglottic or pharyngeal residual
The patient presents with pharyngeal dysphagia characterized by impaired UES opening in the presence of substantial anterior hyoid movement resulting in: (implies intrinsic cricopharyngeus abnormality or timing issue)	
Pre-swallow	• None
During the swallow	• Impaired bolus transport through cricopharyngeus
Post-swallow	• Post-swallow pyriform sinus residual (>vallecular residual) • Supraglottic penetration of residual • Aspiration of supraglottic or pharyngeal residual
The patient presents with pharyngeal dysphagia characterized by poor pharyngeal motility resulting in:	
Pre-swallow	• None
During the swallow	• Impaired bolus transport throughout the pharynx • Nasal redirection • Supraglottic penetration
Post-swallow	• Diffuse (non-specific) pharyngeal residual • Nasal residual • Supraglottic penetration of residual • Aspiration of supraglottic or pharyngeal residual

Note. UES = upper esophageal sphincter.

[1,2]The biomechanical abnormality results in a symptom during the swallow that consequently results in another symptom post-swallow.

PHARYNGEAL PHASE

Pre-Swallow Pooling

A common sign of dysphagia in stroke is the presentation of **pre-swallow pooling** in the pharynx. Table 16–3 presents this sign, as well as aspiration and penetration, which are produced by the sensory deficit of delayed pharyngeal swallowing. At first glance, this appears rather straightforward; however, working from the signs of pre-swallow pooling to delayed pharyngeal swallowing, in practice, is quite complicated.

The conclusion of oral parameters of swallowing is marked by volitional transfer of the prepared bolus into the oropharynx, thereby outside the reach of voluntary control. The transition between oral and pharyngeal components of the swallowing process is heavily influenced by the integrity of neurosensory response systems and subsequent timing of onset of pharyngeal swallowing in relation to voluntary transfer. The videofluoroscopic swallowing study (VFSS) can provide an image of bolus transfer and swallowing onset marked by hyoid movement. However, VFSS cannot provide specific measures of sensory thresholds; for diagnosis of pharyngeal onset disorders, the clinician must infer the physiologic sensory deficit based on biomechanical data. This is a difficult and perhaps imprecise task. Cough reflex testing is emerging as a means for evaluation of the sensory system (see Chapter 6 for review); however, this test evaluates laryngeal, rather than pharyngeal, sensitivity. The clinical technique of assessing gag reflex and sensation is considered to be a direct evaluation of glossopharyngeal sensory integrity; however, as previously discussed in Chapter 6, it lacks diagnostic sensitivity.

One complication in diagnosing delayed pharyngeal swallowing arises from the fact that the primary sign of this disorder, pre-swallow pharyngeal pooling, is shared by the biomechanical abnormality of poor orolingual control. Differential diagnosis of these two disorders is difficult based on VFSS and has substantive clinical consequences. A misdiagnosis may result in the clinician providing a sensory-based treatment for a motor-based disorder, or vice versa, with consequent treatment failure. This represents a waste of health care resources, and frustration for both patient and clinician. Several observations, summarized in Table 16–4, may guide the clinician toward a diagnosis based on the sign of pre-swallow pooling; however, none of these in isolation can be considered an undisputed feature of either diagnosis. There exists no peer-reviewed research to document the sensitivity and specificity of these radiographic features, in part because we lack reliable sensory data on which to validate the observations.

The second major complication inhibiting accurate assignment of a diagnosis of delayed pharyngeal swallowing is the innate variability in temporal relationships in non-impaired individuals and the associated flexibility provoked by consistency adaptation. Specific measures of swallowing onset include the temporal measures of stage transit duration (STD), which is measured from the point where the bolus head reaches the ramus of the mandible to the onset of maximum hyolaryngeal elevation. Strict interpretation of STD is discouraged, as this may lead to overdiagnosis. As discussed in Chapter 3, research has

Table 16–4. Differential Diagnosis of the Etiology of Pre-Swallow Pharyngeal Pooling: Delayed Pharyngeal Swallowing versus Poor Orolingual Control

Clinical Question	*Poor Orolingual Bolus Control*	*Delayed Pharyngeal Swallowing*
As the bolus approaches the oral cavity (pre-oral), what does the base of tongue do?	Does not approximate soft palate for protective glossopalatal seal	Arches to approximate soft palate for protective glossopalatal seal
How does the bolus enter the pharynx?	In non-cohesive, unformed bits as it falls off of base of tongue during bolus preparation	As a cohesive, single bolus unless the patient volitionally segments the transfer
Is there a pronounced drop of the base and push of the blade of the tongue to transfer the bolus?	No	Yes, although there will be a significant temporal delay between this movement and onset of pharyngeal swallow
On which consistency is the pooling most pronounced?	Heavier consistencies, solids	Liquids

indicated that the bolus may be inferior to the ramus of the mandible at onset of maximum hyolaryngeal elevation during sequential swallowing and single swallows in healthy adults (Chi-Fishman & Sonies, 2000; Daniels et al., 2004; Daniels & Foundas, 2001; Martin-Harris, Brodsky, Michel, Lee, & Walters, 2007; Stephen, Taves, Smith, & Martin, 2005). This indicates that hypopharyngeal bolus location at onset of pharyngeal swallowing cannot be interpreted as abnormal if all other physiologic components of swallowing are intact. That is, clinicians must understand that although onset of pharyngeal swallowing may occur deep in the pharynx, for this to be classified as "normal" swallowing, airway protection must be maintained and risk of pulmonary invasion must be consistently low.

Post-Swallow Residual

Pharyngeal swallowing is signaled by onset of hyolaryngeal excursion, particularly anterior movement of the hyoid, which plays an important role in pharyngeal dynamics, as discussed in Chapter 3. As such, inadequate anterior hyoid movement is a common sign of dysphagia in stroke and can lead to a cascade of pharyngeal events and signs, as outlined in Table 16–3. Of note is that the impaired anterior hyoid movement is the etiology of other impaired biomechanical events, which subsequently cause other observable signs. Working backward from the signs (see Table 16–2), the presentation of post-swallow vallecular residual is a consequence of: (1) decreased epiglottic deflection, thus "trapping" the bolus in the superior pharynx, or (2) decreased base of tongue (BOT) to posterior pharyngeal wall (PPW) approximation with resulting inadequate positive pressure to drive the bolus into the hypopharynx. VFSS is not the appropriate instrument to comment directly and objectively on BOT to PPW pressure generation; pharyngeal manometry would be the technique of choice. Thus, observation of epiglottic deflection and a diagnosis by exclusion is the more usual course of clinical problem solving for determining the source of vallecular residual. If epiglottic deflection has failed, then the etiology of this biomechanical movement must consequently be questioned. Failure to deflect the epiglottis may be a consequence of either: (1) intrinsic tissue changes in the cartilaginous tissue of the epiglottis, as in irradiated patients or those with connective tissue disease, or (2) inadequate anterior hyoid movement, which fails to pull the base of the epiglottis anteriorly and shift the apex over the airway. Tissue characteristics cannot be directly evaluated with our clinical tools and in uncomplicated stroke are unlikely. Therefore, observation of hyoid movement is imperative for understanding the underlying basis of epiglottic deflection.

Decreased anterior hyoid movement also contributes indirectly to the sign of post-swallow pyriform sinus residual. Again working backward from the sign, if a patient presents with pyriform sinus residual greater than vallecular residual, this would typically signal an isolated impairment of upper esophageal sphincter (UES) opening. Impaired UES opening can logically be a consequence of: (1) decreased anterior hyoid movement, (2) intrinsic structural functional changes of the cricopharyngeus muscle, or (3) a mistiming of biomechanical events with neurophysiologic relaxation of the muscle. Of these three potential etiologies, VFSS is the technique of choice to visualize hyoid movement. Pharyngeal manometry with or without intramuscular EMG may be required to optimally evaluate the other two possible sources of pyriform sinus residual. Manometry will aid in documentation of the relationships between pressure in the pharynx and cricopharyngeus and the amplitude of pressure drop in the cricopharyngeus. EMG will provide specific objective information about cricopharyngeal activation and deactivation.

Nasal Redirection

The presenting sign of nasal redirection of the bolus is controversial, as we lack substantive data to guide our practice. Invasion of the bolus into the nasal cavity is not simply an issue of impairment of velopharyngeal closure, but this sign, more importantly, requires impairment of pressure systems that provide the driving force behind the bolus. Therefore, this is likely to be presented in cases of pharyngeal dysmotility, where pressure systems are disrupted or mistimed. Although VFSS reveals bolus flow patterns, more specific information about pharyngeal pressure systems would best be obtained through pharyngeal manometry. Using this instrumentation, the clinician may obtain objective measures of dysmotility patterns that underlie the sign of nasal redirection.

Reduced Pharyngeal Motility

In the prior section, specific biomechanical characteristics that are subject to impairment in stroke and a method for problem solving from sign to specific biomechanical cause were discussed. In many individuals with stroke, the dysphagic presentation is much more extensive, with multiple components of impairment with diffuse post-swallow residual. The categorical term of poor pharyngeal motility may be applied when either all components of the process are collectively impaired or a specific etiology is not able to be identified. Poor motility may be a result of any number of neuromuscular or temporal deficits, characterized with terms such as weakness, spasticity, slowness, reduced pharyngeal shortening, or discoordination. Again, VFSS reveals bolus flow patterns and allows for assessment of timing measures; pharyngeal manometry would be required to provide specific objective measures of pressure systems or very detailed pressure sequences. Neuromuscular substrates such as weakness and spasticity are only presumed in our current practice due to inadequately developed clinical instrumentation.

Airway Invasion

Supraglottic penetration can be a sign of any number of biomechanical abnormalities and can occur pre-swallow from pooled material, post-swallow from oral or pharyngeal residual, or during swallowing secondary to either impaired epiglottic deflection and pharyngeal/supraglottic shortening or overflow of pooled material that enters the airway as the larynx elevates. Aspiration, as well, can occur before or after pharyngeal swallowing, but only occurs during swallowing in the case of specific impairment of either the degree or timing of vocal fold closure. It is not an uncommon finding for patients with stroke to present with supraglottic penetration during pharyngeal swallowing and then proceed to aspirate on postprandial glottic opening. VFSS and videoendoscopy will allow for detection of supraglottic penetration and aspiration. Videoendoscopy may more optimally visualize vocal fold closure and identify impairments of adduction. Multimodality assessment using more standard techniques paired with respiratory airflow will be required to evaluate swallowing respiratory coordination.

ORAL AND PHARYNGEAL DYSMOTILITY IN STROKE

Given this overview of diagnosing dysphagia, what can research and clinical observation teach us about swallowing after stroke? Any clinician who has worked with patients who have sustained a stroke knows there is no "prototypical" swallowing pattern in this population, aside perhaps from patients with lateral medullary syndrome (LMS). Research findings (Table 16–5) when integrated with clinical observations can, however, help focus clinicians on particular patterns of pathophysiology that may be evident following stroke.

To facilitate discussion, stroke is discussed in terms of supratentorial (cortical, subcortical) and brainstem lesions. Research has suggested that dysphagia following stroke primarily is secondary to large, predominantly cortical lesions—for example, middle cerebral artery territory infarcts (Alberts, Horner, Gray, & Brazer, 1992; Robbins et al., 1993), particularly to the right hemisphere (Falsetti et al., 2009). Other studies, however, have demonstrated that changes in swallowing can occur with small, isolated subcortical lesions (Cola, Daniels, et al., 2010; Daniels & Foundas, 1999; Logemann et al., 1993), with some proposing that swallowing generally is functional with small subcortical lesions, albeit different from age-matched controls (Logemann et al., 1993). While many recent studies, some including more exact measures of lesion volume, have suggested that larger strokes are associated with dysphagia and airway invasion (Galovic et al., 2013; Suntrup, Kemling, et al., 2015, Wilmskoetter et al., 2018), decreased cough response (Suntrup-Krueger et al., 2017), feeding tube dependency (Galovic et al., 2016), and pneumonia (Minnerup et al., 2010), others have suggested the size of the infarct does not influence dysphagia characteristics (Steinhagen, Grossman, Benecke, & Walter, 2009) or outcomes such as pneumonia (Steinhagen et al., 2009; Suntrup-Krueger et al., 2017). While controversy remains concerning the influence of lesion size effects on swallowing and outcomes, it is clear that both cortical and subcortical brain regions influence swallowing. As no study has identified specific dysmotility patterns distinguishing swallowing between cortical and subcortical lesions, cortical and subcortical lesions are discussed under the umbrella term "supratentorial."

Table 16–5. Research Detailing Dysphagia in Patients with Stroke Using Objective and Subjective Measures

Authors	*Subjects*	*Time Post-Onset or Admission*	*Trials/Stimuli*	*Techniques*	*Measures*	*Results*
Butler, Stuart, Pressman, Poage, & Roche, 2007	26 stroke with dysphagia (11 aspirators, 15 non-aspirators) 20 healthy adults	N/A	Two trials: 5, 10 15, 20 mL thin and thick liquid	Simultaneous VFSS and respiratory measure	Objective	• ↑ SAD and variability of duration in stroke patients as compared to controls • ↑ SAD in aspirators as compared to non-aspirators • ↑ in I-I respiratory pattern in aspirators and greater dysphagia severity
Chen, Ott, Peele, & Gelfand, 1990	46 stroke	1 month	3 and 5 mL thin and thick liquid; 3 mL paste; ¼ cookie	VFSS	Subjective	• 39 oral and pharyngeal dysmotility • 5 isolated pharyngeal dysmotility • 2 isolated oral dysmotility • 18 mild dysphagia • 23 moderate dysphagia • 5 severe dysphagia • Dysmotility pattern not associated with hemisphere
Daniels, Brailey, & Foundas, 1999	59 stroke	5 days	Two trials: 3, 5, 10, 20 mL liquid; 1 tsp paste; ½ cookie	VFSS	Subjective and Objective	• Equal incidence of lingual discoordination in RHD and LHD

Authors	Subjects	Time Post-Onset or Admission	Trials/Stimuli	Techniques	Measures	Results
Daniels & Foundas, 1999	54 stroke	5 days	Two trials: 3, 5, 10, 20 mL; 1 tsp paste; ½ cookie		Subjective and Objective	• Equal incidence of dysmotility patterns (subjectively measured) and aspiration between in LHD and RHD • 19 oral and pharyngeal dysmotility • 20 isolated pharyngeal dysmotility • 3 isolated oral dysmotility
Daniels et al., 2006	13 healthy adults 9 stroke	2 days 33 days	Two trials: 5 mL liquid	VFSS	Objective	• Dysphagia defined as dysfunction on 2 of 6 swallowing measures: OTT, STD, PTT, P-A Scale, vallecular residual, pyriform sinus residual • 2 SD above normal means to determine dysfunction • 5 stroke patients presented with dysphagia acutely • 2 presented with continued dysphagia at 1 month.

continues

Table 16–5. *continued*

Authors	***Subjects***	***Time Post-Onset or Admission***	***Trials/Stimuli***	***Techniques***	***Measures***	***Results***
Daniels et al., 2017	80 stroke	5 days	Two trials: 5 mL, self-regulated cup sip liquid; 1 tsp paste; ½ cookie, 90 mL liquid	VFSS	Objective	• ↑ PA scale score for infratentorial stroke compared to RHD • No difference in oral and pharyngeal impairment scores based on hemisphere or lesion location
Irie & Lu, 1995	74 stroke	2 to 59 days	3 mL liquid and paste; mouthful liquid	VFSS	Objective	• 33 oral and pharyngeal dysmotility • 8 isolated pharyngeal dysmotility • 24 isolated oral dysmotility • stroke isolated oral dysmotility in LHD • ↑ in both oral and pharyngeal dysfunction in RHD
Jeon et al., 2014	178 stroke	31-175 days	2, 5 mL liquid, yogurt, thick gruel, wafer	VFSS	Objective	• ↓ laryngeal elevation and ↑ pharyngeal delay time associated with brainstem stroke

Authors	Subjects	Time Post-Onset or Admission	Trials/Stimuli	Techniques	Measures	Results
Leslie, Drinnan, Ford, & Wilson, 2002	18 stroke patients with clinically determined dysphagia 50 healthy adults	4 to 28 days	5, 20 mL liquid; 5 mL pudding	Simultaneous VFSS and respiratory measure	Objective	• ↑ inspiration after swallow in stroke group
Logemann et al., 1993	8 LHD (basal ganglia /internal capsule) 8 healthy adults	21 to 28 days	Two trials; 1, 3, 5, 10 mL liquid; 1 mL paste; ½ cookie	VFSS	Subjective and Objective	• ↑ OTT • ↓ OPSE* • ↓ PRT
Mann, Hankey, & Cameron, 2000	128 stroke	10 days	5, 10 mL thin liquid, thick liquid, paste; 20 mL thin liquid	VFSS	Subjective and Objective, ordinal scale for severity; weighted median score determined dysphagia and severity	• 36 oral and pharyngeal dysmotility • 22 isolated pharyngeal dysmotility • 3 isolated oral dysmotility • 37 mild dysphagia • 39 moderate dysphagia • 6 severe dysphagia

continues

Table 16–5. *continued*

Authors	***Subjects***	***Time Post-Onset or Admission***	***Trials/Stimuli***	***Techniques***	***Measures***	***Results***
Nilsson, Ekberg, Bülow, & Hindfelt, 1997	33 neurologically impaired (including stroke) patients with clinically determined dysphagia	N/A	Mouthful thick liquid barium	Simultaneous VFSS and respiratory measure	Objective	• Airway invasion associated with lower SSI** • Post-swallow respiratory phase not associated with airway invasion
Perlman, Booth, & Grayhack, 1994	330 (101 stroke)	N/A	N/A	VFSS	Subjective and Objective	• Deviant epiglottic inversion, delayed pharyngeal swallow, vallecular residue, hypopharyngeal residue, decreased hyoid elevation; Linear trend between incidence of aspiration and severity of post-swallow residual and delayed pharyngeal swallow
Robbins & Levine, 1988	8 LHD 8 RHD 8 healthy adults	3 wks	Two trials: 2 mL liquid and paste	VFSS	Objective	• ↑ OTT and "apraxia of swallowing" in LHD • ↑ PTT and aspiration in RHD

Authors	Subjects	Time Post-Onset or Admission	Trials/Stimuli	Techniques	Measures	Results
Robbins, Levine, Maser, Rosenbek, & Kempster, 1993	20 LHD 20 RHD 20 healthy adults	3 wks	Two trials: 2 mL liquid and paste	VFSS	Objective	• ↑ OTT and "apraxia of swallowing" in LHD • ↑ STD, PTT and aspiration in RHD
Robbins, Coyle, Rosenbek, Roecker, & Wood, 1999	15 multi-infarct 98 healthy adults	mean: 146 days	Two trials: 3 mL liquid	VFSS	Objective	• ↑ in P-A scale scores • ↑ silent aspiration • ↑ within subject variability
Selley, Flack, Ellis, & Brooks, 1989b	21 neurologically impaired patients with complaints of dysphagia (11 stroke)	N/A	5 mL liquid	Nasal airflow	Subjective and Objective	• ↑ inspiration after swallow
Smithard et al., 1997	121 stroke (only 95 had VFSS	3 days 29 days	Thin and thick liquid	VFSS	Objective	• ↑ aspiration acute LHD/RHD • ↑ aspiration RHD at 1-month

continues

Table 16–5. *continued*

Authors	***Subjects***	***Time Post-Onset or Admission***	***Trials/Stimuli***	***Techniques***	***Measures***	***Results***
Suntrup, Kemling, et al., 2015	200 stroke	4 days	Saliva, puree, liquid, bread	VEES	Objective based on airway invasion and residue	• ↑ airway invasion and dysphagia severity in RHD
Suntrup-Krueger et al., 2017	200 stroke	4 days	Saliva, puree, liquid, bread	VEES	Objective	• ↑ pharyngeal residue and pneumonia rate in RHD • ↓ pharyngeal swallow response in RHD • No difference cough response in RHD and LHD
Teasell, Foley, Fisher, & Finestone, 2002	20 medullary stroke (only 9 had VFSS) 8 healthy adults	4 to 77 days	Thin and thick liquid, pudding, solids	VFSS	Subjective and Objective	• Post-swallow residual • Delayed pharyngeal swallow • Aspiration • Reduced epiglottic deflection • Reduced hyoid movement

Authors	*Subjects*	*Time Post-Onset or Admission*	*Trials/Stimuli*	*Techniques*	*Measures*	*Results*
Theurer et al., 2008	6 RHD	5 to 22 days	Two trials: 2 and 5 mL thin and thick liquid, pudding	VFSS	Subjective and Objective	• Oral stage impairments > pharyngeal stage impairments
Veis & Logemann, 1985	38 stroke	<1-4 months	Two trials: 1/3 tsp liquid and paste	VFSS	Subjective and Objective	• Delayed onset of the pharyngeal swallow • Reduced pharyngeal peristalsis • Reduced lingual control
Wilmskoetter, Martin-Harris, et al., 2018	45 unilateral stroke	0-23 days	Thin, nectar, honey thick liquid, paste, cookie	VFSS	Objective	• ↑ pharyngeal impairment scores and P-A scale scores in RHD • Impaired laryngeal vestibule closure in RHD • No difference in oral impairment scores between RHD and LHD

Note. ↑ = increased, > = greater than, I-I = inspiration-inspiration, LHD = left hemisphere damage, N/A = not available, OPSE = oropharyngeal swallowing efficiency, OTT = oral transit time, P-A = penetration-aspiration, PRT = pharyngeal response time, PTT = pharyngeal transit time, RHD = right hemisphere damage, SAD = swallowing apnea duration, SSI = swallowing severity index, STD = stage transit duration, VEES = videoendoscopic evaluation of swallowing, VFSS = videofluoroscopic swallowing study.

*OPSE calculated by dividing the percentage of the bolus swallowed (minus percentage of oral residue, pharyngeal residue, and aspiration).

**SSI = SAD/PTT.

Dysphagia in Supratentorial Stroke

Oral dysmotility is a common problem following supratentorial stroke, characterized by longer transfer and possibly discoordination in oral transfer. Stroke research has focused on defining oral stage impairment primarily by measuring oral transit time (OTT). This is defined as the time from onset of bolus movement to the point where the bolus head reaches the ramus of the mandible. OTT is increased for patients with stroke compared with healthy controls (Robbins & Levine, 1988; Robbins et al., 1993). "Apraxia of swallowing" also has been described in a subset of patients with left hemisphere damage (LHD) and has been characterized by a "lack of labial, lingual, and mandibular coordination" with OTT of over 10 seconds (Robbins et al., 1993, p. 1298).

Daniels and colleagues (1998) describe lingual discoordination in patients with LHD as well as right hemisphere damage (RHD) ranging from durations of 1 to 3 seconds (mild), to 4 to 10 seconds (moderate), to greater than 10 seconds (severe). Verbal cue to swallow has been reported to exacerbate this oral dysmotility pattern (Logemann, 1998; Robbins & Levine, 1988; Robbins et al., 1993) with resolution of oral dysfunction during the normal mealtime environment. Conversely, others note persistent oral dysmotility in the natural environment in patients with LHD as well as RHD (Daniels et al., 1998).

Although pre-swallow pooling is common following supratentorial stroke, research has not attempted to identify whether the etiology of the pooling is more related to oral dysmotility or delayed initiation of pharyngeal swallowing. As noted previously, oral dysmotility yielding pre-swallow pooling is prominent following stroke. Individuals with stroke, however, frequently demonstrate increased STD (Daniels, Foundas, Iglesia, & Sullivan, 1996; Robbins & Levine, 1988; Robbins et al., 1993), which yields pharyngeal pooling. Increased STD has been identified as an independent predictor of aspiration, with increased delay associated with an increasing likelihood of aspiration (Perlman, Booth, & Grayhack, 1994). In this study, STD was rated on a Likert scale from 1 (STD between 1 and 2 seconds) to 3 (STD >5 seconds). Although this study consisted of a heterogeneous population, one-third of the patients had a stroke etiology.

Recent research had found decreased swallowing response, i.e., delayed onset of pharyngeal swallowing, to be associated with right parieto-temporal infarction (Suntrup-Krueger et al., 2017). It is important to note, however, that swallowing was evaluated with videoendoscopy, thus the oral phase could not be observed, and decreased swallowing response was based on the duration of pharyngeal pooling. Given the evaluation techniques and methods, it would be difficult to discern whether delayed onset of pharyngeal swallowing or decreased orolingual control produced the pooling.

The study of bolus flow has been the primary focus in stroke research; however, pharyngeal biomechanics can be impaired. No study has compared objective temporal and spatial structural measures in patients with supratentorial strokes and age-matched healthy participants. Only one study has detailed pharyngeal biomechanical events in a homogeneous cohort that included patients with stroke (Perlman et al., 1994); however, the measure of these events was qualitative more than quantitative. This study, however, focused on the relationship between swallowing biomechanics and aspiration. Dichotomous yes/no scores were used to define abnormal structural movement, whereas depth of post-swallow residual was measured on a scale of 1 (mild) to 3 (severe). Abnormal epiglottic inversion and reduced hyoid elevation as well as bolus flow measures of vallecular residual and diffuse hypopharyngeal residual were strongly related to aspiration. As with STD, as severity of the residue increased, the number of patients who aspirated increased. As discussed earlier, reduced extent of structural movement can lead to post-swallow residual. Patients with supratentorial stroke may present with unilateral pharyngeal hemiparesis, which yields post-swallow residual on the contralesional side of the pharynx.

Increased airway invasion (laryngeal penetration and aspiration) has been documented in patients with supratentorial stroke (Alberts et al., 1992; Mann, Hankey, & Cameron, 2000; Robbins et al., 1993). When using the Penetration-Aspiration Scale to rate airway invasion, patients with stroke generally have higher scores compared with healthy controls (Robbins, Coyle, Rosenbek, Roecker, & Wood, 1999). Aspiration in patients with stroke, particularly those with supratentorial stroke, may not be hallmarked by a cough or voice change and is frequently termed as "silent." In a study of consecutive patients admitted with acute stroke, aspiration was identified in 38% of the patients, with 33% of these patients aspirating overtly, that is, coughing, and 67% aspirating silently (Daniels et al., 1998). Although lesion location (supratentorial or brainstem) was not specified, the increased incidence of inspiration after swallowing in patients with stroke (Leslie, Drinnan, Ford, & Wilson, 2002; Selley, Flack, Ellis, & Brooks, 1989b) has been shown to be associated with increased aspiration in this population (Butler, Stuart, Pressman, Poage, & Roche, 2007).

Although stroke can impact all phases of swallowing, the clinician must also consider the impact of reduced cognition on swallowing. Cognitive deficits, particularly neglect, have frequently been correlated with dysphagia. Hemispatial inattention has been associated with increased non-oral intake in patients with acute stroke (Schroeder, Daniels, McClain, Corey, & Foundas, 2006). Reduced awareness of dysphagia results in lack of self-modification of swallowing behavior and increased medical complications compared with patients who are aware of dysphagia signs (Parker et al., 2004). Moreover, rehabilitation of swallowing is longer in patients with neglect following stroke (Neumann, 1993). It should be noted that recent research did not identify hemispatial neglect, as measured by line bisection, to be associated with dysphagia; however, aphasia was associated with pyriform sinus residue (Jeon, Park, Lee, Jeong, & Sim, 2014). It is unclear how aphasia would affect the occurrence of residue. More research is warranted to confirm this finding and to discern the rationale for this effect should it prove consistent.

Although hemispatial inattention and other cognitive disorders are not totally lateralized (e.g., Steinhagen et al., 2009), they generally occur more frequently in patients with RHD compared with patients with LHD (Heilman, Watson, & Valenstein, 2011). These cognitive deficits may yield greater functional impairment in patients with RHD even though swallowing pathophysiology may be similar in patients with RHD and LHD. Greater functional impairment may lead the clinician to impose greater restrictions on oral intake for patients with RHD. Thus, in addition to rehabilitating swallowing, it is critical that clinicians address cognitive deficits in treatment.

Dysphagia in Brainstem Stroke

Research is limited concerning swallowing in brainstem stroke. Studies are generally limited to single case reports that have outlined the progression of swallowing recovery in patients with brainstem stroke (Logemann & Kahrilas, 1990; Martino, Terrault, Ezerzer, Mikulis, & Diamant, 2001; Robbins & Levine, 1993) or focused on aspiration in case series (Kim, Chung, Lee, & Robbins, 2000; Teasell, Foley, Fisher, & Finestone, 2002). Clinicians, however, are probably aware of patients with LMS presenting with classic features. These are the patients who in the acute stage are expectorating saliva into a container due to an inability to swallow. The clinical swallowing examination generally is characteristic of intact cognition and language and the presence of dysphonia and dysarthria. Unilateral true vocal fold paresis is not uncommon in patients with LMS. Patients are fully aware of swallowing deficits with intact sensation and immediate coughing with attempts to swallow the smallest of volume.

The pre-oral and oral stages of swallowing generally are intact. Although attempts at initiation of pharyngeal swallowing are present (on the clinical swallowing evaluation, the clinician may palpate multiple lingual hyolaryngeal gestures), pharyngeal swallowing is frequently never elicited or, if initiated, is significantly delayed, with limited extent of superior and anterior hyolaryngeal movement and UES opening (Aydogdu et al., 2001; Logemann, Kahrilas, Kobara, & Vakil, 1989; Martino et al., 2001; Steinhagen et al., 2009; Teasell et al., 2002). Unilateral pharyngeal hemiparesis is not uncommon in patients with LMS and is characterized by post-swallow residual on one side of the pharynx (Logemann & Kahrilas, 1990; Logemann et al., 1989). Airway invasion may be evident before, during, or after the pharyngeal swallow. Although swallowing is severely impaired in patients with LMS and recovery frequently is slow, they make the ideal clients for swallowing rehabilitation due to intact sensation, cognition, and motivation.

Patients with brainstem stroke not involving the lateral medulla or with pontine stroke also may present with dysphagia, but characteristics are not as circumscribed as those with LMS. Given the close proximity to the medullary swallowing center and the multiple neural networks involved with swallowing, these patients warrant swallowing evaluation.

SUMMARY

The analysis of swallowing biomechanics and physiology is a complex process of integrating what is known of normal swallowing processes, paired with amalgamation of both subjective and objective evaluation of instrumental and clinical data. Given the complexity of this task and the substantive consequences of inaccurate or incomplete diagnosis, the astute clinician will develop a methodical approach for problem solving relying on the easily observable signs to lead to the biomechanical source of the impairment. Future research into diagnostic techniques should lead us one step deeper—to identify the underlying physiologic abnormality that leads to impaired biomechanics.

17 Diet Considerations: To Feed or Not to Feed

AN OVERVIEW OF OPTIONS FOR FEEDING THE PATIENT WITH DYSPHAGIA

Management of the patient with stroke and dysphagia should reflect several primary goals: to ensure pulmonary safety, to promote nutritional integrity, to normalize swallowing physiology, and to maximize quality of life. Certainly, one would hope in the best circumstance for a resolution of dysphagic signs and symptoms and a return to a full, satisfying oral diet that realizes these goals. However, in the short term, and unfortunately for some in the long term, alternative routes of nutritional intake are required to address the goals of management.

Wise decisions regarding the route of nutritional intake are multifaceted and complex and demand an interdisciplinary approach. Although the speech pathologist may be in a position to understand oropharyngeal ingestion and risks of aspiration better than many others on the team, the complexities of pulmonary clearance and resilience to infection as well as the intricacies of nutritional digestion, absorption, and assimilation generally are well beyond standard clinical training. Historically in dysphagia management, our strong focus has been on prevention of aspiration, almost to the neglect of all else. Fortunately for our patients, we are learning that inhibition of aspiration may not be the key to the effective management of the patient with dysphagia. Langmore and colleagues (1998) published a landmark study that has served our clinical thinking well. In an effort to identify true risk factors for development of pneumonia, this research group followed 189 elderly patients for 4 years to monitor for the outcome of pneumonia as it related to a variety of risk factors. The best predictors of pneumonia were dependence for feeding, dependence for oral care, number of decayed teeth, tube feeding, more than one medical diagnosis, number of medications, and current smoking.

Dysphagia, although identified as posing some risk, was not sufficient to cause pneumonia unless other risk factors were present as well.

Using this information, clinicians may develop a more intelligent approach that weighs the hazards of aspiration more realistically against other consequences of diet manipulation. A thoughtful balance of risks to the pulmonary system, the nutritional system, and the sociocultural systems that underlie oral intake may not always have pulmonary safety as the priority. With increased attention to patient rights and quality of life, this may be particularly true in the elderly patient with substantial disability.

Thus, decisions regarding route of oral intake should be made through collaborative discussion among the patient, family, and a variety of skilled health care professionals. In most clinical settings, this is the standard of practice, but unfortunately this is not the case in all. Relative to percutaneous endoscopic gastrostomy (PEG) tube insertion, Sinha, James, and Hasan (2001) documented that 87% of physicians they surveyed always involved speech pathology input. However, Hasan, Meara, Bhowmick, and Woodhouse (1995) reported that the decision to use PEG feedings was reached through a multidisciplinary team approach in only 64% of respondents. Worryingly, Hanson and colleagues (2008) found, in response to asking "Who ultimately made the decision to place the feeding tube," only 10% of individuals reported shared decision making, with the patient deciding in only 11% of circumstances, the family in 18%, and the physician in 62% of cases ($n = 288$).

There are data which suggest that these decisions should be made sooner rather than later. An interesting study by Davalos and colleagues (1996) sought to determine the prevalence of malnutrition after 1 week of hospitalization for acute stroke. Of significant concern was the finding that malnutrition increased progressively during hospitalization, evident in 16.3% at admission, 26.4% after 1 week, and 35% after 2 weeks. Certainly, many factors would be predicted to contribute to this trend, but it is suggested that nutrition, in whatever form, should be addressed promptly after admission. This finding was replicated in a study of 62 patients with stroke, most of whom demonstrated marked and significant deterioration in nutritional status within four weeks of hospitalization (Gariballa, Parker, Taub, & Castleden, 1998). After adjusting for an array of logical covariates, low serum albumin (a measure of protein) was a strong and independent predictor of death following acute stroke. Kokura, Maeda,

Wakabayashi, Nishioka, and Higashi (2016) reported that in elderly adults recovering from stroke ($n = 540$), suboptimal nutritional status predicted less improvement as rated by the Functional Independence Measure (FIM). Further, Finestone, Greene-Finestone, Wilson, and Teasell (1996) evaluated 49 consecutive patients admitted to an inpatient rehabilitation unit and similarly found overall nutrition was an independent predictor of length of stay and functional improvement. They concluded by commenting that nutrition is "likely the most potentially modifiable variable relating to length of stay and functional outcome" (p. 340).

NON-ORAL, ENTERAL FEEDING OPTIONS

Adaptation of diet consistency for both food and liquid is a common approach in dysphagia management and is discussed at length in Chapter 18. The decision to withhold oral feeding leaves the patient and medical team with several options. The primary decision most often is a selection between nasogastric tube (NGT) feeding and gastrostomy tube feeding. A less frequently utilized non-enteral feeding option for patients with dysphagia following stroke is total parenteral nutrition, where nutritional elements are provided intravenously. However, this approach has been linked with atrophy within the digestive tract and is linked with increased gastric dysmotility compared with NGT and PEG feeding (Ono et al., 2003). Regardless of the route, all non-oral nutrition options carry with them risks of mechanical complications (e.g., tube obstruction, displacement, ulceration), infection (e.g., tube site, gastric, pulmonary), and metabolic complications (Blumenstein, Shastri, & Stein, 2014).

Nasogastric Tubes

NGTs provide enteral nutrition and hydration via a flexible tube that enters through the nasal cavity (or oral cavity in the case of an orogastric tube), passes through the pharynx and upper esophageal sphincter (UES), and enters the stomach. NGT is generally considered to be a short-term option. Although this approach is widely used, there is risk of inappropriate insertion (e.g., into lungs) in approximately

5% of cases (Roe, Harris, Lambie, & Tolan, 2017), dislodgement during use, as well as accidental or purposeful extubation (McFarland, 2017). Provision of feeding following inappropriate insertion (e.g., into lungs) has, understandably, been found to have significant respiratory complications and has been defined as a "never event" by organizations such as the National Health Service National Patient Safety Agency (Roe et al., 2017). Published guidelines recommend that an NGT should be assessed with pH testing and/or radiography after insertion as well as after any episode that may have impacted positioning (e.g., emesis) (McFarland, 2017). Dziewas, Warnecke, Hamacher, et al. (2008) evaluated patients following stroke (n = 100) with videoendoscopy following NGT insertion. Their results indicated that 5% of patients had misplaced NGT, either looping around the epiglottis (n = 3) or crossing the laryngeal vestibule (n = 2).

The effect of an NGT in situ on pharyngeal swallowing has been studied, with conflicting results. Huggins, Tuomi, and Young (1999) compared the conditions of no NGT, a small-bore NGT, and a large-bore NGT on swallowing function in young healthy participants. The large-bore NGT was found to significantly alter several temporal features of swallowing, including stage transition, pharyngeal response, and UES opening. Similar, although nonsignificant, trends were seen for the small-bore tube. This study presents an important question: Are we creating an iatrogenic dysphagia through our management approaches?

This study was followed by a videofluoroscopic swallowing study (VFSS) of 22 patients with stroke by Wang, Wu, Chang, Hsiao, and Lien (2006). These researchers reported that transit times were reduced between 0.2 to 0.6 seconds after removing the tube. However, in contrast to the study by Huggins and colleagues (1999), this finding was not significant, and indeed, no other temporal or spatial measures were found to be significantly impacted by the presence of the tube. Using videoendoscopy, Fattal, Suiter, Warner, and Leder (2011) evaluated swallowing in patients before and immediately after NGT placement (n = 21) as well as before and immediately after NGT removal (n = 41). Presence or absence of aspiration was evaluated following provision of three puree and three liquid boluses of approximately 5 mL volume. Results indicated that the presence of an NGT did not affect aspiration status, regardless of the NGT diameter. Similarly, Dziewas, Warnecke, Hamacher, et al. (2008) evaluated patients with stroke using videoendoscopy with and without an NGT (n = 25); all videos were randomized and analyzed offline. Results indicated no significant difference in airway invasion with or without the NGT present.

In contrast, Pryor and colleagues (2015) completed a randomized, controlled crossover study with healthy elderly ($n = 15$; age range 60–81 y) using large-bore NGTs, small-bore NGTs, and no tube as a control. All participants were assessed using VFSS; specific measurements included the Penetration-Aspiration (P-A) Scale, pharyngeal residual, and duration of pharyngeal transit. All VFSS images were analyzed by trained raters independent of the study; intra- and interrater reliability were high (98% and 96%, respectively). Results indicated increased airway penetration, pharyngeal residual, and delayed pharyngeal transit as a response to the presence of an NGT. Interestingly, however, results varied depending on small- versus large-bore NGTs. For example, increased P-A Scale scores were found with use of a small-bore NGT. Yet, swallowing duration was found to increase with a larger-diameter NGT. Both small- and large-bore NGTs increased vallecular residual compared with the control condition. Taken together, it appears that the larger-diameter NGTs have increased likelihood to worsen signs of dysphagia, including residual and increased transit time. While ongoing research continues regarding iatrogenic dysphagia as a result of NGT placement, it is important to bear in mind there may be some patients in which the NGT indeed leads to further complication.

A broader range of complications were reported by Ciocon, Silverstone, Graver, and Foley (1988). Seventy tube-fed patients were followed across 11 months. Early complications of NGTs included agitation and self-extubation in 67% and a notable 43% with aspiration pneumonia. Late complications were the same, but with aspiration pneumonia at 44% and agitation seen in 39%. Mullan, Roubenoff, and Roubenoff (1992) evaluated 276 patients who were tube fed over a 6-month period. Twelve aspiration events were documented (prevalence 4.4%, incidence 2.4 per 1,000 tube-feeding days); however, no increase in mortality was associated with aspiration. The major risk factors for aspiration were patient age and hospital location, with more frequent development on the wards rather than in the intensive care unit.

Gastrostomy Tubes

Gastrostomy tube feeding consists of enteral nutrition and hydration via surgically placed tubing through the abdominal wall and directly into the stomach. Surgical gastrostomy has largely been replaced (except when contraindicated) by percutaneous procedures, achieved through endoscopic or radiologic imaging (Yuan, Zhao, Xie, & Hu, 2016). PEG is a procedure in which a gastrostomy tube is placed through the abdominal wall using endoscopic guidance. A percutaneous radiological gastrostomy, also known as radiologically inserted gastrostomy (RIG), uses fluoroscopic guidance for gastrostomy tube insertion. Despite the differences in imaging method, PEG and RIG procedures result in the same gastrostomy tube, and there are as yet no randomized controlled trials comparing efficacy between these insertion procedures.

Sinha and colleagues (2001) investigated practice patterns surrounding PEG tube insertion using a questionnaire completed by 88 physicians. NGT was reported typically to precede PEG placement in 76% of respondents, with 45% waiting more than two weeks before PEG insertion. The use of PEG was strongly preferred by the surveyed physicians, with only 7% preferring long-term NGT feeding to PEG. Delaying gastrostomy tube insertion until at least 14 to 28 days is advocated internationally by groups such as the American Stroke Association, the United Kingdom National Collaborating Centre for Acute Care, and the German Society for Clinical Nutrition (Wilmskoetter, Simpson, Simpson, & Bonilha, 2016). Other societies, such as the European Society for Clinical Nutrition and Metabolism, advocate for a further delay of greater than 28 days. However, with pressure to shorten length of hospitalizations, the insertion of gastrostomy tubes is becoming increasingly rapid. In a retrospective review of the timing of PEG administration in patients with stroke from 2002–2012, Wilmskoetter, Simpson, Simpson, and Bonilha (2016) found an average PEG insertion time of 7 days following admission, with only 14.1% of PEG tubes placed on or after the 14-day international recommendation. These results were mirrored in a large retrospective study of over 34,000 hospital admissions; results indicated that 53% of all individuals received a PEG within 7 days of admission, with an overall range of 3 days to over three weeks (George, Kelly, Albert, Hwang, & Holloway, 2017). In a follow-up study, Wilmskoetter, Simpson, and Bonilha (2016) reported that in patients with stroke and a PEG tube, the likelihood of hospital readmission within 30 days was higher for patients with gastrostomy tube insertion during an initial length of stay of less than 11 days.

PEG has historically been considered the procedure of choice when the non-oral status of the patient is considered to be longer term or permanent. However, it should be clear from the following studies that placement of a PEG does not implicate permanence. Based on a review of retrospective studies, Wilmskoetter, Simpson, Simpson, and Bonilha (2016) reported PEG tubes are removed in 16.3% to 75% of patients with dysphagia following stroke. More specifically, James, Kapur, and Hawthorne (1998) completed a retrospective review of 126 patients fed via PEG for dysphagia secondary to stroke. Median duration of PEG across all participants was 127 days; however, for patients with PEG inserted within 2 weeks of onset, the average duration of placement was 52 days. At long-term follow-up, 29% of patients had the PEG removed, 57% had died, and only 12% continued with PEG feedings. Aspiration pneumonia was found to be the most common complication in patients fed via PEG. This is a critical finding when considering the appropriateness of PEG placement to avoid aspiration risk.

A study by Yim, Kaushik, Lau, and Tan (2000) consisted of a clinical audit of 50 PEG placements to evaluate practice patterns. Stroke was the etiology for placement in 80% of the population. PEG was placed within the first month in 46% of the population and within 1 to 2 months in another 16%, with the final 38% receiving their tube more than 2 months post-onset. Post-PEG infection was documented in 14% of patients receiving routine antibiotics and in 39% not provided antibiotics. Infection was also found to be a complication in a study by Anis and colleagues (2006); however, this was reported in only 3% of 191 patients. Late complications of PEG were infection at the tube site in 15% and dislodgement or blocking of the tube in 13.6%. Ciocon and colleagues (1988) also reported on complications with placement of PEG. Early complications included 56% of patients developing aspiration pneumonia, 50% with tube dysfunction, and 44% with agitation and self-extubation.

DECISION MAKING FOR NON-ORAL NUTRITION

Oral versus Non-Oral Intake

As discussed in Chapter 19, one of the 10 principles of neural plasticity (Robbins, Butler, et al., 2008), termed "use it or lose it," has important implications in the discussion of oral versus non-oral intake. It is believed that continued activation of neural substrates involved in feeding can aid in preventing disuse, thereby contributing to stimulation of the sensorimotor system involved with swallowing (for a review, see Robbins, Butler, et al., 2008). Importantly, clinicians should educate patients and family members that provision of alternate nutrition does not in any way restrict the ability to provide rehabilitation or oral trials (see Chapters 18–22).

Several studies have sought to identify characteristics of patients requiring non-oral feeding. Wojner and Alexandrov (2000) evaluated clinical differences in age, stroke severity scores, length of stay, and cost per case between the tube-feeding and control groups. Seven dependent risk factors were identified; four were found to be independent risk factors. These included wet voice after swallowing water, hypoglossal nerve dysfunction, National Institutes of Health Stroke Scale score, and incomplete oral labial closure. A subsequent study by Lin and associates (2005) identified biomechanical features of swallowing on VFSS that were associated with feeding dependency at discharge in 189 patients with dysphagia subsequent to stroke. In the final logistic regression analysis model, advanced age, recurrent stroke, confinement to a wheelchair at discharge, long duration from stroke onset to VFSS, and stasis in valleculae or pyriform sinuses and aspiration on VFSS were independently associated with tube-feeding dependency at discharge. This finding is critical, as research indicates nutritional status is related to ability to resume oral rehabilitation in patients with stroke who are dependent on tube feeding. This is echoed by Nakadate et al. (2016), who investigated predictors of resuming oral intake in patients who were dependent on tube feeding following stroke (n = 107). Their results suggested that having two out of three of the following criteria was a significant predictor for a patient's ability to return to oral feeding: age less than or equal to 80 years, a body mass index greater than 20.0 kg/m^2, and low white blood cell count.

The assumption that feeding tube placement attenuates the risk of aspiration and subsequent pneumonia has been evaluated by several research groups. As referenced earlier in this section, seminal work by Langmore and colleagues (1998) identified tube feeding as one of the highest predictors of aspiration pneumonia in a group of 189 elderly patients of mixed etiology followed for 4 years. This assumption was also questioned in individuals with stroke by Nakajoh et al. (2000). They studied three groups of patients with stroke: those who were orally fed without dysphagia ($n = 43$), those on oral feeding with dysphagia ($n = 48$), and those with NGT feeding and with dysphagia ($n = 52$). Patients underwent cough reflex testing and assessment of swallowing physiology on initial evaluation, and documented pneumonia development within the first year post-onset was identified. Results of this study support that non-oral feeding may reduce pulmonary complications. The incidence of pneumonia was found to be related to suppressed cough and was higher in patients with oral feeding than in those with tube feeding.

Dziewas and colleagues (2004) also sought to address this question, but with conflicting results. They evaluated 100 patients with acute stroke fed via NGT secondary to dysphagia. Logistic regression was used to identify variables significantly associated with the occurrence of pneumonia and those related to a poor outcome at 3 months. Pneumonia was diagnosed in 44% of the patients who were tube fed, with most acquiring pneumonia within 3 days of onset. Independent predictors for the occurrence of pneumonia were a decreased level of consciousness and severe facial palsy. The authors concluded that NGTs offer only limited protection against aspiration pneumonia in patients with dysphagia from acute stroke; however, this study did not offer a comparison group to those without NGT. Mamun and Lim (2005) supported these data with a comparative study of 122 patients in two groups: those with NGT feedings and those orally fed. The rates of aspiration pneumonia and death were greater in patients fed via NGT than in those who were orally fed. However, the authors concede that patients requiring an NGT were more cognitively and functionally impaired than those on an oral diet; indeed, when they compared those receiving nutrition via NGT with those who were recommended for NGT but refused, no statistically significant differences were identified.

Yet again, the concern for increased pneumonia risk was documented in another prospective cohort study of 330 patients with ischemic stroke, followed for 30 days post-insult (Langdon, Lee, & Binns, 2009). Within this group, 22% of patients were exclusively tube fed; of these patients, 40% developed respiratory infections compared with respiratory infections in only 8% of patients who were fed orally. Logistic regression analysis identified tube feeding during admission to be a significant predictor for respiratory infection. Taken together, these studies emphasize the need for careful consideration of the balance between risk and benefit of non-oral feeding.

The question of increased rate of pneumonia in patients who receive nutrition orally versus non-orally is further complicated by oral care status, as alternate feeding can predispose patients to increased risk of oral colonization, as discussed later in this chapter. In addition to chemical and mechanical cleansing from the provision of oral care, mastication, which is reduced in patients with non-oral routes of intake, aids in reducing oral colonization. In a study comparing patients with NGT ($n = 78$), PEG ($n = 57$), and oral intake ($n = 80$), Leibovitz et al. (2003) took oral samples to identify rates of gram-negative bacteria and *Staphylococcus aureus*, both of which are linked to the development of aspiration pneumonia. Interestingly, results revealed a higher rate of colonization in the NGT (81%) and PEG (51%) groups compared with the control group (17.5%), with specific bacteria found exclusively in the non-oral intake groups.

A retrospective case-matched study compared morbidity, mortality, and functional recovery of patients admitted to rehabilitation with a PEG tube (Iizuka & Reding, 2005). Patients with a PEG admitted for stroke rehabilitation ($n = 193$) were matched with case controls without PEG ($n = 193$). Participants were within 90 days of stroke onset and were matched for age, sex, type of stroke, FIM score, duration from onset to stroke unit admission, and year of admission. Patients with PEG more often required transfer back to acute hospital and had a poorer survival status, supported by recent research (Wilmskoetter, Simpson, Logan, Simpson, & Bonilha, 2018). However, patients with PEG who survived were no different relative to length of rehabilitation admission, improvement in total FIM score from admission to discharge, and final discharge destination (home versus institution) compared with those with poor survival.

Perhaps the most comprehensive approach to addressing decision making relative to provision of nutrition was completed by researchers in the United Kingdom. The FOOD trial (Dennis, Lewis, Cranswick, & Forbes, 2006) consisted of three randomized controlled trials that recruited over 5,000 patients from 131 hospitals. The first study evaluated the benefits of nutritional supplements when added to a normal hospital diet and identified a reduction in risk of death of 0.7% as well as an increase in the risk of "death or negative outcome" of 0.7%; thus, the recommendation for oral supplements is ambiguous. The second study investigated whether early tube feeding within the first week of admission compared with whether holding tube feeding for one week improved outcomes in patients with stroke-related dysphagia.

Early tube feeding was associated with a reduction in risk of death of 5.8%. This provides clear evidence in a large population of patients that early tube feeding may substantially decrease mortality. The third investigation compared the method of NGT with PEG placed during the first 30 days on patient outcomes. PEG was associated with an increase in absolute risk of death of 1.0% and an increased risk of "death or poor outcome" of 7.8%. This finding is contrary to other studies comparing PEG with NGT as outlined below.

NGT versus PEG Tube

Park and colleagues (1992) evaluated 40 patients with dysphagia of at least 4 weeks duration who were randomized to receive either NGT or PEG. No complications occurred in the NGT group, but 3 (16%) individuals in the PEG group developed what the authors considered to be minor problems—aspiration pneumonia (2 patients) and wound infection (1 patient). However, the patients with PEG received a significantly greater proportion of their prescribed nutritional intake (93%) compared with those receiving NGT (55%) and consequently gained significantly more weight after 7 days of feeding. The average duration of NGT feeding was quite brief (5.2 days); thus, longer-term comparisons were not possible.

Norton, Homer-Ward, Donnelly, Long, and Holmes (1996) evaluated 30 patients with acute stroke who were randomized to receiving gastrostomy or NGT feedings at 14 days post-onset. Contrary to the FOOD trial results, mortality at 6 weeks was significantly lower in the gastrostomy group, with two deaths (12%) compared with eight deaths (57%) in the NGT group. Patients with an NGT received a significantly smaller proportion of their prescribed nutrition (78%) compared with the gastrostomy group (100%). In the gastrostomy group, the mean albumin concentration increased, whereas there was a reduction of albumin in patients fed via NGT. Six patients from the gastrostomy group were discharged from hospital within 6 weeks of the procedure compared with none from the NGT group.

Bath, Bath, and Smithard (2000) completed a review of the literature to assess the effect of different management strategies for patients with stroke-related dysphagia, in particular how and when to feed, whether to supplement nutritional intake, and how and whether to treat dysphagia. Based on their review through March 1999, it was concluded that PEG reduces end-of-trial case fatality and treatment failures and improves nutritional status, including weight, mid-arm circumference, and serum albumin compared with NGT feeding. This overall conclusion is supported by Hamidon and colleagues (2006), who published a small randomized study of 22 patients that compared NGT and PEG for nutritional outcomes. PEG tube feeding was found to be more effective than NGT feeding in improving the nutritional status (in terms of the serum albumin level) of patients with stroke-related dysphagia. As with the study by Norton and associates (1996), NGT feeding resulted in decreased serum albumin level within 4 weeks of initiation of tube feedings.

Kostadima, Kaditis, Alexopoulos, Zakynthinos, and Sfyras (2005) evaluated differences in frequency of ventilator association pneumonia in a randomized controlled trial comparing use of early gastrostomy tubes ($n = 20$) versus a control group who received an NGT ($n = 21$), consistent with usual care. There were no significant differences between the groups regarding age, diagnosis, or severity of neurologic impairment or medical treatment regimen (e.g., antibiotic and H2 receptor antagonist treatments). Patients were admitted following either stroke or head injury and were reliant on mechanical ventilation; patients with respiratory disease, thoracic trauma, or multiple traumatic injuries were excluded. All individuals received either a PEG or NGT within 24 hours of intubation. Two patients (10%) developed ventilator associated pneumonia in the PEG group versus eight patients (38.1%) in the NGT group ($p = 0.04$). While the findings of this randomized controlled trial are informative, the authors caution that replication with larger sample size in varying severities of patients following neurologic impairment is indicated.

A meta-analysis of 11 randomized controlled studies ($n = 735$) evaluated PEG versus NGT feeding in adults with dysphagia (Gomes et al., 2015). Results indicated that intervention failure was significantly less frequent in participants with PEG compared with NGT. Further, there was no statistically significant difference between the groups for secondary outcomes of mortality, adverse events, aspiration pneumonia, or weight change. However, the meta-analysis revealed individuals with a PEG had improved nutritional metrics, including arm circumference and levels of serum albumin compared with the NGT group. Additionally, quality of life was significantly higher in individuals with a PEG tube with regard to themes such as convenience, comfort, and social interaction. These randomized studies tend to support PEG feedings over NGT. Importantly, however, this is in stark contrast to the very large FOOD trial (Dennis et al., 2006), and ongoing research is needed to weigh the risks and benefits of PEG versus NGT feeding.

Ethical Considerations

Much of the research relative to risks and benefits of non-oral feeding in patients with stroke has addressed nutritional and pulmonary safety. Much less has been written regarding the ethical and quality-of-life dilemmas that emerge when approaching decisions regarding non-oral feeding in the patient with stroke-related dysphagia. Studies have sought to evaluate the perception of patients and caregivers in regard to PEG placement. Anis and colleagues (2006) studied a mixed population of patients who had undergone PEG. Using a questionnaire to address psychological, social, and physical performance status of health-related quality of life issues, they interviewed 126 patients/caretakers. Sixty percent of those surveyed would agree to have the PEG tube again if required; 83% felt ease in feeding, and 60% felt that the PEG tube helped in prolonging their survival. Regarding negative opinions, 39% felt that the feeding was too frequent, 36% felt apprehensive about dependency for feeding, and 49% were concerned about the cost of care.

Callahan, Haag, Buchanan, and Nisi (1999) gathered information from patients or surrogate decision makers through face-to-face interview; in addition, 82 primary care physicians completed a written questionnaire. Although not limited to stroke, the most common etiology necessitating the need for PEG was stroke. Several adverse factors were reported by patients or their surrogates, including the confusion of having multiple discussants, incomplete information, and considerable distress in arriving at the decision to proceed with artificial feeding. According to these consumers, the decision for gastrostomy often appeared to be a "non-decision" in the sense that decision makers perceived few alternatives. In a systematic review of attitudes and barriers to PEG feeding, Jaafar, Mahadeva, Morgan, and Tan (2016) similarly found most publications report themes of poor understanding and knowledge of the contraindications, insufficient time to make a decision, and fear/anxiety regarding making a choice with "life or death" implications.

Physicians also reported considerable distress in providing recommendations for PEG, including perceived pressures from families or other health care professionals. Although most health care workers reported having a clear method for selecting patients appropriate for PEG tube placement, the assumptions underlying clinical practice were not well supported by the medical literature. Research has shown that families overestimate tube feeding benefits (Carey et al., 2006); this may be a by-product of physician beliefs. In a survey of physicians (n = 173), medical professionals similarly anticipate benefits more readily than negative consequences. Physicians reported an expectation that the majority (76%) of patients with stroke will have reduced risk of aspiration following tube feeding compared with estimates of 31% to 44% for other diagnoses (Hanson et al., 2008). This is in stark contrast to the literature and may reflect inadequate training in non-oral feeding outcomes in dysphagia following stroke. Critically, multidisciplinary input is needed to reach a joint consensus with patient and family participation, clearly explaining the possible risks and benefits.

Due to the risk of tube removal or dislodgement, NGT and PEG have also been associated with increased use of restraints, such as nasal loop or hand mittens. It is important to keep in mind that while these methods may temporarily improve nutritional intake, they do so at a substantial ethical cost. Mahoney and Veitch (2018, p. e435) comment that "by their very nature, [they] restrict freedom of choice and can result in potential physical and psychological harm."

FREE WATER

The use of free water has been recommended for patients with liquid aspiration who are either on tube feeding or receiving thickened liquids and was initially put forth by the Frazier Rehabilitation Institute in Louisville, Kentucky (for review, see Panther, 2005). The premise behind the free water protocol is that water has a neutral pH, which is innocuous to the lungs if aspirated in small amounts. The free water protocol is suggested to promote compliance, improve hydration, and increase quality of life.

The guidelines for the Frazier free water protocol include the following:

- Water access is unrestricted for patients on oral diets—water pitchers are in the room (successful compensatory strategies are encouraged during ingestion of water).
- Patients with cognitive deficits such as impulsiveness or excess coughing during water ingestion are provided water under supervision.
- Patients with significant choking during water ingestion are not eligible to receive water.
- Water intake is discontinued for 30 minutes after a meal to allow clearing of post-swallow residual.
- Aggressive oral care is undertaken.
- Medications are not provided with water.

It is noted that use of a water protocol should be tailored for individuals in acute care settings, as the original protocol is designed for patients in a rehabilitation unit (Panther, 2005).

Several studies have evaluated the free water protocol (Bernard, Loeslie, & Rabatin, 2016; Carlaw et al., 2012; Frey & Ramsberger, 2011; Garon, Engle, & Ormiston, 1997; Karagiannis, Chivers, & Karagiannis, 2011; Karagiannis & Karagiannis, 2014; Murray, Doeltgen, Miller, & Scholten, 2016; Pooyania, Vandurme, Daun, & Buchel, 2015). In the first free water protocol study, 20 patients in a stroke rehabilitation unit who had documented aspiration of thin liquids were recruited and randomized to one of two groups: (1) thickened liquids only or (2) thickened liquids with free access to water (Garon et al., 1997). Patients were within 3 weeks of stroke and were followed until resolution of thin liquid aspiration. Slightly different than the Frazier protocol, participants completed a pre-rinse prior to water ingestion and had to request water; it was not available for uncontrolled access. Results revealed that no patient in either group developed dehydration or pneumonia. Patients with thickened liquids only averaged approximately 1 week longer to resolution of thin liquid aspiration compared with the patients receiving free water. In addition, patients in the thickened liquid group averaged slightly less fluid intake (1210 mL) per day compared with the thickened liquid plus free water group (1318 mL). As expected, patient satisfaction was higher in those receiving free water compared with those who received only thickened liquids. Although results of this study are positive, the reader must look closely at the study methods to fully interpret results, particularly in regard to patients with stroke. Exclusion criteria for the study included poor cognition, severe coughing on aspiration, aspiration of thickened liquids or food, inability to rinse and expectorate, inability to hold a cup or self-feed, and impulsive behavior. With these stringent criteria, only 17.5% of patients were eligible for inclusion in the study, representing a fairly small proportion of rehabilitation patients and perhaps a small proportion of acute patients with dysphagia, yet these are frequently the patients who present with stroke-related dysphagia. This limits generalizability. Additionally, the patients assigned to the group ingesting thickened liquids only may have represented a great level of physiologic impairment, with 5 patients aspirating on greater than 50% of swallows, compared with only one patient in the free water group. Finally, patients had to request water, suggesting that patients involved in this study were on the milder end of the severity spectrum.

A broader study was conducted by Karagiannis et al. (2011), who report on lung-related complications and hydration levels and assessed quality of life in patients with dysphagia in a general medical population. The control group (n = 34) was allowed only thickened fluids, and patients in the intervention group (n = 42) were allowed access to water for 5 days. Those patients given access to water presented a significantly increased risk of respiratory infection (14.3%) compared with the control group (0%). With a more varied population group and fewer exclusion criteria, information relative to etiology could be identified. Those who developed pneumonia in the intervention group had neurodegenerative disease and/or reduced mobility. These authors further evaluated fluid intake and identified increased intake in the patients allowed access to water.

The finding of increased fluid intake with a water protocol has been further documented (Carlaw et al., 2012). Fifteen patients were recruited to this within-subject, crossover design study, with all participants completing the water protocol either immediately or after a 14-day delay. All participants aspirated thin liquid on the instrumental assessment with either nil per os/nothing by mouth or thickened liquid recommendations. Results revealed that all patients remained free from adverse events. Increased liquid intake of up to 10% was documented in 11/15 patients during the water intake phase compared with the control phase without water access. Additionally, quality of life measures were found to improve.

Increased fluid intake in the access to water group, however, is not uniformly evident in all studies. In a small randomized control trial of 14 patients with stroke-related dysphagia and aspiration in rehabilitation facilities, no difference in fluid intake was identified between the group receiving only thickened liquids and the group with additional access to water (Murray et al., 2016). Of note, 71% of the participants were identified with dehydration prior to beginning the study. While not statistically significant, individuals in the water protocol group demonstrated a trend toward improved hydration, whereas individuals in the thickened liquid group showed no improvement. Also, urinary tract infections were significantly more frequent in the thickened liquid group. Unlike findings from previous studies (Carlaw et al., 2012; Garon et al., 1997), satisfaction in liquid intake was the same across groups. As with earlier studies (Carlaw et al., 2012; Garon et al., 1997), it is difficult to comment on the influence of water protocols on pulmonary outcomes when the outcome of interest is not observed in either group.

A systematic review and meta-analysis of free water protocol studies has recently been completed (Gillman, Winkler, & Taylor, 2017). Results revealed low-quality evidence supporting a reduced likelihood of pulmonary complications with a water protocol and low-quality evidence of increased fluid intake with a water protocol. In previous editions of this book, we suggested that until large randomized controlled studies are completed that incorporate patients with stroke in various care settings (e.g., acute care, rehabilitation) who have thin liquid aspiration, an individualized approach must be undertaken in recommending free water to people with stroke-related dysphagia and aspiration. Gillman et al. also suggest this, stating that individuals must be carefully selected adult rehabilitation inpatients who are cognitively intact or with appropriate supervision, generally mobile, and without progressive neurological disorders.

ORAL HYGIENE[1]

Regardless of the decision concerning oral or non-oral intake, oral hygiene should be addressed in all patients with stroke-related dysphagia. As is evident from the section on free water, implementation of an oral hygiene program is integral to the protocol. The oral cavity

[1]Portions of this section were developed after review of the thesis from Sarah Davies, PhD.

contains various types of bacteria, including innocuous bacteria which can provide a defense against respiratory pathogens (Jenkinson & Lamont, 2005) as well as pathogenic bacteria. In unhealthy oral cavities, however, there is no longer equilibrium between harmless and harmful bacteria which can subsequently serve as a precursor to the development of aspiration pneumonia. Factors that may disturb this equilibrium include advancing age, dental status, dependence level, and oral hygiene, all of which may be evidenced with stroke.

Aging is associated with illness, lowered immunity, salivary hypofunction, decreased mobility, increased use of dental prosthesis, reduced ability to perform dental care as well as access to dental services (Carter et al., 2004; Wilson, 2005). The number of decayed teeth is significantly associated with the development of aspiration pneumonia (Langmore et al., 1998; Terpenning et al., 2001), and respiratory infection is reported to be more common in dentate (40%) versus edentulous (27%) individuals (Mojon, Budtz-Jørgensen, Miche, & Limeback, 1997). Specific pathogens, nevertheless, are associated with denture plaque and can contribute to aspiration pneumonia (Sumi, Miura, Sunakawa, Michiwaki, & Sakagami, 2004). Furthermore, denture wearing during sleep in elderly individuals was shown to significantly increase the risk of pneumonia as well as oral cavity plaque, gum inflammation, and positive culture for *Candida albicans* (Iinuma et al., 2015). Dependence level may lead to decreased ability to provide self-care of the oral cavity and/or a need for assistance with oral hygiene. Both can result in poor oral hygiene and increased risk of aspiration pneumonia (Langmore et al., 1998).

Systematic literature reviews of randomized controlled trials have identified positive results in reducing morbidity and mortality with the implementation of oral hygiene interventions in nursing home facilities (Sjögren, Nilsson, Forsell, Johansson, & Hoogstraate, 2008; van der Maarel-Wierink, Vanobbergen, Bronkhorst, Schols, & de Batt, 2013). Based on these reviews, brushing teeth following meals, daily denture cleaning, and weekly professional oral health care is suggested. The optimal regime of oral care is unclear, as frequency and duration of tooth brushing varied from no formal protocol (Bassim, Gibson, Ward, Paphides, & Denucci, 2008) to tooth brushing of unspecified duration after every meal (Yoshino, Ebihara, Ebihara, Fuji, & Sasaki, 2001) or 5 minutes of tooth brushing after every meal (Watando et al., 2004; Yoneyama et al., 2002). In these studies, oral care was provided by health care staff. Individuals randomized to the control group in the Yoshino et al. study performed their own dental care. While this finding may suggest that oral hygiene must be performed by health care providers, at least in residents in nursing homes, it is important to note that the cognitive status in both the control and experimental groups was notably low, with a mean of 14 on the Mini-Mental State Examination. Thus, it is unclear if more cognitively intact individuals can independently complete adequate oral hygiene. Additionally, many studies incorporated weekly professional health care (Ishikawa et al., 2008; Watando et al., 2004; Yoneyama et al., 2002), which may not be feasible in many settings.

Potential secondary benefits from implementing oral hygiene programs are reported as well. These benefits include reduced swallowing latency hypothesized to be the result of sensory stimulation of the oral cavity yielding increased neuropeptide release (Yoshino et al., 2001) and increased cough reflex sensitivity measured by a citric acid cough reflex test (Watando et al., 2004).

Stroke can impact an individual's independence, mobility, and swallowing. Thus, individuals who have premorbid history of good dental hygiene may suddenly become dependent for oral care. Individuals who had a history of poor oral hygiene but no occurrence of pneumonia may now have, for example, limited mobility, dependence for feeding, and/or poor secretion management, which may increase the likelihood of development of pneumonia. In either scenario, facilitating oral hygiene during hospitalization for stroke appears imperative. Implementation of an oral hygiene program to reduce risk of pneumonia is suggested in the American Heart Association/American Stroke Association guidelines for management of acute ischemic stroke (Powers et al., 2018). While the delegation of dental care is frequently relegated to nursing staff, multidisciplinary collaboration between nursing, speech pathology, and additional disciplines such as occupational therapy and dental hygiene is required to develop and implement effective education and adherence to a targeted oral care program.

SUMMARY

Our approaches to diet manipulation in patients with swallowing impairment are maturing. Clinicians are now in a better position to more intelligently judge the real risks of developing pneumonia, and therefore can more judiciously balance the needs of pulmonary safety, nutrition, and patient quality of life. Certainly, there will be times when complete non-oral nutrition is the only wise option either in the short term until rehabilitative potential is reached or in the long term for patients with poorer prognosis. Maintaining adequate oral hygiene regardless of mode of nutritional intake is imperative.

18 Compensatory Management of Oropharyngeal Dysphagia

Compensatory management does not change the physiology of swallowing; rather, bolus flow is altered. Compensatory strategies provide immediate benefit by eliminating the patient's signs or symptoms—for example, aspiration or post-swallow residual. Benefits are seen immediately but are not permanent. That is, when the compensatory strategy is removed, the previously noted swallowing dysfunction prevails. These strategies are frequently manipulated by the clinician. While many compensatory strategies are relatively simple and may not require comprehension of compound or complex directions to complete, they all require good cognitive ability such as attention and memory to consistently implement with every swallow for the particular consistency in which they were recommended. Compensatory strategies should be thought of as short term to maintain oral intake with long-term management focusing on rehabilitative intervention, which changes swallowing physiology. Only in those patients with significant cognitive or language deficits should management stop with compensatory strategies, but this should be temporary until cognition or comprehension improves to the point where the patient can participate in rehabilitation.

Before implementing compensatory strategies, most should be determined effective during the instrumental examination (e.g., during the videofluoroscopic swallowing study [VFSS], pre-swallow aspiration is eliminated with a chin tuck posture). When attempted during the clinical swallowing examination (CSE), the clinician cannot be certain that a compensatory strategy is needed or that it accomplished its goal. That is, thickened liquids are employed based on a patient's cough with liquids; however, aspiration may not be occurring. In another clinical scenario, a patient may no longer cough when a thickened liquid is employed, but the clinician does not know if aspiration actually ceased or if it is no longer overt. Research has shown that some individuals may cough with thin liquid aspiration, but these same individuals do not cough with aspiration of thickened liquids (Miles, McFarlane, Scott, & Hunting, 2018). Although not addressing thickened liquids as a compensatory technique, Daniels and colleagues (1998) noted increased silent aspiration with barium during VFSS as opposed to overt aspiration with water in these same patients during the CSE. This may suggest that lack of cough cannot be equated with resolution of aspiration. Two studies have highlighted the importance of confirming the effect of chin tuck posture during an instrumental examination. In a cohort of patients with acute stroke, clinicians demonstrated limited ability to accurately predict aspiration and its resolution using a chin tuck posture during the CSE compared with VFSS (Baylow, Goldfarb, Taveria, & Steinberg, 2009). Moreover, Fraser and Steele (2012) found reduced airway invasion with liquid aspiration when using the chin tuck posture with cup drinking but not with teaspoon administration of a thin liquid bolus, further supporting the need to confirm success of compensatory strategies using an instrumental examination. Other types of compensatory strategies, such as those for airway management, may require additional training outside the instrumental evaluation with subsequent re-evaluation to determine effectiveness.

It is not the role of the clinician to instruct implementation of the compensatory strategy at every meal. Rather, the clinician should apply the best compensatory strategy based on the sign(s) observed in the instrumental evaluation, and the patient's cognitive and language abilities. The clinician must instruct and document competency in implementation by either the patient or caregiver and reassess as indicated. Once the compensatory strategy is effectively employed, the clinician should devote management to rehabilitative techniques. Observed VFSS signs, the physiological abnormalities which may produce the signs, and the multiple compensatory strategies which can be implemented for a specific sign are listed in Table 18–1. This is the approach that most clinicians would use based on the results of the instrumental examination. Of note, effortful swallowing and Mendelsohn maneuver, which can be used as compensation or for rehabilitation, are discussed in Chapter 20.

The astute reader will note a wide range of evidence for the compensatory strategies discussed. This holds true for rehabilitative management strategies discussed in subsequent chapters. Outcomes vary for many studies for which the same compensatory strategy is studied.

Table 18–1. Sign Approach for Application of Compensatory Strategies

Occurring	***Sign***	***Secondary to***	***Compensation Technique***
Pre-Swallow	Anterior leakage	Poor orolingual control	Thickened liquids
	Poor bolus preparation		Chopped/puréed solids
	Discoordinated bolus transfer		3-second prep
	Pooling	Poor orolingual control	Volume regulation 3-second prep Chin tuck* Thickened liquids
		Delayed pharyngeal swallow	Volume regulation 3-second prep Chin tuck* Carbonation Thickened liquids Sour bolus
	Airway invasion (penetration/aspiration)	Pooling due to above underlying impairments	(above 6) PLUS Supraglottic swallow Super-supraglottic swallow
During	Penetration	Reduced laryngeal valving	Chin tuck* Super-supraglottic swallow
	Aspiration	Reduced true vocal fold adduction	Head turn (weaker side) Supraglottic swallow
	Nasal regurgitation	Poor pharyngeal motility Reduced BOT retraction Decreased anterior HLC movement Decreased UES relaxation	Volume regulation Change consistency

continues

Table 18–1. *continued*

Occurring	*Sign*	*Secondary to*	*Compensation Technique*
During *continued*	Inadequate epiglottic deflection	Decreased HLC movement	Effortful swallow**^ Mendelsohn maneuver^
		Intrinsic tissue changes	None
Post-Swallow	Oral residue with/without airway invasion	Poor orolingual control	Dry swallow Cyclic ingestion Carbonation Sour bolus
	Vallecular residue with/without airway invasion	Decreased BOT to PPW contact	Dry swallow Cyclic ingestion Chin tuck* Carbonation Sour bolus Effortful swallow**^
	Vallecular residue with/without airway invasion	Inadequate epiglottic deflection due to decreased HLC movement	Dry swallow Cyclic ingestion Carbonation Sour bolus Effortful swallow**^ Mendelsohn maneuver^
	Vallecular residue with/without airway invasion	Inadequate epiglottic deflection due to intrinsic tissue changes	Dry swallow Cyclic ingestion Carbonation Sour bolus
	Inadequate opening of the UES	Decreased anterior hyolaryngeal movement OR intrinsic cricopharyngeus changes	Head turn to either side Mendelsohn maneuver^

Table 18–1. *continued*

Occurring	*Sign*	*Secondary to*	*Compensation Technique*
Post-Swallow *continued*	Unilateral pyriform sinus residue with/without airway invasion	Unilateral pharyngeal hemiparesis	Dry swallow Cyclic ingestion Head turn to weaker side
	Bilateral pyriform sinus residue with/without airway invasion	Inadequate UES opening due to decreased anterior hyolaryngeal movement OR intrinsic cricopharyngeus changes	Dry swallow Cyclic ingestion Carbonation Sour bolus Head turn to either side Mendelsohn maneuver^

Note. BOT = base of tongue, HLC = hyolaryngeal complex, UES = upper esophageal sphincter, PPW = posterior pharyngeal wall.

*Precaution: Use with pooling inferior to the valleculae may increase risk of airway invasion. Of note, chin tuck does not prevent pooling, rather, it maintains the bolus in the pharyngeal space prior to swallowing, thus preventing airway invasion.

**Ensure that negative effects on hyolaryngeal elevation, pharyngeal shortening, and/or nasal redirection are not evident.

^Discussed in Chapter 20, Rehabilitation.

Furthermore, subject selection varies across studies, with many investigations including participants who did not demonstrate the physiological impairment or resulting sign for which the compensation is targeting, thus limiting the strength of available evidence.

POSTURAL CHANGES

Compensatory swallowing postures are designed to change pharyngeal dimensions and redirect bolus flow. Specific postures have been designed for specific motility disorders (see Table 18–1). As with thickened liquids, a specific posture must be evaluated during an instrumental evaluation to determine effectiveness prior to implementation. Posture compensation should not be randomly applied but should be attempted for the specific dysmotility pattern for which it was designed. As with bolus modification, the use of a posture should be considered short-term, with rehabilitative management targeting the underlying pathophysiology.

Although posture is generally recommended over strict diet modification, many factors in addition to swallowing must be considered. Comprehension, attention, memory, and awareness of deficit are critical for the patient to execute a posture adjustment. If a patient cannot independently implement a posture or any compensatory strategy during mealtime, recommendation for its use is questioned even if it is shown to prevent aspiration during the instrumental examination. In a heterogeneous cohort of patients with aspiration, including those with a stroke diagnosis, Rasley et al. (1993) noted that postures were less effective in prevention of aspiration for patients with cognitive deficits. Moreover, honey-thick liquid was more effective than nectar-thick liquid and chin tuck posture with thin liquids in preventing immediate aspiration on VFSS in patients with dementia and/or Parkinson disease (Logemann et al., 2008).

The two most common postures used, chin tuck and head turn, are reviewed in this chapter. Although other postures and various combinations of these postures are available (see Logemann, 1998 for review), the chin tuck and head turn postures are the most clinically relevant in terms of management of patients with stroke-related dysphagia.

Chin Tuck Posture

The chin tuck posture was designed to facilitate swallowing in patients with delayed onset of the pharyngeal swallow or reduced orolingual control with resulting pre-swallow pharyngeal pooling and aspiration (Logemann, 1983). The initial notion behind the use of this posture was that it would widen the valleculae. This, in turn, would yield a larger space for material to pool prior to pharyngeal swallow initiation, thereby decreasing aspiration. The initial research was completed to determine pharyngeal dimensions with the head in a neutral position and with the chin tucked (Welch, Logemann, Rademaker, & Kahrilas, 1993). Although results did not reveal a significant increase in vallecular width with the chin tuck posture, they did reveal narrowing of the laryngeal entrance and closer approximation of the laryngeal surface of the epiglottis with the posterior pharyngeal wall (PPW), which would yield improved airway protection. Reduced depth of airway invasion was demonstrated in patients using the chin tuck posture (Bülow, Olsson, & Ekberg, 2001), probably due to the identified decreased distance between the thyroid cartilage and hyoid. While timing of airway invasion can be assumed to be before or during the swallow in this study as participants swallowed liquids, it is important to note that this was not explicitly stated. Increased duration of laryngeal vestibule closure was more recently identified with the chin tuck posture (Macrae, Anderson, & Humbert, 2014) which further supports the notion of using the chin tuck to facilitate airway protection during the swallow.

An additional study to determine the effects of chin tuck posture on aspiration was completed in a group of patients with neurogenic dysphagia and pre-swallow aspiration (Shanahan, Logemann, Rademaker, Pauloski, & Kahrilas, 1993). Results revealed the chin tuck to be effective in preventing pre-swallow aspiration when pooling was limited to the valleculae. Aspiration persisted in patients with pooling to the pyriform sinuses. It was suggested that aspiration persisted due to laryngeal elevation and shortening of the pharynx at onset of the pharyngeal swallow, which caused hypopharyngeal material to enter the airway. As discussed earlier, this further supports the need to use an instrumental examination to identify location of pooling and effects of implementation of a compensatory strategy.

Given posterior movement of the epiglottis in the chin tuck posture, Welch et al. (1993) suggested that the base of tongue (BOT) also moved closer to the PPW, and thus, chin tuck could be used to facilitate BOT-PPW contact and reduce valleculae residue. However, it is important to note that BOT-PPW approximation was not directly studied. The epiglottic base was also used as a surrogate marker for BOT movement by Leigh et al. (2015), who identified closer approximation of the epiglottis and PPW in the chin tuck position compared with head neutral. Manofluoroscopy was used in the study by Bülow et al. (2001) discussed earlier. While pharyngeal pressures were measured, they did not measure BOT-PPW contact pressures, thus an opportunity to potentially identify increased pressure with a chin tuck posture in patients with dysphagia was missed. High-resolution manometry (HRM) (McCulloch, Hoffman, & Ciucci, 2010) and solid-state intraluminal manometry (Balou et al., 2014) have been used to measure pressure changes in healthy young adults; however, no increase in BOT-PPW pressure with a chin tuck posture was identified in either study. While increased pressure using a chin tuck posture would appear required to reduce vallecular residue, Knigge and Thibeault (2016) found no significant differences in tongue base peak pressure in patients with or without vallecular residue. While the chin tuck was not evaluated in this study, it suggests that factors other than pressure are important in vallecular clearance. Thus, while chin tuck is suggested as a compensatory strategy for vallecular residue due to decreased BOT-PPW contact, empirical studies are required to determine its effectiveness.

The clinician may attempt the chin tuck posture as a compensatory strategy in patients presenting with the following signs: (1) airway invasion occurring pre-swallow or during the swallow resulting from a delayed pharyngeal swallow or poor orolingual control resulting in pooling to the level of the valleculae, (2) vallecular residual with or without post-swallow airway invasion resulting from reduced BOT retraction, and (3) airway invasion during the swallow due to reduced laryngeal closure. While the chin tuck generally does not prevent pharyngeal pooling, it serves to keep the bolus in the valleculae until elicitation of pharyngeal swallowing. Thus, a clinician may trial the posture if hypopharyngeal pooling is observed in an attempt to maintain the bolus in the valleculae. However, the astute practitioner should not be surprised if aspiration occurs if the bolus is not contained in this pharyngeal space.

With the chin tuck posture, the aim is for the patient to touch the chin to the chest. The spine should stay stable as the patient rotates his/her neck forward to look at his/her chest. The patient should assume this posture prior to oral transfer. Many patients with stroke-related dysphagia, however, have problems with bolus control or have cognitive deficits and cannot adequately coordinate timing to assume the posture prior to bolus entry into the pharynx. In these patients, the use of straw delivery of a liquid bolus may improve effectiveness of the technique, if the straw is positioned to where the patient must first assume the posture before ingestion.

Head Turn

A head turn posture, generally to the weaker side, was designed to clear unilateral pharyngeal residue in patients with pharyngeal hemiparesis. It was suggested that by closing off the weaker side, the bolus would travel down the unaffected side of the pharynx (Kirchner, Scatliff, Dey, & Shedd, 1963; Logemann, 1983). This was demonstrated in healthy participants with the bolus traveling through the pharyngeal side opposite the head turn (Logemann, Kahrilas, Kobara, &

Vakil, 1989). In addition, upper esophageal sphincter (UES) diameter increased and intrabolus pressure decreased in the healthy participants. In this same study, patients with lateral medullary stroke were evaluated with and without the head turn posture. Results revealed improved oropharyngeal swallowing efficiency and increased UES diameter with head turn; pressure was not studied. In a single descriptive case report using computed tomography, pyriform sinus closure at the level of the hyoid with dilation of the hypopharynx opposite from the turned side was demonstrated (Tsukamoto, 2000).

Research using HRM and solid-state intraluminal manometry has been completed to determine the pressure changes with the head turn posture in a small sample of healthy adults. Head turn significantly lowered pre-swallow UES pressure compared with head neutral UES pressure (McCulloch et al., 2010). While duration of UES opening was increased, it was not statistically significant. Balou et al. (2014) identified increased duration of UES relaxation with the head turn posture; however, they found no change in pharyngeal pressures and a decrease in the duration of inferior pharyngeal pressure. Thus, these data partially support the use of a head turn posture to facilitate bolus clearance.

For the clinician completing a videoendoscopic evaluation of swallowing (VEES), bilateral or unilateral pyriform sinus residue may easily be identified. When post-swallow residual is identified in the pyriform sinus in the VFSS lateral view, a static anterior-posterior image should be obtained to identify whether retention is bilateral or unilateral. When unilateral residue is noted, the patient should turn his or her head to the affected side. Although residual present from prior swallows may or may not clear on the affected side with implementation of this posture, there should be improved bolus flow with minimal residual during subsequent swallows. When bilateral pyriform sinus residue is identified, head turn to either side can be attempted to determine whether a posture change to one side or the other facilitates bolus flow.

SENSORY ENHANCEMENT

Compensatory sensory techniques involve heightening sensory input and include such things as temperature and taste. Many sensory enhancements involve chemesthetic properties which stimulate the trigeminal nerve (Slack, 2016). Oral chemestesis is the detection of chemical irritants through activation of temperature or pain receptors and results in perceptions of cooling, burning or heat, stinging, or tingling. Thermal-tactile application (TTA) is reviewed in this section, as research has not identified long-term effects of this strategy.

Temperature

Numerous research studies have been undertaken to determine the effects of bolus temperature on swallowing. Most research has focused on cold temperature, with studies generally concentrated on healthy geriatric participants. The majority of results suggest that temperature does not impact swallowing. In a series of studies from the Shaker lab, no effects of temperature were found on pharyngeal motility (Shaker et al., 1993), duration of true vocal fold (TVF) closure (Ren et al., 1993), or threshold volume required to evoke a pharyngeal swallow (Shaker et al., 1994) in healthy young and older adults. In a study in which a tasteless, odorless material was ingested by healthy young adults, results suggested that the warmer food at 50°C was subjectively judged to be easier to swallow than colder food (5°–35°C) (Miyaoka et al., 2006). No significant differences in durations of the oral and oropharyngeal phases were identified with the various temperatures; however, reduced suprahyoid amplitude as measured by surface electromyography (sEMG) was evident with 50°C compared with 20°C. The authors concluded that the higher temperature of 50°C may facilitate swallowing, as they surmised that greater suprahyoid activity indicates increased effort required for laryngeal elevation. This notion seems counterintuitive as rehabilitation is frequently geared to increase distance, force, and speed of muscle movement. In somewhat contradictory findings, cold water compared with room temperature water and hot water resulted in a significantly faster swallow reaction time, which was the latency between cue to swallow and onset of pharyngeal swallowing (Michou, Mastan, Ahmed, Mistry, & Hamdy, 2012).

Limited effects of temperature on bolus flow measures have been reported by Bisch, Logemann, Rademaker, Kahrilas, and Lazarus (1994). This study revealed no differences between cold and room temperature liquids on swallowing measures in patients with stroke-related dysphagia. Longer pharyngeal response time and duration of laryngeal elevation were identified for the 1 mL volume in healthy participants.

A series of studies has been completed testing the effects of a cold bolus and cold plus sour bolus on swallowing timing measures in patients with acute or sub-acute stroke (Cola, Gatto, et al., 2010; Cola et al., 2012; Gatto et al., 2013). Patients were evaluated using VFSS as they ingested in a non-randomized fashion a single 5 mL pudding bolus trial in each of the following conditions: natural, cold, sour, cold-sour. Results revealed faster oral transit times (OTTs) for the cold-sour bolus compared with the untreated pudding stimulus (Gatto et al., 2013) and faster pharyngeal transit times (PTTs) for cold-sour compared with all other pudding stimuli (Cola, Gatto, et al., 2010; Cola et al., 2012). Cola and colleagues (2012) also evaluated PTT in a separate cohort when the stimuli were presented in a randomized order. No significant effect between stimuli conditions was identified; in fact, the randomized group appeared to have significantly shorter PTT in all conditions compared with the non-randomized group. The authors suggested that the results were due to the influence of the cold-sour bolus on subsequent swallows; however, in the randomized group, the various presentation orders of stimuli were not indicated. Of note for all three studies, it is unclear if the individuals determining transit times were blinded to stimuli conditions, as this was not explicitly stated. There is no discussion of clearing the oral cavity after each swallow in order to prevent effects on subsequent swallows. Last, it is questioned if a single trial of each stimulus provides stable results.

Carbonation

Carbonation is a common chemesthetic agent that has been studied in healthy adults and patient populations. No effects with carbonation were identified for timing and amplitude of contraction for the orbicularis oris, submental, and infrahyoid muscles using sEMG in healthy individuals (Ding, Logemann, Larson, & Rademaker, 2003). More recent research has revealed a larger number of swallows successfully completed within a pre-determined time window with carbonated liquids compared with plain water (Elshukri, Michou, Mentz, & Hamdy, 2016; Michou et al., 2012) and increased corticobulbar excitability for up to 60 minutes following ingestion of the carbonated beverage (Elshukri et al., 2016).

Improvements in swallowing with carbonated liquids have been identified in individuals with dysphagia. The use of carbonation to facilitate swallowing was first reported by Jennings, Siroky, and Jackson (1992) in patients who underwent skull base tumor resection. Six of the 12 patients benefited from the use of a carbonated beverage to clear or reduce the amount of post-swallow residual. Further evaluation of carbonation in a cohort of patients with neurological impairment revealed that carbonated liquids reduced airway invasion and post-swallow residual and decreased PTT compared with noncarbonated thin liquids (Bülow, Olsson, & Ekberg, 2003). However, the interested reader should review the methodology of this study before assuming ready translation to clinical practice. Non-carbonated liquids were swallowed on cue, whereas carbonated liquids were swallowed without verbal cue. Only participants who were able to sit upright and who could follow instructions were offered the opportunity to swallow the carbonated liquid.

One additional study has been completed testing the effects of carbonation in a patient population. The effects of carbonation were evaluated during VFSS in 17 individuals with neurogenic dysphagia (stroke = 13) and VFSS confirmation of delayed onset of pharyngeal swallowing (Sdravou, Walshe, & Dagdilelis, 2012). The effects of carbonated liquid barium on temporal measures, residue, and airway invasion were compared with non-carbonated liquid barium. No significant differences between carbonated and non-carbonated liquids were identified for timing measures (OTT, PTT) or residue and bolus location at swallowing onset. There was, however, a significant decrease in the Penetration-Aspiration Scale scores with the carbonated stimulus. Furthermore, stage transition duration (STD) was significantly longer with carbonated liquids at the 25 mL volume compared with non-carbonated liquids, but no differences in STD between the stimuli were evident with smaller volumes. Given the intersubject variability of this measure, the clinical significance of this finding is questionable. Moreover, while subjects were required to have a delayed pharyngeal response to be eligible to participate, the authors noted that many of the participants had normal STD times, thus creating a floor effect which limits the ability to detect change.

Recent systematic review and quality assessment of the available literature concerning the use of carbonation as a compensatory strategy suggest weak evidence, due in part to the various study methodologies which limit the ability to compare findings (Turkington, Ward, & Farrell, 2017). The authors note that it remains unclear as to what signs evident on the VFSS are best targeted with carbonation, what physiological changes would be expected, and how best to implement carbonation in the clinical setting. These factors affect clinicians' practice patterns in implementation of carbonation as well as other sensory stimuli in VFSS (Turkington, Nund, Ward, & Farrell, 2017).

Certain considerations must be made before employing carbonation as a compensatory strategy during VFSS. Unless mixed with barium, a carbonated liquid such as cola will not be visualized. Mixing the cola with barium will decrease and possibly neutralize the effects of the carbonation. If the clinician is interested in the ability of carbonation to clear pharyngeal residue, plain cola may be administered, and although it will not be visualized, the clearing of post-swallow retention will be evident if this strategy is effective. If the clinician is interested in increasing swallowing speed or reducing airway invasion, a method described by Bülow and colleagues (2003) may be used. They added sodium bicarbonate to barium and thus were able to view bolus flow of the carbonated liquid.

Taste

The impact of taste on swallowing physiology and the potential of taste to facilitate disordered swallowing is the focus of many research studies. The notion behind this line of research is twofold. First, it has been suggested that increasing sensory input may facilitate disordered swallowing (Logemann, 1998). Second, taste sensitivity decreases with advancing age (Schiffman, 1993). Thus, findings from this line of research have increased clinical relevance for the stroke population, as dysphagia is prominent in this group and the incidence of stroke increases with advancing age.

As reviewed in Table 3–1 in Chapter 3, taste may impact many aspects of swallowing in healthy adults, including timing and/or amplitude of submental muscle contraction (Ding et al., 2003; Leow, Huckabee, Sharma, & Tooley, 2007; Pelletier & Steele, 2014), lingual-palatal pressure (Abdul Wahab, Jones, & Huckabee, 2011; Nagy, Steele, & Pelletier, 2014; Palmer, McCulloch, Jaffe, & Neel, 2005; Pelletier & Dhanaraj, 2006; Pelletier & Steele, 2014), number of swallows and volume swallowed per second (Chee, Arshad, Singh, Mistry, & Hamdy, 2005), and oral preparation time (Leow et al., 2007). In addition to immediate effects of stimulation, Abdul Wahab et al. (2011) identified long-term stimulation effects, including decreased lingual-palatal pressures 30 to 60 minutes post-stimulation, suggesting maintenance of increased oral phase efficiency. Long-term effects on motor evoked potentials which represent neural excitability and transmission have also been identified (Abdul-Wahab, Jones, & Huckabee, 2010). Research has also indicated that taste does not impact swallowing apnea duration (Butler, Postma, & Fischer, 2004; Hiss, Strauss, Treole, Stuart, & Boutilier, 2004), duration of tongue movement (Steele, van Lieshout, & Pelletier, 2012), and onset of pharyngeal swallowing when liquid is infused into the valleculae (Pouderoux, Logemann, & Kahrilas, 1996).

Most studies have focused on sour taste with a few studies focused on sweet, bitter, and salty in addition to sour (Chee et al., 2005; Ding et al., 2003; Leow et al., 2007; Pouderoux & Kahrilas, 1995; Pouderoux et al., 1996). Two recent studies evaluated the combination of sour taste plus sour smell, that is, flavor (Abdul Wahab et al., 2010, 2011).

Research on the effects of taste on swallowing in the neurogenic population has also demonstrated changes in swallowing physiology and supports the notion that heightened sensory stimulation may facilitate certain aspects of swallowing. In the first study to examine the effects of a sour bolus on swallowing pathophysiology, a cohort of patients with dysphagia post-stroke as well as patients with other neurogenic disorders were studied (Logemann et al., 1995). All individuals were diagnosed with delayed onset of oral transfer and/or delayed pharyngeal swallowing on VFSS. Barium (1:1 barium to water) was compared against a sour bolus (1:1 barium to ReaLemon brand lemon juice). The patients with stroke demonstrated a significant reduction in oral transfer onset, OTT, STD, and PTT, and a significant increase in oropharyngeal swallowing efficiency with the sour bolus. In the group with other neurogenic etiologies, the sour bolus resulted in faster onset of oral transfer, later onset of BOT retraction, and shorter duration of BOT to PPW contact. Although the effects of the sour bolus on swallowing physiology were significant, the patients reported the taste to be unpleasant, thus negating its implementation as a functional compensatory strategy.

As discussed earlier in this chapter, positive swallowing effects using a sour plus cold bolus were identified in patients with stroke-related dysphagia (Cola, Gatto, et al., 2010; Cola et al., 2012; Gatto et al., 2013). Limitations of these studies were previously discussed. The intensity and the palatability of sour taste were not detailed in these studies.

Due to its high citric acid content, a sour bolus may be considered a chemesthetic agent. In addition to acid or sour, other chemical agents such as capsaicinoid, piperine, and menthol have been studied to determine their effects on swallowing. Capsaicinoids produce a heat-related sensation and are found in ginger and capsicum. Piperine is in black pepper and responsible for the strong, pungent burning sensation. Menthol, which is in peppermint, produces a cooling sensation.

The effect of carbonation plus gingerol was recently studied in healthy, young adults (Krival & Bates, 2012). The carbonation plus gingerol beverage resulted in significantly increased lingual-palatal pressure compared with carbonation alone or water; however, it was significantly less palatable than the other two beverages. In patient populations, capsaicinoids have been shown to decrease the incidence of airway invasion, reduce residue, shorten time to onset of laryngeal vestibule closure and UES opening (Rofes, Arreola, Martin, & Clavé, 2013), and increase onset of pharyngeal swallowing (Ebihara et al., 2005). Rofes et al. (2013) evaluated a capsaicinoid concentrate mixed with Gastrografin plus thickening agent, whereas Ebihara et al. used a capsaicinoid lozenge which dissolved in the participants' mouths prior to a meal. Piperine concentrate was also mixed with Gastrografin plus a thickening agent and resulted in significantly reduced airway invasion and shortened time to onset of laryngeal vestibule closure (Rofes, Arreola, Martin, & Clavé, 2014); however, unlike capsaicinoid, no effect on residue was identified. Last, the effects of menthol were evaluated via injection of a 1 mL menthol solution into the pharynx of older individuals and resulted in faster onset of pharyngeal swallowing (Ebihara et al., 2006).

Mixture suppression has been studied in an attempt to make a sour bolus more palatable while maintaining the positive physiologic effects demonstrated by Logemann and colleagues (1995). Mixture suppression involves the addition of a second taste (e.g., sweet) to the mixture to inhibit the impact of the first taste (e.g., sour). Pelletier and Lawless (2003) studied the impact of mixture suppression on 11 residents of a skilled nursing facility, 10 of whom had a neurogenic etiology (7 with dementia). All participants were previously diagnosed with dysphagia and were receiving thickened liquids. Participants swallowed water, high sour, and sour-sweet liquids. The high sour liquid was associated with decreased airway invasion compared with water. Both the high sour liquid and the sour-sweet liquids were associated with an increase in spontaneous dry swallows. More work is required to determine the correct balance of mixtures to maintain improved swallowing function with high-intensity sour while achieving palatability. This type of research is also required for chemesthetic agents and until then, the functional use of sour taste or other chemicals on swallowing management strategy is limited.

Thermal-Tactile Application

TTA is designed to heighten sensitivity in the central nervous system to increase the speed at which pharyngeal swallowing is evoked and was first described by Logemann (1983). Hence, TTA is recommended for patients with delayed onset of pharyngeal swallowing. The clinician is reminded from Chapter 3 that the concept of "delay" has evolved with research showing that the bolus may be in the pharynx prior to onset of pharyngeal swallowing with both single and sequential swallows in healthy adults (Chi-Fishman & Sonies, 2000; Daniels et al., 2004; Daniels & Foundas, 2001; Martin-Harris, Brodsky, Michel, Lee, & Walter, 2007; Stephen, Taves, Smith, & Martin, 2005). The presence of the bolus in the distal pharynx should be considered abnormal only when the duration of pooling affects the efficiency of the swallow or if the pooling impacts swallowing safety.

Traditionally, TTA involves the vertical rubbing of the anterior faucial arches with a chilled laryngeal mirror (Logemann, 1998), although frozen ice sticks have been used (Rosenbek et al., 1998). Ice sticks have been suggested due to the rapid temperature acceleration of a cold laryngeal mirror (Selinger, Prescott, & Hoffman, 1994). The back of the cold mirror, or ice stick, is initially placed at the base of the anterior arch, and brisk vertical up-and-down rubbing along the arch is completed five times. Both faucial arches are stimulated in this manner, followed by the swallowing of a small amount of liquid or saliva if the patient cannot have oral intake. Three to four 5- to 10-minute daily treatment sessions have been recommended (Logemann, 1998).

Research on the effects of TTA in healthy adults is contradictory, with some studies reporting no change in elicitation of the pharyngeal swallow after TTA (Ali, Laundl, Wallace, deCarle, & Cook, 1996; Bove, Mansson, & Eliasson, 1998), while another study identified increased timing of the swallow response as well as the number of swallows following stimulation (Kaatzke-McDonald, Post, & Davis, 1996).

Initiation of pharyngeal swallowing may be at its peak in healthy adults with little room for improvement; therefore, study of participants with disordered swallowing may be best to determine the effectiveness of TTA. Lazzara, Lazarus, and Logemann (1986) were the first to report on the immediate effects of TTA on faster initiation of pharyngeal swallowing in neurologically impaired patients (one-half with stroke). TTA was completed in the radiology suite with immediate rescanning of the participant to determine improvement. Results revealed improvement in the majority of patients for at least one swallow. Four patients were further studied to probe impact of TTA on subsequent swallows. Results of this pilot study suggested that the influence of TTA may last for two to three swallows. Findings of positive immediate effects of TTA in shortening the time to onset of pharyngeal swallowing were supported by Rosenbek, Roecker, Wood, and Robbins (1996). Participants were 1 month to more than 1 year post-stroke. In a treatment trial to investigate more long-term effects of TTA, a single-subject A-B-A-B (treatment-withdrawal) design was completed in seven patients with stroke who demonstrated delayed pharyngeal swallowing and airway invasion (Rosenbek, Robbins, Fishback, & Levine, 1991). Each treatment period was for 1 week, with participants receiving on average 18 trials in each of the five daily sessions. Results revealed reduced STD without change in penetration or aspiration in two participants, thus offering weak support for sustained effects of TTA. In the last of the series of studies on TTA, Rosenbek et al. (1998) studied treatment intensity ranging from 150 to 600 TTA trials distributed across 3 to 5 days. Results revealed that no one intensity level was more therapeutic than another.

Currently, results support only immediate effects of TTA, which would place it under a compensatory strategy; however, the clinician must consider the feasibility of implementing TTA during a meal before recommending it as a compensation technique. Until appropriate and feasible treatment intensity is identified and applied in a research trial, the long-term rehabilitative effects of TTA remain elusive.

VOLITIONAL CONTROL OF ORAL TRANSFER

By volitionally delaying the onset of oral transfer, swallowing is changed from an automatic behavior to a more volitionally controlled action. This is the notion behind the 3-second prep as described by Kagel in the 1980s and reviewed by Huckabee and Pelletier (1999). In the 3-second prep technique, the patient silently counts to three prior to onset of oral transfer to facilitate organized execution of oral transfer and initiation of pharyngeal swallowing. This strategy does not have direct empirical evidence to support it, but the concept has been indirectly supported by other studies with preliminary favorable results. Although they did not study the 3-second prep, Ludlow and colleagues (2005) suggested that the self-initiated coordination of a button press with onset of swallowing may improve swallowing due to central volitional control. Moreover, Daniels, Schroeder, DeGeorge, Corey, and Rosenbek (2007) evaluated the effects on bolus flow of a clinician-controlled verbal cue to swallow in healthy older adults. The participant was provided a verbal cue to swallow after placing the bolus in the oral cavity. Findings from this study as well as preliminary findings in patients with mild Alzheimer disease (Daniels, Corey, Schulz, Foundas, & Rosenbek, 2007) revealed shorter OTT and STD with a cue to swallow. Verbal cue affected bolus position at onset of timing measures, thereby influencing duration. The bolus was positioned more posterior in the oral cavity at onset of oral transit, and the leading edge of the bolus at onset of pharyngeal swallowing was superior in the pharynx for cued compared with non-cued swallows. Anecdotal reports have suggested that verbal cue to swallow may increase OTT and produce "apraxia of swallowing" in patients with a left hemispheric stroke (Logemann, 1998; Robbins & Levine, 1988; Robbins, Levine, Maser, Rosenbek, & Kempster, 1993). Thus, results must be replicated in individuals with stroke to determine whether the effects of cued swallowing, either self-initiated or clinician initiated, are beneficial or deleterious. Furthermore, 3-second prep must be directly studied in a patient population to determine the effects, if any, on specific swallowing signs of uncoordinated oral transfer or pharyngeal pooling.

BREATH-HOLDING TECHNIQUES

The supraglottic and super-supraglottic swallow maneuvers are two techniques designed to facilitate airway protection (Logemann, 1998). Airway protection is at the level of the TVF for the supraglottic swallow and at the level of the laryngeal vestibule for the super-supraglottic swallow. Breath-holding strategies may be implemented to prevent aspiration (supraglottic swallow) and/or penetration (super-supraglottic swallow) before or during swallow. In addition to airway protection, these breath-holding maneuvers can impact temporal relationships and biomechanical events during swallowing. In a study of healthy adults comparing swallows with breath-hold maneuvers to swallows without, onset of hyoid, laryngeal, and BOT movement, laryngeal closure, and BOT-PPW contact occurred significantly later with either maneuver (Ohmae, Logemann, Kaiser, Hanson, & Kahrilas, 1996). In addition, onset of airway closure at the level of the arytenoids and the TVF was significantly earlier with either maneuver compared with swallows without the maneuver; the duration of laryngeal closure and UES opening also significantly increased. In a case study of three patients with head and neck cancer treated with surgery and/or radiotherapy, BOT-PPW pressure and contact duration increased with the super-supraglottic swallow maneuver (Lazarus, Logemann, Song, Rademaker, & Kahrilas, 2002). Although impacting more than just laryngeal valving, the effects of these two breath-holding techniques have been shown to be immediate. No study has been completed to determine whether repeated use produces long-term changes in swallowing physiology.

In the supraglottic swallow, patients are instructed to hold their breath, swallow during breath-holding, and cough immediately after the swallow but before inhalation. For the super-supraglottic swallow, patients are instructed to hold their breath, bear down (this provides closure of the laryngeal vestibule), swallow while breath-holding and bearing down, and cough immediately after the swallow. It should be noted that for both maneuvers, patients are instructed to take a deep breath prior to holding their breath in the directions provided by Logemann (1998). The degree of laryngeal valving is influenced by the techniques, and instructions appear to be a critical component in attaining airway protection. A "hard" breath hold has been shown more likely to achieve maximum laryngeal valving (TVF and false vocal fold adduction, arytenoid adduction and tilting) than an easy breath hold (Martin, Logemann, Shaker, & Dodds, 1993; Mendelsohn & Martin, 1993). Further research has suggested that inhaling prior to the breath hold was least effective in attaining TVF adduction (Donzelli & Brady, 2004). The authors reported that participants abducted their TVF to take the deep breath and that although they stopped breathing, they never adducted the TVF. To ensure that the patient is achieving maximum TVF adduction, the clinician can ask the patient to phonate "ah." If vocalization is evident, the TVFs are not completely adducted.

VEES may also be used as visual feedback to achieve laryngeal valving with either breath-holding technique.

The "hard" breath hold is frequently effective in achieving laryngeal valving, as it may create a Valsalva maneuver. The Valsalva maneuver has been associated with adverse events such as cardiac arrhythmia (Metzger & Therrien, 1990). As cardiovascular disease is associated with stroke, it is important to understand the impact of using breath-holding swallowing maneuvers in patients with stroke. Chaudhuri et al. (2002) studied three groups of patients: 11 patients with a recent stroke, dysphagia, coronary artery disease (CAD); 4 patients with a recent stroke, dysphagia, no CAD; and 8 orthopedic patients, no dysphagia, no CAD. Cardiac status was monitored for 4 hours. During this time period, subjects completed a swallowing treatment session involving performing either the supraglottic swallow or the super-supraglottic swallow, a regular therapy session, and a meal. In the swallowing session, a minimum of eight swallows were completed using either technique. For the two groups with a stroke diagnosis, 87% of participants demonstrated arrhythmia during the swallowing session. The arrhythmia subsided after completion of the treatment and did not occur with other activities such as walking. In the orthopedic group, one participant exhibited bradycardia. Abnormal cardiac findings were equally evident with either maneuver. Although a Valsalva effect is created when lifting a heavy box or straining to have a bowel movement, it is brief and not repetitive, whereas with swallowing using a breath-holding technique, the Valsalva effect may be slightly more sustained and repeated over the course of therapy or a meal. Thus, it is important for the clinician to review the medical history and discuss the treatment plan with medical staff prior to implementing breath-holding techniques in patients with stroke.

BOLUS MODIFICATION

Bolus modification may involve thickening liquids or pureeing solids. The volume that a person swallows as well as the speed of bolus delivery may be controlled. In addition, the order in which different consistencies of a bolus are swallowed may be used to immediately improve swallowing. Many of these strategies are implemented due to disordered swallowing physiology; thus, effectiveness should be evaluated during the instrumental examination. On the other hand, other strategies are implemented secondary to the cognitive deficits often seen following stroke and may not require study during the instrumental evaluation. In order to identify the level of diet modification and restriction concerning oral intake recommendations, various scales are available which can be used to measure progress. These include the American Speech-Language-Hearing Association's National Outcome Measurement System (http://www.asha.org), the Functional Oral Intake Scale (Crary, Mann, & Groher, 2005), and the International Dysphagia Diet Standardization Initiative (IDDSI) Functional Dysphagia Diet (Steele et al., 2018).

Standardization of Bolus Modification

The IDDSI was recently developed to provide a global framework for dysphagia diet uniformity (Cichero et al., 2017). It involves a continuum of eight levels from liquid to solid and a standardized measurement method to ensure consistency in terms of flow and texture (http://www.iddsi.org). There are five liquid thicknesses ranging from thin liquid to extremely thick liquid and five food categories ranging from liquidized (moderately thick liquid) to regular food.

Thickened Liquids

Increased viscosity reduces bolus speed (Dantas et al., 1990). This decrease in speed should lead to improved bolus control, thereby reducing pharyngeal pooling and the depth to which a bolus travels in the pharynx until the pharyngeal swallow is elicited. This may serve to explain the evidence of reduced airway invasion during VFSS with thick liquids compared with thin liquids (Clavé et al., 2006; Clavé et al., 2008; Kuhlemeier, Palmer, & Rosenberg, 2001; Leonard, White, McKenzie, & Belafsky, 2016; Vilardell, Rofes, Arveola, Speyer, & Clavé, 2016). Thickening a liquid, however, may also increase the occurrence of residue, particularly with spoon-thick or pudding-type consistencies (Clavé et al., 2006 Clavé et al., 2008; Rofes et al., 2013; Vilardell et al., 2016). The type of thickener, xanthan gum or cornstarch, may impact swallowing safety and efficiency. Recent research suggests that gum-based thickeners may reduce the occurrence of airway invasion compared with starch-based thickeners (Leonard et al., 2016). While Vilardell et al. (2016) reported no difference in airway invasion when comparing the two types of thickening agents, they did note significantly increased oropharyngeal residue with starch-based thickeners. The interested reader is referred to a white paper from the European Society for Swallowing Disorders which provides an extensive summary of safety, efficiency, and physiological changes in swallowing with increased viscosity (Newman, Vilardell, Clavé, & Speyer, 2016).

Clinicians frequently use thickened liquids in the management of their patients with dysphagia (Garcia, Chambers, & Molander, 2005). One study evaluated the immediate effect of three compensatory strategies (nectar-thick liquid, honey-thick liquid, and chin tuck with thin liquids) in patients with VFSS-confirmed aspiration (Logemann et al., 2008). Patients were diagnosed with dementia and/or Parkinson disease. Results indicated that the honey-thick liquid was significantly more effective than either nectar-thick or thin fluids with chin tuck posture in preventing thin liquid aspiration during the VFSS. However, an equally important finding was that one-half of the patients aspirated on all three compensatory interventions. How these results translate to patients with stroke is unclear and requires further research; however, it does add even further support for using an instrumental examination to determine if a compensation technique is effective and if it has any negative effects such as increased residue.

In deciding to recommend thickened liquids, clinicians must consider three key points:

1. *Patient satisfaction/quality of life:* Patient dissatisfaction with food preparation, that is, thickened liquid or pureed diet, has been identified as highly related to patients' lack of compliance (Colodny, 2005) and reduced quality of life (Swan, Speyer, Heijnen, Wagg, & Cordier, 2015). Moreover, patients with dysphagia expressed preference for postural strategies over liquid alteration and preference for nectar-thick liquids over honey-thick liquids (Logemann et al., 2008).
2. *Risk/benefit ratio:* Concerning the risks and benefits of thickened liquids, the clinician must consider aspiration, dehydration, and fatigue. As previously discussed, aspiration occurs less often with thickened liquids compared with thin liquids with greater immediate elimination of aspiration using honey-thick liquids compared with nectar-thick and chin tuck posture management (Logemann

et al., 2008). However, no change in immediate aspiration status was evident in one-half of the patients studied. A companion study revealed a slight but non-significant increase in the incidence of pneumonia in patients randomized to receive honey-thick liquids for 3 months as compensation for thin-liquid aspiration compared with patients randomized to receive nectar-thick liquids or chin tuck posture with thin liquids over the same length of time (Robbins, Gensler, et al., 2008). Additional adverse events such as fever, dehydration, and urinary tract infection occurred more often in patients assigned to thickened liquids compared with the chin tuck, thin liquid group, but again, the differences were not statistically significant. A recent systematic review confirms that thickened liquids are not significantly associated with increased incidence of pneumonia (Kaneoka et al., 2017). The type of thickener, however, was not considered in this systematic review. Recently, researchers evaluated the effects of high volume aspiration of water, gum-based thickened liquids, and starch-based thickened liquids in an animal model (Nativ-Zeltzer et al., 2018). Significantly decreased survival rates were documented in the animals receiving the starch-based thickened liquid. Furthermore, greater pulmonary injury was evident in animals aspirating the thickened liquids, regardless of the type of thickener, compared with animals aspirating unthickened liquids. While this study involved injection of large quantities of liquid into the trachea, and thus cannot be directly compared with the occurrences of aspiration in humans, this finding taken in conjunction with less reduction in aspiration with starch-based thickeners (Leonard et al., 2016) as well as increased residue (Vilardell et al., 2016) should make clinicians strongly consider the type of thickening agent if recommending a thickened liquid.

While aspiration is associated with the development of aspiration pneumonia in patients with stroke (Holas, DePippo, & Reding, 1994; Johnson, McKenzie, & Sievers, 1993), other factors such as dependency for feeding and oral care, the number of decayed teeth, and tube feeding are more predictive of aspiration pneumonia (Langmore et al., 1998). Although an important clinical concern is prevention of aspiration, an additionally important concern is prevention of dehydration. Dehydration is not due to the thickening agent, as it does not compromise free-water content or absorption. Rather, dehydration may ensue due to palatability, with patients drinking lesser amounts of the thickened liquid compared with thin liquids (Murray, Miller, Doeltgen, & Scholten, 2014). Many foods have a high water content which can facilitate obtainment of adequate hydration; however, this must be closely monitored in patients receiving thickened liquids. Last, thickened liquids increase intrabolus pressure (Dantas et al., 1990), leading to increased effort and strength to swallow (Miller & Watkin, 1996; Nicosia et al., 2000; Reimers-Neils, Logemann, & Larson, 1994) and possibly fatigue over the duration of a meal with an overall decrease in oral intake. Thus, strong collaboration between the speech pathologist and dietician is essential if thickened liquids are recommended.

3. *Variations in thickened liquids across manufacturers, thickening agents, and VFSS liquids:* Currently, thin and thick liquids ingested during mealtime and those used in the VFSS are not correlated in terms of rheologic properties (viscosity, density, yield stress). The interested reader is referred to Bourne (2002) for a review of rheology. Findings on lack of correlation apply when barium was used as the base and material was added to achieve the desired consistency (Cichero, Hay, Murdoch, & Halley, 1997) as well as to when the mealtime liquid (i.e., water, thickened liquid) served as the base and barium was added to create a radiopaque fluid (Cichero, Jackson, Halley, & Murdoch, 2000). Both strategies are used in the clinical setting. Since these studies were completed, standardized Varibar® barium in thin liquid, nectar, thin honey, and thick honey consistencies is available in many countries. Each of these barium consistencies was shown to correlate with an IDDSI liquid classification (Steele, 2017). The IDDSI syringe flow test can be used to evaluate the characteristics of non-standardized contrast agents. While many clinicians may add thickening agents to non-standardized contrast material, many limitations of this method have been identified (Popa Nita, Murith, Chisholm, & Engmann, 2013; Steele, Molfenter, Péladeau-Pigeon, & Stokely, 2013). Moreover, it is important to note that the rheologic properties between commercially prepared pre-thickened liquids are not consistent across manufacturers or matched with Varibar® products. Given this, it would seem critical for the clinician to implement the IDDSI flow test on liquids to be ingested during mealtime if thickened liquids are recommended. As the method is quite simple, patients and/or caregivers can complete it as well.

As discussed earlier in this section, most compensatory strategies, including thickened liquids, must be evaluated for effectiveness during the instrumental evaluation (Logemann et al., 2008). Use of a thickened liquid should begin at the volume at which consistent aspiration of a thin liquid is observed. The remainder of the evaluation for liquids, including sequential swallowing, should proceed with thickened liquid consistency, as the clinician must ensure that the compensatory strategy would be effective in normal mealtime situations of self-regulated liquid volumes. The clinician should start with a nectar consistency and only proceed to thin honey and finally honey thick liquid as indicated.

Due to reduced patient acceptance and the associated increased swallowing effort with potential for fatigue, the use of thickened liquids is frequently considered a last option in swallowing management. Generally, other compensatory strategies such as chin tuck, if shown effective in the instrumental evaluation, are recommended prior to implementing thickened liquids. However, the clinician must also consider the patient's language or cognitive status, which may be severely impaired in individuals with a stroke. If the clinician is resolute that a patient's safety and oral intake is compromised without employment of a compensatory strategy for aspiration and if a patient's language or cognitive status precludes the use of compensatory postures—for example, the patient cannot consistently remember to use the posture—thickened liquids may be the only option for maintaining oral liquid intake. However, the goal should be to initiate rehabilitation to ameliorate pathophysiology and remove any restrictions as quickly as possible.

Modification of Food

A patient's ability to manipulate dense foods and solids can be evaluated with the CSE and VFSS. If mastication is poor, yielding an inability to break down food, or lingual strength is reduced and yields notable oral and pharyngeal post-swallow residual, diet alteration generally is considered. From the previous review of thickened liquids, the clinician will note that increased consistency requires increased muscular strength to propagate the bolus through the oral cavity and pharynx. Likewise, efficient mastication requires a functional set of teeth (or tough gums as is the case with some patients) and good lingual strength and movement. As with thickened liquids, diet modification is generally the last strategy implemented and if possible initiated with the least restrictive diet. Using the IDDSI framework for modifying food texture, the order of least to most restrictive would be: (1) soft and bite-sized, (2) minced and moist, (3) pureed, (4) liquidized (http://www.iddsi.org). The IDDSI website describes various tests to determine food categories. Especially when more restrictive diets, such as pureed or liquidized, are recommended, the clinician must be concerned about decreased acceptance, which may lead to reduced intake.

When post-swallow residual in the oral cavity or pharynx is the sign observed, the use of a dry swallow or cyclic ingestion would be a more optimal compensatory strategy compared with diet alteration. In the instrumental evaluation, the clinician should note the patient's spontaneous initiation of a dry swallow to clear residual prior to asking the patient to swallow his or her saliva. If this does not clear the residue, cyclic ingestion, which involves alternating ingestion of liquids and semisolid/masticated solid consistencies to facilitate clearing of post-swallow residual, should be attempted.

Volume and Rate of Delivery

The evaluation of swallowing generally is initiated with small liquid volumes to prevent aspiration of large quantities. If aspiration is consistent with a certain volume, compensatory intervention generally is initiated before increasing the volume. However, the reader may recall from earlier chapters that increased volume is associated with decreased OTT and STD in healthy adults (see Table 3–1) and provides increased sensory input. No study has been completed to determine whether increased volume can have a therapeutic benefit for specific swallowing pathophysiology.

Current practice frequently regulates volume of liquid ingestion for delayed pharyngeal swallowing or reduced oral control if preswallow pooling with airway invasion is observed. Volume regulation may be completed on a global level with recommendation for small sips or it may be more exact by recommending a prescribed volume. Commercially available cups and straws that allow regulation of the volume ingested are available. These cups and straws have not been studied in terms of maintenance of volume over time, prevention of aspiration, or patient acceptance. In patients with a stroke who may be too cognitively impaired to self-regulate volume, volume regulation cups and straws may be helpful.

Impulsive behavior, which is frequently evident in patients with right hemispheric or frontal stroke, may impact the pre-oral and oral phases in that the patient takes too large a bite of a solid or continually stuffs food into the oral cavity without swallowing between each bite. This may lead to more concerns of asphyxia versus aspiration. With patients such as this, the underlying issue is cognition, not impaired swallowing physiology. For these patients, a team approach to patient management is critical. Mealtime supervision may be recommended, but this should not be considered treatment that is provided by the clinician. Rather, the dysphagia team must review and agree on eating/feeding strategies, and appropriate staff, such as the nursing assistant, should provide supervision and daily monitoring of the meal. If swallowing pathophysiology is not identified in a patient such as this, then the clinician can concentrate solely on cognitive deficits, which in time should impact eating behavior.

Rate of presentation may include single versus sequential swallowing. Currently, it is unclear whether sequential swallowing may improve certain dysmotility patterns evident with single swallows. By sequential swallowing, it is meant that a person continuously completes multiple swallows of a larger volume (e.g., 50–100 mL) as described by Chi-Fishman and Sonies (2000) and Daniels et al. (2004). Although these studies identified longer STD and PTT compared with single swallows, a cyclic elevation and partial lowering of the hyolaryngeal complex between swallows was identified for many participants. Chi-Fishman and Sonies suggested that as sequential swallowing has distinct biomechanical and sensorimotor properties such as bolus flow momentum, prolonged sensory stimulation, and heightened motor responsiveness, it may serve as a compensatory strategy. Research is indicated to identify whether specific types of swallowing disorders are facilitated by sequential swallowing. If implemented for the wrong disorder, the risk of aspiration could be greater, as the patient is self-administering large liquid volumes.

19 Principles of Rehabilitation for Oropharyngeal Dysphagia

The evolution of our clinical approaches to the management of dysphagia is bringing us to a point of exciting discoveries. Initially, as we struggled in both clinical practice and research to understand fundamental swallowing biomechanics, we developed a series of compensatory techniques that allowed for an immediate reduction in risks. As discussed in Chapter 18, these techniques are valuable for short-term risk management and will continue to hold an important place in the clinical armamentarium.

The rehabilitation of swallowing pathophysiology, although not new, has finally come into prominence in research and clinical practice. In the first edition of this text in 2008, we allocated 48 pages to rehabilitation. This increased to 60 pages in the second edition, published in 2014. Finally, in this third edition, 4 chapters and 84 pages are required to satisfactorily cover the topic of rehabilitation. Rehabilitation has finally come into a place of prominence in our practices.

As we develop greater sophistication in our understanding of dysphagia, both at a biomechanical level and at a neural level, we ultimately develop greater specificity in patient management. We are understanding that all dysphagia is not due to weakness and that the pharyngeal "reflex" is actually more of a response that can be manipulated and modulated by volitional, cortical control. Thus, in this third edition of *Dysphagia Following Stroke*, the subsequent chapters reflect rehabilitation modalities that target the peripheral sensorimotor system (Chapter 20), including widely used strengthening and the newer albeit controversial peripheral stimulation techniques, and the central control system (Chapters 21–22), detailing exciting new developments that are emerging into clinical practice. Central change will be discussed through the lens of extrinsic modulation, with stimulatory approaches such as repetitive transcranial magnetic stimulation and transcranial direct current stimulation (Chapter 21) as well as intrinsic modulation, including behavioral approaches classified as

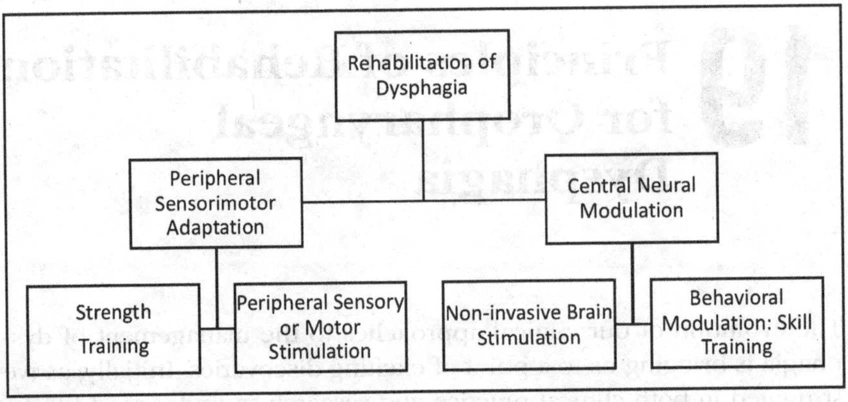

Figure 19–1. Framework for classification of rehabilitation approaches.

the broad description of skill training (Chapter 22) (Figure 19–1). This chapter will review current thoughts on concepts impacting rehabilitative effectiveness, including the need for refinement of differential diagnosis, treatment dose, and perhaps more relevant to the chapters on central change, concepts of neural plasticity.

DIAGNOSTIC PRECISION FOR REHABILITATIVE EFFECTIVENESS

For any given treatment, some patients with swallowing impairment may not respond with improved function. There is often a presumption that the lack of progress is patient centered, e.g., the patient "failed" to respond to treatment, by virtue of degree or nature of impairment, lack of capacity, or lack of motivation. However, perhaps the error lies not in the patient, but in the clinician and the clinical inaccuracy of diagnosis. This would consequently lead to improper selection of rehabilitation approaches. Emerging research in the rehabilitation of the patient with dysphagia is making it increasingly clear that diagnostic precision is a mandate for rehabilitative effectiveness. Greater diagnostic specificity, therefore, may ultimately lead to improved patient outcomes. However, our classification system of pathology in dysphagia diagnosis is rudimentary compared with other areas of rehabilitation medicine, where pathology can be classified by the nature of underlying impairment, such as a spastic dysarthria or an ataxic gait.

The videofluoroscopic swallowing study (VFSS) is largely considered the gold standard in evaluation of deglutition as it can visualize all stages of swallowing as an integrated process (Rugiu, 2007) and has been utilized in research and clinical practice for over 30 years (Logemann, 1998). Although impaired biomechanics may be dynamically observed, this technique cannot provide information on the underlying nature of impairment, such as weakness, spasticity, apraxia, or other neuromuscular change. Timing can be precisely measured, but we have no methods to delineate if errors in timing are centrally generated—a disorder of motor programming—or if timing errors reflect inadequacy in peripheral execution—the central command is executed without flaw but peripheral motor deficits restrict timely recruitment of muscle activation. This lack of specificity is also problematic in understanding mechanisms of peripheral force generated on the bolus. A failure to generate adequate force for bolus propulsion does not automatically equate to peripheral muscle weakness but may reflect peripheral muscle *hyper*function that inhibits range of motion or a central motor planning deficit in activating end-point muscle recruitment. Unfortunately, we have no clinically practical method of differentially diagnosing peripheral weakness versus neural activation for motor execution, thus we rely solely on surrogate measures, such as observation of bolus flow on VFSS or pressure measures from pharyngeal manometry. These do not measure muscle contraction directly but rather are produced from muscle contraction.

The expansion of diagnostic modalities may provide some clarification, if not to rule out weakness as much as to rule in another underlying etiology. Huckabee, Lamvik, and Jones (2014) reported a manometric investigation of 16 patients presenting with diffuse pharyngeal residue, routinely interpreted as a symptom of weakness when swallowing. Manometry identified mis-sequenced timing of pressure generation in the pharynx, despite relatively normal generation of force, as measured by amplitude of pressure generation. This impaired sequencing of force generation occurs within a 200-msec time frame, and thus cannot be visualized on VFSS alone. Although undoubtedly a valuable tool, the widespread dependence on VFSS in isolation appears to impose a bias toward misinterpretation of pharyngeal bolus residual to be a consequence of "weakness" and, therefore, development of a preponderance of strength-based rehabilitation options.

To further complicate matters, much of the research that evaluates the effectiveness of rehabilitation strategies has initially, and sometimes exclusively, been conducted in healthy participants. As a first step, this is critical, so that we can evaluate relative safety and understand adaptability of biomechanics under optimal conditions before we seek to understand the influence of impairment of biomechanical flexibility. Clearly, in rehabilitation of the patient following stroke, optimal conditions are rarely encountered. Patients admitted following stroke are frequently unwell, easily fatigued, and cognitively compromised and present with lesions that disrupt motor planning and neural transmission. Consequently, much of our rehabilitation research never transitions to scrutiny in the population for whom it was intended. As such, there is a limited evidence base for many of our commonly used treatment options. Further, many rehabilitation practices presumed to be well established in our field have been investigated by only one research group, without replication, or did not specify or include subjects to demonstrate only the physiological impairment or resulting sign for which the intervention is targeting. It is, therefore, no surprise that these trends are mirrored in clinical practice. In a survey of dysphagia rehabilitation practices in the United States (Carnaby & Harenberg, 2013), responses from speech pathologists (n = 254) provided with clinical and instrumental data revealed that five of the seven most recommended swallowing techniques could be classified as strengthening exercises. Importantly, only 3.9% of respondents reported deriving recommendations from a physiologic abnormality.

Refinement of our rehabilitation approaches, the research that supports them, the scientists that explore them, and the clinicians that use them is critical. There are data to suggest that both compensatory and rehabilitative techniques have substantial potential for both benefit and harm. The technique of effortful swallowing has certainly seemed benign enough and has been applied regularly as both a compensation to facilitate bolus clearance during swallowing and a rehabilitative exercise to strengthen pharyngeal contraction. However, multiple studies have identified mixed outcomes for the effect of effortful swallowing on pharyngeal pressure generation, and research has offered the suggestion that this technique may inhibit anterior hyoid movement (Bülow, Olsson, & Ekberg, 1999, 2001, 2002) as well as increase pharyngeal residual (Molfenter, Hsu, Lu, & Lazarus, 2018) and contribute to disrupted timing in swallowing (Huckabee et al., 2014). It is critical to understand the impact that targeted rehabilitation has on the pharyngeal swallowing response overall. As pharyngeal swallowing is a highly orchestrated response, isolating targeted aspects can have unintended effects on the gestalt, as reported, for example, with increased nasal redirection as a presumed result of an effortful swallowing paradigm (Garcia, Hakel, & Lazarus, 2004). Although replication of this work is needed, these data suggest the need for caution and careful evaluation before implementation of rehabilitation plans. We are learning that swallowing does not require maximal muscle contraction and may not need significant unused muscle reserve; in some patients, strengthening may be the wrong approach.

Expansion of rehabilitation approaches beyond peripheral muscle change then requires consideration of the possibility of central change. If we question the role of peripheral muscle weakness in producing swallowing impairment, we might alternately speculate that impaired biomechanics would be considered a deficit of swallowing motor control and generated from compromise in the central nervous system. A growing corpus of research is emerging regarding the use of techniques in swallowing rehabilitation that can be classified as neuro-modulatory; this will be further discussed in Chapters 21 and 22. These central approaches target a change in the brain in a very specific manner, but the consequent effects on swallowing are a nonspecific by-product of altered neural function. For example, there is no specific protocol or approach to specifically address delayed pharyngeal response that is different from an approach for reduced upper esophageal sphincter opening. Appreciating the complexity of the oropharyngeal swallowing response, this leads to a further question. Can we develop options that change swallowing behavior first, in a physiologically specific manner, with a consequent effect on the brain that will ensure a neurophysiologic change which encodes and sustains improved function such that it is resistant to detraining?

PRINCIPLES OF NEURAL PLASTICITY

As discussed in Chapter 2, neural plasticity and potential maladaptive cortical plasticity are receiving increased attention (Humbert & German, 2013; Kleim & Jones, 2008; Malandraki, Johnson, & Robbins, 2011; Martin, 2009; Robbins, Butler, et al., 2008; Takeuchi & Izumi, 2012). Neural plasticity refers to the adaptive capacity of the central nervous system to reorganize its neural circuitry as a result of experience (Kleim & Jones, 2008). This is critical when developing rehabilitation approaches designed to modulate cortical responses to neurological impairment. There are 10 principles of neural plasticity, itemized in Table 19–1. For a comprehensive discussion, the reader is encouraged to review Kleim and Jones (2008) or Robbins, Butler, et al. (2008). While all principles impact rehabilitation of oropharyngeal dysphagia, select key principles will be discussed in greater detail below.

Use and Specificity of Practice

Three key principles of neural plasticity include the concepts of "use or lose it," "use it and improve it," and "plasticity is experience specific" (Robbins, Butler, et al., 2008). As discussed in Chapter 17, patients experiencing a period of non-use, such as patients deemed unable to eat safely by mouth, may have reduced motor recovery after stroke for that function (Takeuchi & Izumi, 2012). Simply put, if a neural substrate is not active, its function can degrade. Thus, limited use of the oropharyngeal swallowing mechanism after neurologic impairment may reduce activation of neural substrates, thereby potentially impeding long-term outcomes, contrary to the principles promoting neural plasticity (Robbins, Butler, et al., 2008).

Table 19–1. Principles of Neural Plasticity

1. Use It or Lose It
2. Use It and Improve It
3. Specificity
4. Repetition Matters
5. Intensity Matters
6. Time Matters
7. Salience Matters
8. Age Matters
9. Transference
10. Interference

Source: Kleim and Jones, 2008.

What we know from these principles is that not only should we be "using" swallowing but attempting to improve it as well. While simply swallowing may prevent against loss of function, it may not necessarily improve swallowing in a person with dysphagia. Indeed, it may do little more than reinforce an abnormal behavior pattern. As stated by Robbins, Butler, et al. (2008) "although neural plasticity may result in a behavioral change, not all behavioral change necessarily involves neural plasticity" (p. S277). Goals for improvement should center on maximizing cortical activation. With a preponderance of intervention approaches that target increasing strength of the peripheral muscles, we need to look to novel methods that focus on central change to remediate oropharyngeal dysphagia and inhibit the development of maladaptive patterns. Strengthening exercises will likely still have a place in patients with weakness or in patients who need to acquire a baseline level of strength to perform a skill. However, tasks focused on skill-based elements of swallowing, such as improving the timing or accuracy of task, may be more in line with the "use it and *improve it*" principle of neural plasticity. With ongoing research, we may find further refined methods to establish greater potential for skill, with specific swallowing skill exercises rather than typical strengthening-based approaches. This will be further discussed in Chapter 22.

Dose: Repetition, Time, and Intensity Matter

A subset of the principles of neural plasticity center on dose, or the specific elements structuring rehabilitation, including frequency of trials, intensity of input, and duration of intervention. Historically, in clinical training, the issue of treatment intensity is given little attention. A cursory review of several texts on the provision of clinical service in speech pathology reveals no mention of dose issues or treatment intensity. However, the issue of "dose" of service delivery in all rehabilitation domains is critical. For example, limb literature has revealed that it is possible to "overuse impaired extremities in a manner that worsens function. This seems to require both an extreme amount of use and that the overuse occur during an early vulnerable period" (Kleim & Jones, 2008, p. S230). However, there also appears to be a threshold of intensity to induce plasticity. Low-intensity treatment is unlikely to result in optimal results (Robbins, Butler, et al., 2008). Even within-treatment intensity is a seldom-discussed aspect of rehabilitation. Clinicians are encouraged to count the number of trials completed in a single session—the results may surprise you! Due to typical scheduling constraints and low-intensity repetitions during sessions, it may be subsequently difficult to determine if a patient is deemed a treatment failure—perhaps this is actually a service delivery failure. Did the treatment not work, or was it not executed frequently enough to manifest clinical change? It is well understood that resource allocation may hinder the provision of intensive treatment (Robbins, Butler, et al., 2008). However, short bursts of intensive treatment may indeed produce more favorable outcomes and, therefore, decreased costs compared with protracted treatment offered at a much lower intensity. It becomes an issue of prioritization and scheduling. This issue translates to research activity as well. There is pressure to document efficacy of dysphagia management practices using randomized controlled trial studies. However, the evaluation of treatment efficacy is inherently encumbered by the evaluation of treatment intensity. One cannot assess efficacy without attending to dose. Although we have a string of studies, outlined below, that document positive effects of treatment, these studies were conducted at a set dose level; generally, all were completed at a fairly intensive level of treatment. Adequate studies have yet to be published to compare intensities and determine whether positive effects can be gained from a less intensive approach.

There is a pronounced lack of data regarding optimal dose of rehabilitation. However, the fundamental tenets of intensive rehabilitation utilizing the principles of neural plasticity are supported by rehabilitation research, with reports of positive clinical outcomes (Kleim & Jones, 2008; Murray, Ashworth, Forster, & Young, 2003; Robbins, Butler, et al., 2008). A systematic review revealed intensive multidisciplinary rehabilitation was associated with reduced odds of mortality (odds ratio, 0.66), institutionalization (odds ratio, 0.70), and dependency (odds ratio, 0.65) (Langhorne & Duncan, 2001). Despite this, evidence from McNaughton, McRae, Green, Abernethy, and Gommans (2014) revealed only 50% and 51% of rehabilitation units in their study achieved 1 hour per weekday of direct therapist-patient contact time and stated "few services . . . provide community or outpatient rehabilitation more than 2 or 3 days per week" (p. 17). This is in stark contrast to evidence-based recommendations for rehabilitation to have a minimum intensity of 45 minutes per day, for each discipline.

Not only is rehabilitation typically offered with insufficient intensity, there is often little guidance in the research or justification for

Table 19–2. An Informal Survey of Dysphagia Rehabilitation Session Frequency

Health Care Setting	***Average Number Visits per Week and Duration of Sessions (range)***
Acute hospital	Highly variable; as needed for diagnosis and compensation
Post-acute rehabilitation	3.8 sessions at 32 min (3 sessions at 20 min to 5 sessions at 45 min)
Outpatient clinic	1.3 sessions at 43 min (1 sessions at 30 min to 2 sessions at 55 min)
Community therapy	0.06 session at 38 min (1 session every 6 months at 30 min to 1 session at 20 min)

clinicians as to why they develop specific treatment plans. An informal survey of 16 clinicians from 10 regional hospitals and rehabilitation centers in two countries was conducted by one of the authors. Clinicians were asked, "On average, how often do you see your patients for dysphagia intervention?" These findings are summarized in Table 19–2. When consequently asked, "How did you determine this schedule?" the overwhelming response from clinicians was that the treatment schedule was initially determined by administrative issues and resource availability and secondarily by what was thought to be best for the patient. No clinician in this limited sampling referred to the literature as a basis for her/his treatment frequency decisions.

A Look to the Literature

Our colleagues in other areas of physical medicine and rehabilitation also have work to do in investigating dose effects. Remarkably few studies could be identified in a search of the literature. Sterr and associates (2002) evaluated two treatment intensities of constraint-induced movement therapy (CIMT). Fifteen adults with chronic hemiparesis secondary to stroke who were receiving CIMT for 90% of waking hours were randomized to receive CIMT with 6 hours of direct training or 3 hours of direct training per day for 14 days. Both groups demonstrated improved motor function, but the 6-hour training schedule was significantly more effective for improving motor function in this study population.

Coming closer to home, Denes, Perazzolog, and Piccione (1996) evaluated the influence of dose of treatment on language outcomes in 17 patients with global aphasia (>3 months post-onset) randomized to intensive or traditional treatment. Intensive treatment was defined as 5 hours of treatment per week for 6 weeks; traditional treatment was defined as 2.5 hours per week for 6 months. Both treatment groups demonstrated improvement; however, the intensive group demonstrated significantly greater gains in a shorter period of time. However, the intensive group received a greater total number of sessions (130) compared with the traditional treatment group (60). Thus, the positive results are clouded by the inconsistency in design.

A second series of studies was published by Hinckley and Craig (1998). This group evaluated naming skills in 40 individuals with aphasia secondary to stroke using an A-B-A treatment design. Their intensive treatment program consisted of 6 weeks of treatment at 23 hours per week. After establishing the effectiveness of this treatment protocol for improving naming skills compared with no treatment, the researchers then compared this intensive treatment approach with non-intensive therapy, defined as 6 weeks of treatment of 3 hours or less weekly at home. Significant improvements in naming ability were documented after the intensive treatment regimen. Nonsignificant improvements were achieved from the low intensity treatment period, equivalent to the no treatment period. With re-initiation of the intensive treatment regimen, repeated significant improvement in naming skills was documented.

In the dysphagia literature, we are amassing a slowly increasing body of studies to document outcomes of dysphagia intervention (Bartolome & Neumann, 1993; Carnaby, Hankey, & Pizzi, 2006; Crary, 1995; Huckabee & Cannito, 1999; Klor & Milianti, 1999; Neumann, 1993; Neumann, Bartolome, Buchholz, & Prosiegel, 1995; Robbins et al., 2007; Rosenbek et al., 1998; Shaker et al., 2002, 1997). Only two studies have compared treatment outcomes as a function of dose. Carnaby and colleagues (2006) evaluated three randomized levels of management in 306 acute stroke patients: (1) usual care as prescribed by the attending physician, (2) low-intensity intervention provided three times a week, and (3) high-intensity intervention provided at least daily. When comparing the usual care and low-intensity interventions, high-intensity therapy was associated with an increased proportion of patients who returned to a normal diet and recovered swallowing function by 6 months. Rosenbek and colleagues (1998) sought to evaluate the influence in the outcomes of treatment using thermal-tactile application (TTA). This study included 45 patients following stroke who received TTA to the faucial arches using an ice stick. Each trial consisted of stroking one and then the other faucial arch three or more times each, then instructing the patient to "swallow hard." Participants were randomized to one of four treatment groups based on number of trials of stimulation per week across 3 to 5 days for 2 weeks: 150, 300, 450, or 600 trials. Based on this study, no single treatment intensity emerged as superior.

The application of neuromuscular electrical stimulation (NMES) as a treatment for dysphagia is discussed in some detail in Chapter 20. Much of the research on this emerging modality does not address treatment dose as a variable in outcomes. The exception is offered by the Manchester research group, who have systematically evaluated dose effects (Fraser et al., 2002; Power et al., 2004). An important point emerges from this collective work. Dose can be defined by many treatment parameters: frequency, intensity, and duration of the electrical stimulus. Manipulation of all of these treatment parameters influence treatment effect. Critically, the influence can be both positive and negative.

THE TAKE-HOME POINT

Clinicians and researchers alike have considerable ground to cover to untangle the complex issues surrounding service delivery in dysphagia management. Much of our early outcome data suggest that intensive treatment is more likely to have positive outcomes on the biomechanics of swallowing. Limited data from other areas of physical medicine suggest that *more is better*. But we need to be cognizant that more may also be too much. Research on NMES suggests a potential negative influence of treatment at certain stimulation parameters. For neuromuscular strengthening, this could potentially also manifest as muscle fatigue. Very clearly, more systematic randomized controlled trials of specific techniques executed through a range of intensities are needed. Until further data are accrued and the picture becomes clearer, practicing clinicians should always question their provision of services. If outcomes are not favorable, is it the fault of the treatment, the patient, or the way in which the treatment was provided?

20 Rehabilitation of the Peripheral Sensorimotor Swallowing System

Rehabilitation approaches are those interventions which are thought to result in permanent changes in the substrates underlying deglutition when provided over time. Although many of the strengthening and sensory-based approaches in this chapter are considered clinically standard, the reader should remain thoughtful—and indeed critical—of their recommendation and application. Despite much work regarding these peripheral strengthening and stimulation techniques, "to date, the treatment effects in dysphagia are small to moderate in contrast to the much larger effects of spontaneous recovery in acute stroke" (Drulia & Ludlow, 2013, p. 254). What might account for this lack of efficacy in our rehabilitation? It is important to keep in mind that research in this area is predominantly based on studies in healthy young participants with small sample sizes and limited randomization or blinding. Further, reference to "standard dysphagia therapy" or "usual care" is often implemented as a control condition, despite limited to no consensus as what constitutes *typical care* in dysphagia rehabilitation (Carnaby & Harenberg, 2013). Most peripheral exercises or stimulation are provided in a single session or with limited trials to investigate the immediate effects, with reliance on subjective outcome measures that may be subject to bias or placebo. Questions about dose, long-term maintenance, detraining, and treatment specificity based on swallowing biomechanics remain. In the interim, what is a clinician to do? With thoughtful consideration and a close look at the evidence, recommendations can be made that are specific to biomechanics, treating each patient as his/her own case study. A review of our current rehabilitative strategies, such as peripheral muscle strengthening and peripheral sensory stimulation, is outlined below (Table 20–1).

Table 20–1. Proposed Influence of Rehabilitative Strategies for Use with Specific Signs and Underlying Physiologic Abnormalities

The Sign of	***Secondary to Physiological Abnormality of***	***Rehabilitation Approach***	***Other Considerations***
Anterior leakage Inadequate bolus preparation Inadequate bolus formation Oral residue	Poor orolingual control	Oral motor exercises: Tongue to palate pressure Tongue to tongue depressor pressure	Biofeedback devices: IOPI or other oral pressure measurement device, mirror
Pharyngeal pooling to the level of the ______	Delayed pharyngeal swallow	No known rehabilitation technique at this time	Precautions: avoid effortful swallowing
Nasal regurgitation	Poor pharyngeal motility	Skill training—pharyngeal sequencing	Biofeedback device: pharyngeal manometry or sEMG of submental muscle group Precautions: avoid effortful swallowing

The Sign of	*Secondary to Physiological Abnormality of*	*Rehabilitation Approach*	*Other Considerations*
Inadequate epiglottic deflection	Decreased hyoid movement	Head lift exercise Expiratory muscle strength training (EMST)	Head lift targets anterior hyoid movement EMST may only improve superior, rather than anterior, hyoid movement
	Intrinsic structural changes in supportive tissue	No rehabilitation techniques at this time	
Vallecular residue	Decreased base of tongue to posterior pharyngeal wall approximation	Oral motor exercises (e.g., lingual resistance) Recline exercise (unsupported head lift at 45°) Tongue hold (Masako) maneuver Effortful swallowing	Biofeedback device: IOPI or other oral pressure device for lingual resistance; pharyngeal manometry, or sEMG of submental muscle group with effortful swallowing
	Inadequate epiglottic deflection*	See rehabilitation approaches above for physiologic abnormalities resulting in inadequate epiglottic deflection	
Inadequate opening of the UES*	Decreased anterior hyoid movement	Head-lift exercise	

continues

Table 20–1. *continued*

The Sign of	***Secondary to Physiological Abnormality of***	***Rehabilitation Approach***	***Other Considerations***
Inadequate opening of the UES* *continued*	Intrinsic structural and/or functional changes in cricopharyngeus	Mendelsohn maneuver Modified catheter balloon dilatation	Biofeedback device: pharyngeal manometry or sEMG of submental muscle group with Mendelsohn maneuver Precautions: attend to hyoid movement with Mendelsohn maneuver, may wish to add head-lift exercise as prophylactic aid
Pyriform sinus residue	Inadequate opening of the UES*	See rehabilitation approaches above for physiologic abnormalities resulting in inadequate opening of the UES	Precautions: avoid effortful swallowing
Penetration	Pre-swallow pharyngeal pooling*	Refer to rehabilitation approaches associated with physiologic abnormalities underlying aspiration	
	Inadequate epiglottic deflection*		
	Inadequate supraglottic shortening/laryngeal elevation*		
	Oral residue*		
	Pharyngeal residue*		

The Sign of	***Secondary to Physiological Abnormality of***	***Rehabilitation Approach***	***Other Considerations***
Aspiration	Pre-swallow pharyngeal pooling*	Refer to rehabilitation approaches associated with physiologic abnormalities underlying inadequate true vocal fold closure	
	Inadequate true vocal fold closure	Vocal fold adduction exercises EMST Skill training—respiratory-swallowing training	Biofeedback device: nasal airflow monitoring
	Oral residue*	Refer to rehabilitation approaches associated with physiologic abnormalities underlying inadequate true vocal fold closure	
	Pharyngeal residue*		

Note. sEMG = surface electromyography, UES = upper esophageal sphincter, EMST = expiratory muscle strength training.

*Occasionally a sign will be caused by another sign, which requires the clinician to problem solve through the initial presenting physiologic abnormality.

PERIPHERAL MUSCLE STRENGTHENING

Oral Motor Exercises

For as long as speech pathologists have been engaged in the provision of clinical services, there have been concerted therapeutic efforts to increase the strength and efficiency of orolingual structures. Initially these efforts were focused on improved speech articulatory performance, with an inevitable transfer of the developed exercises to the goal of improving oral phase swallowing and presumably tongue driving forces involved in pharyngeal phase swallowing. What is fairly astonishing, however, given the prolonged use of these techniques, is the lack of sound research data to support these practices. In an historical publication on treatment of speech disorders, Van Riper (1954) commented:

> For centuries, speech correctionists have used diagrams, applicators, and instruments to ensure appropriate tongue, jaw, and lip placement. . . . If these devices and instruments have any real value, it seems to be that of vivifying the movements of the tongue and of providing a large number of varying tongue positions, from which the correct one may finally emerge. (pp. 236–238)

Sadly, in the ensuing 60+ years, we have made only small gains in quantifying treatment effects for oral motor therapy. We have many clinical descriptors of what to do but have very few studies that document the clinical outcomes of these treatment approaches.

Robbins and colleagues have initiated a research program designed to methodically address this gap in our knowledge. Using a hand-held, portable manometric device that measures lingual to palatal pressure, the Iowa Oral Pressure Instrument (IOPI), this research group initially investigated the influence of age on oral pressures (Robbins, Levine, Wood, Roecker, & Luschei, 1995). Pressures were recorded at three lingual sites (tip, blade, dorsum) during a maximal isometric task and during saliva swallows in young and elder healthy participants. Results of this work suggest that functional swallowing pressures remain similar across age groups; however, functional reserve declines with age. The authors highlight two implications. First, elderly individuals may have to work harder to produce functional pressures;

second, age-related illness, such as stroke or even systemic infection, may put elder patients at higher risk of functional impairment. These findings were confirmed and elaborated in a study by Nicosia and colleagues (2000) that replicated methods in the prior study but added an analysis of temporal characteristics of pressure generation. Again, swallowing pressures did not differ between younger and elder participants, but elders generated decreased maximal isometric pressure. Additional temporal analysis of these data also suggests that elders require increased time to reach peak pressure. This supports the earlier supposition that elders have to work harder to reach functional swallowing pressures and that they utilize what the researchers refer to as a pattern of "pressure building," in which multiple lingual gestures are recruited to reach peak pressure.

Additional studies by this research group have sought to evaluate the influence of rehabilitative efforts on generating increased functional reserve. In the first study of this kind, Robbins and colleagues (2005) designed a prospective study of 10 healthy elder participants (aged 70–89) who underwent an 8-week progressive lingual resistance exercise program. Using the videofluoroscopic swallowing study (VFSS) to document functional change and measures of oral lingual pressure, researchers documented that all subjects significantly increased both isometric and swallowing pressures. Additionally, a subgroup of 4 participants who underwent magnetic resonance imaging of the tongue produced an increase in lingual muscle volume averaging 5.1%. This study offers encouragement from a small treatment sample that oral-lingual exercises are effective in elderly individuals. Lazarus, Logemann, Huang, and Rademaker (2003) also sought to evaluate the influence of tongue strengthening exercises in healthy participants. However, instead of relying only on the IOPI, this group compared performance in 31 healthy young adults after participating for 1 month in one of three treatments groups: (1) no exercise, (2) standard tongue strength exercises using a tongue depressor, and (3) exercise using the IOPI. Data from this study suggest that both of the active exercise groups demonstrated substantially greater gains in tongue strength compared with the no exercise group but the type of exercise did not significantly influence outcome. Thus, at least in healthy participants, intervention to strengthen oral function does not appear to be dependent on instrumentation.

A further study was completed by Clark, O'Brien, Calleja, and Corrie (2009) to evaluate specific principles of motor learning as they relate to orolingual strength training. Specifically, the authors evaluated translation of strength training in one movement domain to another domain, isolated versus combined exercise, and detraining effects. This randomized trial assigned 39 healthy participants to receive either a sequential or concurrent lingual strength training protocol for a period of 9 weeks. Lingual strength exercises consisted of lingual elevation, protrusion, and lateralization. Data from this study suggest that orolingual exercises increase labial strength, irrespective of the type of task or whether tasks are completed in isolation or concurrently. Within 2 to 4 weeks following termination of the treatment protocol, significant decreases in lingual strength were noted, highlighting a limitation of strengthening approaches.

The influence of lingual exercise has been evaluated with specific reference to patients with dysphagia subsequent to stroke. In an early study, Robbins and colleagues (2007) recruited 10 patients with stroke to an 8-week intervention program of isometric lingual exercises using the IOPI as a biofeedback device. As in healthy elders, patients with stroke in this study increased maximum isometric pressures and increased swallowing pressures for some trials and some bolus conditions. Using VFSS as an outcome measure, oral transit time was decreased and pharyngeal response duration was increased. Postswallow pharyngeal residual was decreased for all textures. However, reductions of residual specifically in the oral cavity, valleculae, and pyriform sinuses were not statistically significant. The Penetration-Aspiration (P-A) Scale (Rosenbek, Robbins, Roecker, Coyle, & Wood, 1996) documented decreased aspiration. These biomechanical changes were associated with reports of improved quality of life measured with the SWAL-QOL questionnaire (McHorney et al., 2002) and increased tolerance of diet textures.

This study was followed by a randomized trial investigating differences in tongue strength and functional swallowing outcomes in patients ($n = 11$) with dysphagia following stroke (Steele et al., 2016). Participants were randomized to one of two treatment groups; no control group was reported in this study. One group received "Tongue-Pressure Profile Training," in which the goal was to improve posterior tongue pressure by swallowing saliva with effort and releasing tongue pressure gradually. The second group received "Tongue-Pressure Strength and Accuracy Training," with treatment tasks divided into a strength goal, namely, generating pressure of at least 80% of their maximum isometric pressure, and an accuracy target, where participants were instructed to hit a pressure goal as close as possible to a randomly chosen target (discussed further in Chapter 22). Both groups were seen intensively with 24 sessions of tongue-pressure resistance training, two to three times weekly, with 60 repetitions in each session of the tongue-pressure task. While tongue pressure was noted to improve as a result of the intervention, there were no significant differences between the two treatment groups. Further, VFSS outcomes revealed no significant difference in stage transition duration on thin liquid trials or measures of the P-A Scale. This highlights another potential limitation of strength training in that increases in strength, in this case measured by pressure, do not necessarily transfer to improved function.

Schaser, Ciucci, and Conner (2016) investigated the impact of intensive lingual exercise on neuroplasticity, as well as de-training effects using a young and old rat model ($n = 80$). In this study, rats were trained to lick an aluminum disk in order to drink water. The disk was fitted with a force transducer that measured tongue strength. The resistance from this disk was incrementally increased as the rats demonstrated improved lingual strength over an 8-week period; they were compared with a control group who used a similar licking maneuver but without resistance. Measures of detraining were collected 2 and 4 weeks following the exercise training. Results indicated that lingual strength increased significantly compared with the control group ($p < 0.001$). Old rats demonstrated significant detraining 4-weeks after the exercise regimen; however, were able to maintain gains above their baseline level. Interestingly, only old rats demonstrated an increase in markers for neural plasticity (e.g., brain-derived neurotrophic factor), which was significantly lower after the 2- and 4-week detraining period. No changes in markers for neural plasticity were seen in young rats. This study has important implications for translation to human populations, such as the development of specific maintenance programs. Further, this highlights the limitation of peripheral muscle strengthening; it is a method to increase muscle hypertrophy but may have limited ability to drive neuroplastic change at a central level.

As lingual strengthening relies on reliable measures of tongue pressure session-to-session, reliability of tongue-pressure measurement is an important concept to explore. While much research has documented acceptable levels of reliability (e.g., agreement greater than 0.75) using the IOPI (Clark, Henson, Barber, Stierwalt, & Sherrill, 2003; Lazarus et al., 2000), there is concern regarding the reliability of this technique in aging and impaired populations. Evidence from patients is limited; Solomon, Clark, Makashay, and Newman (2008) found interrater reliability of the IOPI suboptimal in patients with dysarthria (intraclass correlation [ICC] = 0.54). Subsequent to this, Adams, Mathisen, Baines, Lazarus, and Callister (2015) evaluated the reliability of tongue force and endurance in elderly adults ($n = 30$), aged 79 to 97 years. Results indicated that while posterior tongue strength was the more reliable measure (ICC = 0.77–0.84) compared with anterior strength (ICC = 0.58–0.77), measures of tongue endurance were not reliable. Similar research has identified further differences as a function of sex, bulb placement, and provision of visual feedback of results, so careful clinical application is necessary to accurately utilize existing normative data (Vanderwegen, Guns, Van Nuffelen, Elen, & De Bodt, 2013). These differences, however, are not apparent in all studies (Peladeau-Pigeon & Steele, 2017). Further evaluation of reliability in elderly and impaired populations is indicated to understand the impact of interrater and test-retest reliability with this technique.

It is important to note that while existing studies predominantly train tongue-to-palate contact, clinicians regularly employ a variety of other techniques and use other devices for which no data are currently available. Significant research is needed to document the efficacy of oral lingual exercises on functional swallowing ability in stroke. As with all exercises, larger sample sizes and treatment controls are required to document efficacy. Additionally, the influence of natural recovery needs to be extricated from experimental data. We have no evidence to suggest that the provision of oral lingual exercise can be contraindicated to functional swallowing and may indeed be helpful. However, it is important to bear in mind that "although maximum isometric pressures decline with age, swallowing pressures are preserved. This begs the question whether increasing tongue strength is an optimal treatment goal for tongue-pressure resistance training programs" (Steele et al., 2016, p. 453).

Effortful Swallowing

The effortful swallow was first introduced by Kahrilas and colleagues (Kahrilas, Lin, Logemann, Ergun, & Facchini, 1993; Kahrilas, Logemann, Krugler, & Flanagan, 1991; Kahrilas, Logemann, Lin, & Ergun, 1992) as a compensatory technique. Very simply, the individual is instructed to swallow "with effort." Early work by these researchers suggested that increased effort in swallowing would result in immediate increased pressure on the bolus and thus decreased pharyngeal residual. Thus, this technique was routinely applied as a compensation for patients with pharyngeal motility disorders. In subsequent years, effortful swallowing has been included in routine clinical rehabilitation, despite conflicting reports of its effects on the biomechanics of healthy and impaired swallow function (Bülow, Olsson, & Ekberg, 1999, 2001, 2002; Garcia, Hakel, & Lazarus, 2004; Molfenter, Hsu, Lu, & Lazarus, 2018). Fortunately, a fairly large body of evidence has been acquired to guide our clinical practice and increase our specificity in using this technique.

The first of three research projects by Bülow et al. (1999) suggested a potential complication with this technique. They documented that effortful swallowing resulted in decreased hyomandibular distance *before* the swallow, presumably as a type of preparatory set for increased effort. However, *during* the swallow, this technique resulted in reduced laryngeal excursion and decreased overall anterior hyoid movement for airway protection and upper esophageal sphincter (UES) opening. This potential contraindication biomechanically makes sense and thus raises significant concerns. A relatively small group of floor of mouth muscles (anterior belly of digastric, mylohyoid, geniohyoid) pull the hyoid forward during swallowing, whereas the larger and longer posterior suprahyoids (posterior belly of digastric, stylohyoid) and the bulk of the middle pharyngeal constrictor pull the hyoid posteriorly. Execution of an effortful swallow does not allow increased effort within isolated muscles; rather, all muscles are presumably recruited with increased effort. Thus, the results of Bülow and associates can certainly be explained by posterior suprahyoid muscles overriding the small anterior suprahyoid muscles with a subsequent cumulative decrease in anterior hyoid movement.

Bülow et al. (2001) sought to expand their investigation of effortful swallowing in patients with moderate to severe pharyngeal phase dysphagia. Based on this research, effortful swallowing resulted in no change in the number of misdirected swallows, although depth of penetrated material into the larynx was reduced. In addition, despite the presumed effect of effortful swallowing, they curiously documented no change in pharyngeal retention on VFSS. In an extension of this work, Bülow et al. (2002) evaluated intrabolus pressure in the distal pharynx and identified no significant increase in peak amplitude or duration of intrabolus pressure. No comment was made on hyoid movement in these two subsequent studies.

Certainly, if these studies withstand the scrutiny of replication, the findings may substantially change the way we apply rehabilitation techniques. For example, in the case of vallecular residual, if this sign is caused by decreased base of tongue (BOT) to posterior pharyngeal wall (PPW) approximation, effortful swallowing may be the treatment of choice. However, if the sign is caused by decreased epiglottic deflection secondary to poor anterior hyoid movement, effortful swallowing could potentially exacerbate the underlying physiologic abnormality and worsen the presentation. Additionally, if a patient presents with impaired cricopharyngeal opening secondary to poor anterior hyoid movement, effortful swallowing to increase pharyngeal motility through the distal pharynx may not only hinder hyoid movement but also may not be effective for its proposed intent.

Hind, Nicosia, Roecker, Carnes, and Robbins (2001) contributed different findings to the discussion on effortful swallowing using VFSS and oral pressure measurement with the IOPI in healthy adults. This group documented increased oral pressure with effortful swallowing and a trend toward decreased oral residual; however, they did not evaluate pharyngeal pressure. They also documented increased *duration* of maximal anterior hyoid excursion, laryngeal vestibule closure, and UES opening. Increased superior, but not anterior, hyoid movement was detected with this technique.

A further contribution was offered by Huckabee, Butler, Barclay, and Jit (2005), who evaluated submental surface electromyography (sEMG) and pressure at the proximal and distal pharynx and within the UES in 22 healthy participants. This study documented increased sEMG amplitude in submental muscles and, contrary to the findings of Bülow and colleagues (1999, 2001, 2002), increased pharyngeal manometric pressures with effortful swallows compared with noneffortful swallows. Of particular relevance to the Bülow et al. studies, this finding was more substantial in the lower pharynx compared with the upper pharynx, suggesting that contributions of the pharyngeal constrictors are increasingly responsible for pressure generation under effortful conditions than increased BOT retraction. Additionally, although sEMG and pharyngeal pressure amplitude increased, there was no correlation between these two measures. Recognizing that these two measures evaluate different mechanisms, the authors speculated that instructions for completing effortful swallowing may influence the degree of pharyngeal pressure generation. Bülow and colleagues (1999), who identified no increase in pharyngeal pressure, instructed participants to "swallow very hard while squeezing the tongue in an upward-backward motion toward the soft palate" (p. 69). These instructions are similar to the instructions provided by Hind and researchers (2001), who documented increased oral pressure. Other studies that have documented contradictory increased pharyngeal pressure have used instructions simply to "swallow hard" (Huckabee et al., 2005; Kahrilas et al., 1991, 1992, 1993). The question was raised as to whether targeted increased orolingual pressure occurred at the expense of pharyngeal pressure.

This speculation gave rise to another study, which sought to evaluate the contribution of lingual movement in pharyngeal pressure generation. Huckabee and Steele (2006) not only evaluated submental sEMG and pharyngeal pressure, but also evaluated oral pressure generation in 20 healthy participants who completed non-effortful swallows as well as effortful swallows under two conditions: tongue emphasis and tongue inhibition. The authors hypothesized by emphasizing superior tongue to palate approximation; tongue to pharyngeal wall retraction would be inhibited, thus explaining the controversial finding of Bülow et al. (1999, 2001, 2002). Contrary to expectations, effortful swallowing produced greater measurement at all five sensors (sEMG, two for oral pressure, two for pharyngeal pressure), with the tongue-to-palate emphasis condition producing greater measured amplitude and pressure than the tongue-to-palate inhibition condition. Thus, these data do not contribute to an explanation of discrepancies in pharyngeal pressure data across studies but tend to support the finding that the effortful swallow increases pharyngeal pressure generation and that emphasizing tongue-to-palate approximation appears to increase the motor drive for pharyngeal pressure.

Other data exist that document temporal influences of effortful swallowing on pharyngeal biomechanics. The first research on this topic was a study of 10 healthy participants presented by Olsson, Kjellin, and Ekberg (1996). The primary finding in this study was that duration of pressure at the tongue base was longer than that measured low in the pharynx during execution of this technique. This led the authors to suggest that an individual who is experiencing increased vallecular residue may best benefit from this technique, whereas an individual with pyriform sinus residue may not and vice versa. In the previously discussed study by Hind et al. (2001), effortful swallowing was found to elicit increased duration of pharyngeal response, maximum anterior hyoid excursion, laryngeal vestibule closure, UES opening, and total swallowing duration. These data suggest that effortful swallowing prolongs most swallowing-related events, either as a mechanism to increase strength or as a concomitant process.

Hiss and Huckabee (2005) confirmed the finding of longer duration of pharyngeal pressure with effortful swallowing in healthy participants but with the additional caveat that greater prolongation of pressure was observed in the proximal pharynx compared with the distal pharynx. Additionally, this study identified that onsets of pharyngeal pressures and UES relaxation were delayed relative to the onset of submental sEMG contraction during performance of the effortful swallow and offered the suggestions that effortful swallowing thus should be carefully considered in patients with coexisting delayed onset of the pharyngeal swallow. Steele and Huckabee (2007) clarified this information by peak of sEMG and pharyngeal pressure rather than onset. As before, longer overall durations of oral and pharyngeal pressure events were recorded during effortful swallowing compared with non-effortful. However, shorter (rather than prolonged) latencies were documented from *peak* submental sEMG contraction to *peak* pressures during the effortful swallow. Fritz and colleagues (2014) utilized dynamic magnetic resonance imaging to evaluate specific pharyngeal biomechanics during effortful swallowing in healthy women ($n = 20$). Although this technique required participants to remain in a supine position, thus potentially altering biomechanics, effortful swallowing was found to both significantly reduce pre-swallow pharyngeal area and increase the duration of pharyngeal closure, similar to previous findings (Hiss & Huckabee, 2005; Olsson et al., 1996).

Importantly, reports of negative consequences as a result of effortful swallowing are present in the literature. Garcia et al. (2004) reported a case study of a 12-year-old patient seen following brainstem tumor resection resulting in chronic, severe dysphagia. Eight months post-surgery, the patient was instructed in effortful swallowing. Shortly thereafter, the patient began experiencing significant nasal redirection when swallowing, despite trial use of a palatal lift and adequate velar movement when swallowing on VFSS. Due to nasal redirection on 100% of trials, the effortful swallow maneuver was untrained, with focus on teaching an effort*less* swallow. The authors reported the frequency of nasal redirection steadily declined, observed in less than 10% of trials following two weeks of effort*less* swallowing. The authors caution that signs of dysphagia (e.g., nasal redirection) may not always represent physiologic abnormalities (e.g., reduced velopharyngeal closure) and potential maladaptive applications of compensations and rehabilitation should be considered. Similarly, Molfenter et al. (2018) compared effortful and non-effortful swallowing conditions in healthy elderly individuals, greater than 65 years of age ($n = 44$). VFSS was the primary outcome measure to analyze timing parameters such as UES opening duration, swallowing kinematics including pharyngeal constriction, as well as bolus trajectory including residue and airway invasion. All swallows were coded and randomized for blinded analysis. Result indicated significantly prolonged duration of all temporal variables during effortful swallowing, including laryngeal closure duration, hyoid movement duration, UES opening duration, and pharyngeal transit time. Importantly, the researchers also found increased pyriform sinus residual during effortful swallowing, coupled with reduced pharyngeal shortening. Taken together, the authors summarize their findings by stating "it appears that [effortful swallowing] prolongs the amount of time the bolus is in the pharynx, but not the amount of time for the bolus to be swept through the UES; a phenomenon which may contribute to the manifestation of pyriform sinus residue" (Molfenter et al., 2018, p. 386).

Until clarity is found, there are reasonable data to suggest that effortful swallowing increases pharyngeal pressure, particularly in the distal pharynx, and increases duration of pressure in the upper pharynx. Data suggest that increased pressure may be facilitated by emphasizing tongue-to-palate contact during execution of the maneuver. There are also reasonable preliminary data, paired with a logical biologic plausibility, that effortful swallowing runs the risk of inhibiting anterior hyoid movement and pharyngeal shortening, which may contribute to possible increased pharyngeal residual. A thoughtful rehabilitation program may pair this technique with the Shaker exercise that is designed specifically to increase anterior hyoid movement. The resulting treatment approach would presumably accomplish a goal of increasing pharyngeal pressure generation while concomitantly addressing anterior hyoid movement either prophylactically or as a therapeutic target. Finally, with a documented increased latency of onset and increased duration of pharyngeal pressure, there may be implications against using this technique in patients with delayed pharyngeal swallowing.

Similar to the compensatory breath-holding maneuvers discussed in Chapter 18, Gomes and colleagues (2016) investigated the impact of effortful swallowing on heart rate and cardiac regulation in a group of healthy women ($n = 34$) with no significant cardiac, cardiovascular, respiratory, or medical history. Participants performed effortful swallows in a training protocol for a period of 5 minutes; heart rate variability was compared with a baseline rest period. The researchers found acute increases in sympathetic cardiac activation, which warrant replication in a more diverse sample to further clarify clinical significance of this finding. In the interim, however, as with the breath-holding maneuvers, it may be beneficial for the clinician to discuss an effortful swallowing treatment plan with medical staff prior to implementing in patients with a significant cardiac history.

Mendelsohn Maneuver

As with the effortful swallow, the Mendelsohn maneuver was initially presented as a compensatory mechanism to facilitate bolus transfer through the UES. Execution of the technique requires an individual to initiate a pharyngeal swallow and, at the peak of hyolaryngeal complex (HLC) excursion, maintain suprahyoid contraction before relaxing and completing the swallow. Prolonging suprahyoid contraction presumably prolongs UES opening to facilitate improved bolus flow. In more recent years, this technique has been applied as a rehabilitative maneuver, with the assumption that repetitive exercise results in overall improved cricopharyngeal compliance and more efficient bolus transport. No specific data are available to this effect.

The first published report of this technique was proffered by Logemann and Kahrilas (1990). This case report documented the biomechanical effects of a series of swallowing maneuvers in a single patient with dysphagia subsequent to lateral medullary infarct. Based on this report, execution of a Mendelsohn maneuver improved swallowing efficiency greater than twofold over other techniques. The following year, Kahrilas and researchers (1991) published a manofluorographic investigation of this technique. In a sample of 10 healthy participants, they documented increased duration of anterior and superior excursion of the larynx and hyoid, thereby delaying closure of the UES. This would suggest an increase in duration of HLC displacement, but not an increase in degree of anterior displacement of the HLC. This is an important distinction. Miller and Watkin (1997) confirmed the finding of prolonged contraction using a real-time ultrasound study of lateral pharyngeal wall movement during execution of the Mendelsohn maneuver. This group documented increased duration of lateral pharyngeal wall movement compared with normal swallowing for this technique. In a study by Bodén, Hallgren, and Witt Hedstrom (2006), 10 healthy volunteers with no history of swallowing complaints were evaluated with manofluorography during execution of the Mendelsohn maneuver. With this maneuver, pharyngeal peak contraction and contraction duration were increased, suggesting not only prolonged contraction but also increased contraction of the pharyngeal muscles involved in swallowing.

Much of the research, with the exception of the initial case report offered by Logemann and Kahrilas (1990), evaluates the immediate (e.g., compensatory) influence of the Mendelsohn maneuver on the swallowing of healthy controls. However, McCullough and colleagues (2012) sought to evaluate the long-term cumulative effects of the Mendelsohn maneuver in patients with swallowing impairment. Using a within-subject crossover design, 18 patients with dysphagia secondary to stroke received 2 weeks of twice daily rehabilitation using sEMG as a biofeedback modality to master execution of the Mendelsohn maneuver. Durational measures of swallowing physiology based on analysis of VFSS were used as outcome measures. Spatial measures were not evaluated. Significant changes were documented in the duration and hyoid excursion immediately following 2 weeks of treatment; these changes were not maintained after 2 weeks of no treatment. A nonsignificant increase was noted for the resulting duration of UES opening immediately post-treatment, which diminished following the no treatment period. Although the data tend to suggest positive improvements, it is unclear whether this demonstrates a rehabilitative effect that changes underlying physiology or just sustained execution of maneuver swallowing.

A follow-up analysis of these data was consequently undertaken to evaluate spatial characteristics of swallowing (McCullough & Kim, 2013). Eighteen outpatients between 6 weeks and 22 months post-stroke were enrolled in a prospective crossover design study for 2 weeks of treatment consisting of execution of Mendelsohn maneuvers with sEMG as a biofeedback modality, followed by 2 weeks of no treatment. Rehabilitation effects were evaluated using VFSS. Specifically, data regarding maximum hyoid elevation, maximum anterior HLC excursion, and maximum UES opening were analyzed. Hyoid elevation was the only measure found to significantly change as a function of treatment, although nonsignificant changes were observed for anterior

HLC excursion and UES opening. Of interest, these authors evaluated the correlation between spatial measures and identified that the correlations increased significantly as a function of treatment, which they infer to reflect increased coordination in swallowing (McCullough & Kim, 2013). These data provide some evidence of rehabilitative effect but raise a critical question; namely, did the changes arise secondary to the Mendelsohn maneuver, or did the use of biofeedback as an adjunct to treatment provide a skill-based training effect that extends beyond the exercise itself?

Similar findings were documented by Doeltgen, Ong, Scholten, Cock, and Omari (2017), who investigated pharyngeal and esophageal response to implementation of the Mendelsohn maneuver in healthy participants (n = 12) with simultaneous sEMG and high resolution manometry (HRM). Participants were provided training for completion of the Mendelsohn maneuver using sEMG as visual biofeedback until mastery was evidenced through independent review by two clinicians. Simultaneous sEMG and HRM was recorded during non-effortful swallowing, followed by effortful swallowing and the Mendelsohn maneuver. Peak pharyngeal pressure and pharyngeal contractile integrals were increased in maneuver swallows compared with non-effortful swallows. The duration of UES opening was significantly faster from the onset of swallowing, but, interestingly, UES opening duration was significantly shorter during the Mendelsohn maneuver. Further, there was no change in any other UES measurement, including UES maximum admittance, relaxation pressure or UES peak pressure. Findings from the Doeltgen et al. study were mirrored in an analysis of the effects of the Mendelsohn maneuver using 320-row area detector computed tomography (CT) in healthy young females (n = 9) (Inamoto et al., 2018). This type of CT scanning provides unparalleled spatial and temporal resolution and is the only currently available method for accurately measuring cross-sectional area of the UES. Although the authors found significantly prolonged duration of hyoid excursion, velopharyngeal closure, epiglottic inversion, and closure of the laryngeal vestibule, there were no significant differences in timing measures of UES opening. Further, there was no significant difference in cross-sectional area of the UES during the Mendelsohn maneuver. It appears that previously held beliefs that the Mendelsohn prolongs or enhances UES opening is, at best, only inconsistently supported by the evidence.

This is further complicated by concerns that this maneuver may impede esophageal peristalsis, further impacting bolus flow (O'Rourke et al., 2014). In a group of healthy adults (*n* = 10), assessment of the Mendelsohn maneuver with HRM revealed significantly more failed or non-peristaltic esophageal swallows following the Mendelsohn maneuver (66% of trials) compared with normal swallowing (53%) or effortful swallowing (33%) conditions. Additionally, there was an increase in esophageal intrabolus pressure during Mendelsohn maneuver swallows, creating a temporary outflow obstruction. Similar findings were documented in the abovementioned study by Doeltgen and colleagues (2017). Based on simultaneous sEMG and HRM data, proximal esophageal contractile integrals were significantly lower during Mendelsohn maneuvers in healthy participants compared with both effortful swallowing and non-effortful swallowing conditions. In patients with concomitant reduced esophageal motility or outflow obstructions, the Mendelsohn maneuver may worsen esophageal peristalsis and bolus flow.

Mastering the Mendelsohn maneuver will challenge both the patient and the clinician. The technique is not easy to accomplish; however, implementation of biofeedback modalities may help increase understanding and accurate completion of this task. VFSS appears to be the most effective biofeedback modality for ensuring accurate completion of the Mendelsohn maneuver; however, this approach is rarely feasible given the radiation exposure, cost, and accessibility (Azola et al., 2015). In most research published to date, the Mendelsohn has been taught to patients with sEMG as the biofeedback method of choice. In a recent study, however, Azola and colleagues found no correlation in a small group of three patients with dysphagia following stroke between submental sEMG and hyolaryngeal kinematics as measured by VFSS, and only moderate correlation in a group of healthy participants (*n* = 21), which was variable based on the sampling frequency used with sEMG (e.g., 1–10 Hz). These findings raise concerns that sEMG may not be accurately reflecting the desired motor response when patients are learning or approximating a Mendelsohn maneuver.

Importantly, further research is needed in larger subgroups of patients following stroke to clarify existing clinical practices. Taken in light of the work on effortful swallowing by Bülow and colleagues (1999, 2001, 2002), attention to hyoid movement during execution of this technique will be important. There are no data that implicate reduced degree of hyoid movement; indeed, the data suggest a nonsignificant increase in anterior hyoid movement (McCullough & Kim, 2013) and duration (Inamoto et al., 2017). However, as a type of effortful swallow, this technique is presumed to increase contraction of pharyngeal constrictor muscles. Until more robust data identify that hyoid movement is not susceptible to inhibition from this technique, the prudent clinician will want to consider carefully before prescribing this technique. As with effortful swallowing, a patient with prominent pyriform sinus residual secondary to impaired hyoid movement may be better served with a technique focused on increasing anterior hyoid movement, such as the Shaker exercise. Further, ongoing research is needed to clarify if the Mendelsohn maneuver has any positive impact on UES opening duration. Current evidence supports a more rapid onset of UES opening, yet this is dampened by scant evidence to support increased UES opening duration or diameter, compounded by reductions in esophageal peristalsis (Doeltgen et al., 2017; Inamoto et al., 2017; O'Rourke et al., 2014). Other treatment modalities, such as modified catheter balloon dilatation discussed later in this chapter, may be a more efficacious behavioral intervention for UES opening to facilitate improved bolus flow until further evidence in patient populations becomes available.

Masako Maneuver

Our development of rehabilitation strategies is becoming increasingly intelligent in more recent years as our attention shifts to restoring swallowing function rather than compensating for impairment. To support our more global strengthening techniques of effortful swallowing and Mendelsohn maneuver, clinical researchers have begun a more systematic analysis of impaired biomechanics with techniques designed specifically to address those impairments. The Masako maneuver, or tongue-hold maneuver, is the first of these techniques. The identification of this technique was based on work by Fujiu, Logemann, and Pauloski (1995), who documented that patients who have undergone BOT resection for cancer have consistently greater anterior movement of the PPW as a biomechanical compensation. Based on this finding, Fujiu and colleagues suggested a technique, which mimics this disorder, thereby forcing the PPW to increase activation during swallowing. Individuals are instructed to "protrude the tongue maximally but comfortably, holding it between the central incisors" (p. 24).

In a clinical trial, Fujiu and Logemann (1996) documented that in 10 healthy participants, the technique resulted in significantly increased anterior bulging of the PPW but with no significant change in temporal features of swallowing biomechanics. The authors were careful to advise that use of the technique concomitantly inhibits BOT posterior retraction, thereby resulting in increased pharyngeal residual. Thus, the technique should be considered a targeted exercise for increasing PPW movement, rather than a compensatory technique.

Lazarus, Logemann, Song, Rademaker, and Kahrilas (2002) evaluated the application of this technique in a small population of three patients with BOT resection. In this manofluorographic study, increased BOT-to-PPW contact pressures were recorded during maneuver conditions compared with those during non-maneuver swallows. This increased hypopharyngeal pressure is remarkable given that BOT structures were resected and suggests substantially increased anterior movement of the PPW to approximate residual structures. Doeltgen, Witte, Gumbley, and Huckabee (2009) sought to further clarify pressure generation using this technique. Contrary to the findings seen in the patient population, an evaluation of 40 healthy individuals revealed that the tongue-hold maneuver produced no change in pressure generation at the level of the upper and mid-pharynx, while producing significantly lower pressure in the UES. Hammer, Jones, Mielens, Kim, and McCulloch (2014) analyzed the Masako maneuver using simultaneous intramuscular EMG and HRM in 8 healthy individuals. Though there was no significant increase in pharyngeal pressure on HRM, intramuscular EMG recordings documented increased activation both before and during the swallow in the submental muscles, genioglossus, and superior pharyngeal constrictors. This may provide early proof-of-concept that the Masako maneuver is providing activation of desired muscle groups, but importantly, this study utilized only a single test session to investigate immediate effects.

Oh and colleagues (2012) report a single-blind randomized controlled study of the Masako maneuver as an intensive exercise regimen. Twenty young, healthy volunteers completed a four-week training program completing the Masako maneuver every 5 seconds for 20 minutes. Their progress was compared with a control group who were cued to swallow without a tongue-hold with the same frequency. Interestingly, results indicated no significant change on any outcome measure evaluated by VFSS, including pharyngeal constriction ratio, HLC movement, or movement of the PPW. It will be of substantial interest to the application of this technique in patients with stroke-related dysphagia to elucidate if increased pressure during execution of the technique is a consequence of anatomic change or functional change. To date, this research is not available.

In summary, the Masako maneuver is presented as a focused technique designed to increase contribution of the PPW during swallowing. Evidence does not currently support improvements using this technique in healthy, young volunteers (Oh et al., 2012); however, patients with BOT resection presented with immediate changes in both structure and consequent function (Lazarus et al., 2002). Further research is needed to elucidate the effect of the technique on individuals with impaired swallowing but intact anatomy, as seen following stroke. The identification of techniques that are specific to a given pathophysiology allows for potentially improved patient outcomes; however, care should be taken that in isolating increased function in one aspect of swallowing, we do not inadvertently compromise other aspects in the delicate balance required for swallowing. Given that this technique is specifically designed to increase contribution of the pharyngeal constrictors, and the middle pharyngeal constrictors have attachments to the cornu of the hyoid, attention to hyoid movement will be important.

Head-Lift Exercise

Another example of increased specificity in rehabilitative approaches is seen in the head-lift, or Shaker, exercise. First identified by Shaker and colleagues (1997), this exercise consists of lying supine and completing a series of head lifts three times per day for 6 weeks. Individuals are instructed to raise the head "high enough to observe the toes" and sustain this movement for 1 minute in the supine position. This is repeated three times. This is then followed by 30 repetitions of briefly raising and lowering the head.

Importantly, this exercise is not a swallowing-related task. The head-lift exercise is designed specifically for increasing UES opening through increased strength of the anterior suprahyoid muscle group. Two published EMG studies have documented this effect demonstrating increased amplitude in the supra- and infrahyoid muscle groups

(Alfonso, Ferdjallah, Shaker, & Wertsch 1998) and fatigue in the submental muscle group (Ferdjallah, Wertsch, & Shaker, 2000) suggesting increased work with this exercise.

The initial clinical study by Shaker and colleagues (1997) provided documentation of the effect of the technique in 31 healthy elderly participants. Two treatment groups were enrolled: one group completed a sham exercise, and the other completed the head-lift exercise for 6 weeks. Manofluorographic analysis revealed no change in any dimension of swallowing after the sham exercise; however, those completing the head-lift exercise demonstrated increased laryngeal excursion, increased width and duration of UES opening, and decreased intrabolus pressure within the UES. A crossover design then documented similar findings in those originally assigned to the alternate treatment group.

A subsequent study was completed to evaluate the effects of the exercise in individuals with chronic dysphagia, all of whom were tube fed. Shaker and colleagues (2002) published a clinical report of 27 patients with specific impairment of UES opening using the same research design. After 6 weeks of exercise, significant improvement was noted in UES opening and anterior laryngeal excursion as well as resolution of post-swallow aspiration. All participants were able to resume oral feeding.

Easterling, Grande, Kern, Sears, and Shaker (2005) published a study that was designed to evaluate treatment compliance for a rehabilitation program incorporating the head-lift exercise. A group of 26 older adults without dysphagia were asked to perform the exercise and complete a questionnaire related to their performance. Four participants underwent pre- and post-treatment VFSS. The authors acknowledged that compliance was an issue; only slightly over half of those enrolled were able to complete the program. However, those who stayed in the program attained the treatment goals of increasing anterior hyoid and laryngeal excursion and UES opening.

Research has posited that poor compliance may be related to difficulty performing this maneuver from a supine position, compounded by difficulty performing this exercise in some patients with limited neck mobility (Koshi, Matsumoto, Hiramtsu, Shimizu, & Hagino, 2018; Mishra, Rajappa, Tipton, & Malandraki, 2015). Mishra and colleagues evaluated the efficacy of a 45° position (with the head unsupported) termed "the Recline Exercise" for completion of a 6-week head-lift regimen, as compared with standard supine positioning, in healthy young adults ($n = 40$). There were no differences in the level of adherence, likely due to the sample consisting of a young, healthy cohort. Further, there were no differences in submental sEMG across both groups, but improved lingual strength was identified in the recline group. Koshi and colleagues subsequently evaluated the impact of the head-lift exercise when used with backrests at varying angles, including 0°, 15°, 30°, and 45°. Backrest angles were randomly assigned to a group of young ($n = 10$) and elderly ($n = 10$) women. Participants were asked to complete the head-lift exercise (30 repetitions and a 1-minute isometric hold) at each angle and rate their perceived level of exertion; muscle activation was assessed using sEMG. Interestingly, five elderly women could not complete the desired number of repetitions in a fully supine 0° position, yet 30° appeared to be the most comfortable backrest angle without any significant differences in sEMG activity in the submental muscles or sternocleidomastoid muscle compared with 0°. In contrast to the study from Mishra and colleagues, Koshi et al. found significantly lower muscle activation in the 45° position. Taken together, there may be potential for use of a semi-reclined position (e.g., 30°); however, these results require validation in patient populations prior to broad clinical application.

A recent study evaluated the influence of head-lift exercise specifically on thyrohyoid muscle shortening (Mepani et al., 2009). Sixteen patients with UES dysfunction were randomized to receive traditional swallowing therapy or the head-lift exercise. Thyrohyoid shortening was evaluated using VFSS. In those participants assigned to the head-lift exercise, thyroid distance increased significantly compared with those participants in the traditional therapy group. The authors conclude that UES opening augmentation secondary to the head-lift exercise is the result of combined increased thyrohyoid shortening and suprahyoid strengthening. This was followed by a study from Park, Hwang, Oh, and Chang (2017), who documented improvements in superior hyoid movement and P-A Scale scores in a group of patients with dysphagia following stroke compared with the control condition, following a 4-week head-lift exercise program.

Recent adaptation of the principles of the head-lift exercise has led to the development of chin tuck against resistance (CTAR) exercise (Yoon, Khoo, & Liow, 2014). CTAR uses the resistance provided by an inflated rubber ball during a chin tuck maneuver to aid in strengthening the submental muscle group. Research has shown that during the task itself, the CTAR and the Shaker exercise both activated the submental muscles on sEMG; however, CTAR was found to have significantly greater contraction amplitude in healthy young individuals (Sze, Yoon, Escoffier, & Liow, 2016; Yoon et al., 2014). Importantly, existing evidence of the CTAR reflects single session results from healthy individuals, rather than response to a multi-week exercise regimen in a patient population; therefore, careful ongoing research will be necessary for further validation of this technique.

To summarize, emergence of the head-lift exercise has offered significantly greater options for addressing swallowing pathophysiology than is commonly observed in dysphagia subsequent to stroke: that of decreased anterior hyoid movement. As this exercise is not completed within the context of functional swallowing, concerns are not presented for adverse compensatory biomechanics. Additionally, this exercise does not require substantial cognitive load or motor control to complete, as is the case with the Mendelsohn maneuver. In many cases of dysphagia secondary to stroke, this technique may ultimately be the first-line rehabilitation approach given the importance of adequate hyoid movement on the cascade of pharyngeal biomechanics that follows.

Expiratory Muscle Strength Training

Effective function of the oropharyngeal neuromuscular system is obviously critical for safe swallowing and has thus been the target of rehabilitation efforts. However, other subsystems support the swallowing process either directly or indirectly. A steady stream of research has emerged regarding the clinical application of expiratory muscle strength training (EMST) on swallowing biomechanics. This very promising approach is quickly emerging into widespread clinical use. With a strong foundation of supportive data, it is taking a prominent place in the repertoire of rehabilitation strategies for the patient with dysphagia.

EMST was originally described in the respiratory medicine literature (Gosselink, 2002; Smeltzer, Lavietes, & Cook, 1996), but it has been adapted for speech and swallowing rehabilitation purposes through the efforts of Sapienza and colleagues (Kim & Sapienza, 2005; Sapienza & Wheeler, 2006; Silverman et al., 2006). EMST utilizes a calibrated device consisting of a mouthpiece and a one-way, spring-loaded valve. Although variation exists in the literature, in general the exercise consists of blowing into the device through the mouthpiece with sufficient effort to release the valve; the valve remains opened as long as air pressure continues. These training breaths are typically repeated in 5-breath blocks, 5 times a day, every day for a period of 5 weeks, followed by a maintenance program. The device is calibrated and adjustable, thus resistance can be increased as appropriate to achieve therapeutic goals.

Early work by Sapienza, Davenport, and Martin (2002) focused not on swallowing but on the novel goal of increasing pressure support in high school band students. High-intensity, low-repetition expiratory training was completed daily for 2 weeks using four sets of six breaths with the device set at 75% maximum expiratory pressure. Significantly increased expiratory pressure was reported within 2 weeks of initiating training. Given the confirmation of a positive training effect in this study, further research was conducted on healthy adults to gauge the training and detraining effects relative to treatment dose. Thirty-two participants, divided into two duration-of-treatment groups, underwent EMST with accumulation of outcome measures pre-treatment, immediately post-treatment, and again after 8 weeks without treatment. All participants demonstrated increased maximum expiratory pressure over baseline measures, regardless of treatment duration.

With the goal of direct application of this modality to improving swallowing biomechanics, Wheeler, Chiara, and Sapienza (2007) investigated the activation of the submental muscle group as a function of EMST. Given the importance of this muscle group in anterior hyoid movement and subsequent effects on pharyngeal physiology, increased activation of these muscles would suggest a specific and direct influence of this treatment on swallowing biomechanics. The timing and amplitude of submental muscle activity was evaluated using surface EMG in 20 healthy participants. Participants performed a saliva swallow and a water swallow with expiratory pressure at 25% and 75% of maximum expiratory pressure. As hypothesized, EMST increased activity in the submental muscle complex. Furthermore, detailed study of exercise effects in healthy participants was documented by Wheeler-Hegland, Rosenbek, and Sapienza (2008). This research was followed by evaluation with simultaneous HRM, sEMG, and intramuscular EMG in 2 healthy participants during EMST at three pressure levels, including sham, 50% of maximum expiratory pressure, and 75% of maximum expiratory pressure (Hutcheson, Hammer, Rosen, Jones, & McCulloch, 2017). As the EMST load increased, results indicated there was a similar increase in velopharyngeal closure and pharyngeal EMG, with activation of submental muscles primarily in preparatory activity prior to the EMST task. This provides important proof-of-concept research to further explain observed benefit of this non-swallowing task on pharyngeal biomechanics.

With indication of treatment effects in healthy participants, several research works have addressed application of this technique in patients with neurologic disorders, including the stroke population. A study by Silverman et al. (2006) documented treatment outcomes of 28 patients with moderate to severe Parkinson disease during the "on" state of medication. Data from this pilot study suggest that respiratory muscle weakness may be amenable to EMST with the consequent potential for improved respiration, swallowing, cough, and speech production. An additional study of a single patient with Parkinson disease was conducted by Saleem, Sapienza, and Okun (2005). A 20-week EMST program resulted in increased maximum expiratory pressures of 50% by the fourth week of training, with an eventual increase of 158% over the 20-week treatment protocol. After discontinuation of treatment, total maximum expiratory pressure decreased 16%. A large randomized, blinded, sham-controlled trial of 60 patients with Parkinson disease was conducted by Troche et al. (2010). Those receiving the target intervention of EMST achieved greater post-treatment hyoid movement and reduced P-A Scale scores. Pitts and colleagues (2009) documented improved compression phase duration, expiratory phase rise time, and cough volume acceleration following EMST in patients with Parkinson disease. A second study evaluated the influence of EMST on cough in healthy but sedentary elderly participants (Kim, Davenport, & Sapienza, 2009), with similar findings. Two further studies have evaluated the influence of EMST on cough and speech production in individuals with multiple sclerosis, both demonstrating positive outcomes (Chiara, Martin, Davenport, & Bolser, 2006; Chiara, Martin, & Sapienza, 2007). Of particular relevance to airway protection was the finding of increased maximal voluntary cough in patients with moderate levels of disability.

With regard to stroke, Hegland, Davenport, Brandimore, Singletary, and Troche (2016) evaluated cough and swallowing function in patients with stroke (n = 14) following EMST. Importantly, patients with stroke were excluded if they presented with a stroke etiology of dissection, known cardiac valve thrombosis, or unstable or evolving stroke lesion, as EMST can raise intracranial pressures. The researchers were blinded to whether data were from pre- or post-EMST outcome testing. Results indicated 85.7% of participants completed the EMST home program, and participants demonstrated significant improvements in cough strength. Regarding swallowing, VFSS results revealed improved initiation of the pharyngeal swallow and laryngeal vestibule closure. Interestingly, there were no significant improvements in P-A Scale scores and no change in measures of voluntary cough airflow. Reflexive cough, however, was found to be more sensitive following training as measured by urge to cough in response to capsaicin stimulus following EMST.

Randomized trials have subsequently been completed comparing EMST to "usual dysphagia therapy" (e.g., combination approach implementing an array of strengthening exercises and compensatory techniques) in patients with stroke; yet, these studies appear to be limited by subjective outcome measures and unequal treatment dose (Eom et al., 2017; Moon, Jung, Won, Cho, & Cho, 2017). However, Park, Oh, Chang, and Kim (2016) implemented a sham EMST device in a randomized, controlled trial of EMST in patients with dysphagia following stroke ($n = 27$). Both groups received the EMST (using a loaded device or a sham device) in addition to 30 minutes of "traditional dysphagia therapy" consisting of strengthening exercises and compensatory techniques. The EMST group demonstrated improvements in submental muscle activity as measured by sEMG, alongside improvements in P-A Scale scores for liquids; however, no respiratory outcomes were measured.

In a systematic review of randomized controlled trials investigating respiratory muscle training in patients following stroke, Gomes-Neto and colleagues (2016) reviewed eight studies. Pooled results revealed no serious adverse effects; the majority of studies utilized an inspiratory muscle training paradigm. As above, inspiratory muscle training may be more preferable for use in acute stroke as inspiration is not related to increasing intracranial pressures compared with expiratory strength training. A subsequent meta-analysis of inspiratory and expiratory muscle training after stroke revealed that inspiratory muscle strengthening was able to achieve an increase in maximum inspiratory pressure by 16% compared with sham (Menezes et al., 2016). However, expiratory muscle strength training was able to increase maximum expiratory pressure by 22% compared with sham. Importantly, this meta-analysis found that respiratory training reduced respiratory complications, but there was no mention of neurologic complications in utilizing this approach in acute stroke. Until research can clarify this point, it may be beneficial for the clinician to discuss the treatment plan with medical staff prior to implementation, taking specific caution with acute patients, as well as patients with a stroke etiology of dissection, known cardiac valve thrombosis, or unstable or evolving stroke lesion.

EMST is an exciting development in rehabilitative research for swallowing impairment. With an emphasis on strengthening the respiratory subsystem underlying swallowing, one would anticipate that further research will document improved capabilities for airway protection and clearance in the stroke population, for whom generalized weakness may reflect poorly on airway protection. With positive effects on velopharyngeal closure, pharyngeal EMG, and potentially floor of mouth muscles, future research may also support the use of this approach for other biomechanical deficits in pharyngeal swallowing. Which patient populations and under which conditions these improvements are evident have yet to be fully identified. In the interim, clinicians are well advised to keep an eye on the literature and anticipate further clarification of benefits of this treatment in the management of dysphagia following stroke.

PERIPHERAL SENSORY STIMULATION

Similar to peripheral muscle strengthening, peripheral sensory stimulation seeks to produce lasting change in the oropharyngeal swallowing response through nonelectrical and electrical provision of sensory stimuli. Non-electrical sensory stimulation techniques include novel methods such as modified catheter balloon dilatation of the UES. Sensory enhancement approaches, including temperature, taste, smell and carbonation, are discussed in Chapter 18.

Electrical stimulation approaches have largely utilized application of submental and suprahyoid electrodes, termed neuromuscular electrical stimulation (NMES). Application of NMES as a modality for swallowing rehabilitation perhaps marked the first step down the slippery slope into neural modulation for speech pathologists treating swallowing impairment, discussed further in Chapters 21 and 22. More recently, however, application of intraluminal electrical stimulation through direct contact to the pharyngeal mucosa has been investigated with pharyngeal electrical stimulation (PES). The excitement generated by these electrical stimulation techniques has traveled quickly, and as a result, techniques such as NMES have entered clinical practice well ahead of research to justify its application. This is not an uncommon pattern in clinical service delivery; however, it bears repeating that all neuromodulatory interventions are invasive and have potential contraindications that should be considered (Martino & McCulloch, 2016).

Modified Catheter Balloon Dilatation

As discussed in Chapter 23, dilatation of the UES is a surgical intervention designed to mechanically facilitate increased opening of the UES and/or esophagus during deglutition. The ability of the UES to finely open or close serves critical protective mechanisms both to enable intra-swallow bolus transit in relaxed states and protect against retrograde bolus movement in tonic states. Conventional dilatation is a passive procedure whereby the UES is forcibly stretched open at rest; e.g., while the muscle is contracted. Although this stretching may lower resistance to bolus flow at the level of dilatation, tissues can tear and become scarred, which may prevent adequate closure. This method, however, has been adapted in recent years to more closely align with theoretical understanding of swallowing. Termed "modified catheter balloon dilatation," this approach combines volitional swallowing while a catheter balloon of increasing diameter is pulled through the UES to pair the desired response of UES opening with peripheral sensory feedback. No dilatation should occur when the muscle is in its state of tonic contraction. Lan et al. (2013) first proposed this rehabilitation technique as a means to improve UES opening and coordination of pharyngeal and UES biomechanics in dysphagia following stroke. In early studies, this approach was found to improve UES opening on VFSS and oral intake as measured subjectively using the Functional Oral Intake Scale (Dou et al., 2012; Lan et al., 2013), as well as improvement in manometric parameters including higher pharyngeal pressure and increased duration of UES nadir pressure (Lan et al., 2013). The authors theorize that as the catheter travels through the UES during volitional swallowing, it provides a rehabilitative effect to not only retrain specific swallowing biomechanics but elicit neuroplastic change.

In a prospective, controlled study, Wei et al. (2017) randomized patients with dysphagia as a result of brainstem stroke ($n = 30$) into two treatment groups to investigate changes in excitability of cortical projections as a result of implementation of modified catheter balloon dilatation. The treatment and control groups completed daily rehabilitation for an hour per day, 5 days per week for a total of 3 weeks. The control group intervention consisted of a combination of conventional exercise-based interventions, including effortful swallowing, Mendelsohn maneuver, and supraglottic swallowing. All participants in the control group had a nasogastric tube in situ for the duration of the study. The experimental group completed the modified dilatation program, which consisted of 30 minutes of modified balloon dilatation and 30 minutes of conventional therapy implemented in the control group. To achieve modified dilatation, the catheter balloon was inserted into the nares and swallowed below the level of the UES by the participant. Once the placement was confirmed, the balloon was inflated with 3 mL of water and pulled out slightly so the balloon was noted to have resistance, inferior to the lower margin of the UES. The participant was then instructed to swallow, while the researcher pulled the balloon through the UES during the swallow. This was then repeated five to eight times per session, with the balloon diameter increasing systematically each day by increasing the volume of water by 0.5 to 1 mL daily to a limit of 9 mL. Outcomes included pre- and post-treatment VFSS and bilateral submental motor evoked potentials (MEPs). The MEPs were stimulated by bilateral motor cortex transcranial magnetic stimulations; raters were blinded to participant group. Results indicated no significant pre-treatment differences between the groups; however, there was a significant improvement in UES opening diameter ($p = 0.03$), maximum hyoid displacement ($p < 0.01$), and submental MEP amplitude ($p = 0.02$) in the modified dilatation group compared with controls. These results serve as preliminary evidence that modified dilatation may not only improve specific biomechanical aspects of pharyngeal swallowing in dysphagia following stroke but may be linked with improved neuroplastic change. The peripheral sensory stimulation of the gradually increasing catheter balloon may provide more robust sensorimotor feedback to corticobulbar centers. These results are worthy of replication and further analysis.

Air-Pulse Stimulation

A different type of peripheral stimulation technique under investigation is air-pulse stimulation. The effects of this technique on swallowing have been investigated in a series of studies on healthy adults (Lowell et al., 2008; Sörös et al., 2008; Theurer, Bihari, Barr, & Martin, 2005; Theurer, Czachorowski, Martin, & Martin, 2009). Repetitive air pulses are delivered to the peri-tonsillar region via plastic tubing housed in a silicone mouthpiece that covers the mandibular dental arch. Studies identified increased swallowing frequency of saliva in young (Theurer et al., 2005) and older adults (Theurer et al., 2009) with bilateral stimulation. Air-pulse stimulation is associated with activation of supratentorial neural networks that have previously been implicated with swallowing (Lowell et al., 2008; Sörös et al., 2008). Unlike other types of sensory stimulation (e.g., thermal-tactile application [TTA]), bilateral air-pulse stimulation provides a wider surface area of touch, pressure, and temperature stimulation. Continued research is needed to determine if this type of treatment provides any immediate and/or long-term effects on swallowing recovery in individuals with dysphagia.

Surface Neuromuscular Electrical Stimulation[1]

As our focus in dysphagia management has shifted to rehabilitation, there is a controversial trend toward the utilization of NMES, also known as transcutaneous electrical stimulation, as a therapeutic modality for swallowing impairment. NMES is defined as "the external control of innervated, but paretic or paralytic, muscles by electrical stimulation of the corresponding intact peripheral nerves" (Baker, McNeal, Benton, Bowman, & Waters, 1993, pp. 5–6). This is achieved through the carefully regulated administration of pulsed electrical current to nerves, myoneural junctions, or muscles (Ragnarsson, 1994), which results in changes in the ionic composition of the neural or muscular cell membrane and triggers transmission of a motor unit action potential with subsequent motor response. The clinical benefit arises from skeletal muscle contraction with subsequent effects on strength, reaction time, and stamina (Alon, 1991). The resulting contraction differs from physiologic muscle activity in the ordering of muscle fiber recruitment, the synchronicity of individual motor units,

[1]Portions of this section have been extracted from Huckabee, M. L., and Doeltgen, S. H. (2007). Emerging modalities in dysphagia rehabilitation: Neuromuscular electrical stimulation. *New Zealand Medical Journal*, *120*(1263), 1–9.

and the intensity of stimuli required to produce these changes. These are important distinctions when considering the complex patterned motor event of pharyngeal swallowing.

Not surprisingly, the literature addressing the use of NMES in physical rehabilitation is contradictory, with some reports of a positive influence and other reports of minimal or no effect (Glanz, Klawansky, Stason, Berkey, & Chalmers, 1996). As with any treatment approach, one size does not fit all, and the available literature supports this. Specific to swallowing rehabilitation, many clinical researchers and basic scientists are investigating the safety and efficacy of this technology. The quality of subsequent publications is variable and thus requires careful scrutiny of both experimental methods and interpretation of results before implementing this modality into clinical work. Although some of these data are reviewed below, the reader is directed to intelligent review articles offered by Ludlow (2010), Martino and McCulloch (2016), and Steele, Thrasher, and Popovic (2007).

A Chronology of Surface NMES Literature in Swallowing

Park, O'Neill, and Martin (1997) published perhaps the first report of NMES applications in swallowing rehabilitation. This group investigated the effect of oral electrical stimulation on the physiologic abnormality of "delayed swallowing reflex" in four stroke patients with chronic dysphagia. Stimulation was applied to the posterior soft palate through a custom-designed palatal prosthesis with stimulation parameters set with a duration of 200 μsec, repeated at 1-second intervals and intensity at the patient's individual pain tolerance. Although two of four patients were identified to demonstrate decreased penetration/aspiration, NMES did not facilitate a timelier onset of swallowing, which was the primary target of treatment. Although many methodologic details were unjustified or unexplained, this initial work suggested a positive effect of this modality on at least some biomechanical features of swallowing.

The clinical effects of NMES on 110 patients with dysphagia following stroke were investigated by Freed, Freed, Chatburn, and Christian (2001), who are responsible for development of the VitalStim™ device. Time post-onset was not specified. Eighty-three patients were enrolled in an NMES group, whereas 36 patients received what they considered to be a "standard" treatment, that of TTA. Randomization for treatment group assignment was not applied. Daily treatment for inpatients and thrice weekly treatment for outpatients of 60 minutes in duration was administered by the primary investigator until the participants achieved a swallowing function score of at least 5 out of 6, or progress plateaued. Outcomes were based on a non-standardized scale rating of pre- and post-treatment VFSS that was completed by the primary investigator. Specific biomechanical changes were not evaluated. Ninety-eight percent of patients receiving NMES improved in some way, compared with 69% of patients receiving TTA. Results of this study were promising at first glance; however, the design of this study limits the validity of the results. No justification or experimental control of stimulation parameters was undertaken or reported. TTA is problematic as a comparison treatment because this technique has not withstood the rigors of empirical research on long-term effects. Outcome measures were based on a non-validated rating scale, and ratings were assigned only by the primary investigator, who also provided the treatment. Furthermore, an unspecified number of patients in the NMES group received concomitant dilatation of the upper esophageal sphincter, which is an accepted treatment in its own right. Unfortunately, these methodologic flaws erode the validity of the positive results and illustrate the need to interpret the available research with caution.

Leelamanit, Limsukul, and Geater (2002) evaluated the influence of synchronized electrical stimulation on the pathophysiologic feature of "reduced laryngeal elevation" in 23 patients with time post-onset ranging from 3 to 12 months. Thyrohyoid muscle stimulation was provided through surface electrodes at a frequency of 60 Hz and an amplitude of 100 V, for 3 to 30 treatments of 4 hours per day until they demonstrated improved swallowing. Again, the primary investigator rated treatment outcomes, which were based on a patient's ability to swallow more than 3 mL of water without aspiration, adequate oral intake with weight gain, and improved laryngeal elevation during VFSS. Twenty patients demonstrated clinical improvement, whereas 3 patients had no improvement; 6 patients relapsed on follow-up at 2 to 9 months but regained benefits with another round of treatment. This study has strength in its specific pathophysiologic target; however, no control group was utilized in this project, and as with the prior study, outcomes measures were by the primary investigator with no control for rater bias.

Burnett, Mann, Stoklosa, and Ludlow (2005) investigated self-triggered NMES using hooked-wire electrodes in the mylohyoid and thyrohyoid muscles in nine healthy adults. Stimulation was synchronized with swallowing behavior and delivered at a frequency of 30 Hz and at the highest comfortable intensity level. Objective measures of muscle activity were calculated to document treatment effects, rather than a non-validated subjective scale. No significant change in amplitude or duration of muscle activity was identified after self-triggered, synchronized electrical stimulation.

Subsequent to the questionably positive results reported by Freed and colleagues (2001), other investigations have attempted to more critically evaluate NMES specifically using the VitalStim device. Suiter, Leder, and Ruark (2006) evaluated the influence of VitalStim treatment protocol on submental muscle activity in healthy participants using an AB/BA treatment design. Based on these data, seven of eight subjects exhibited no significant gains in myoelectric activity of the submental muscle group following 10 hours of NMES treatment; two subjects withdrew from the study due to mild skin irritations after treatment. The effects of stimulation on HLC movement in healthy individuals at rest and during swallowing were investigated by Humbert and associates (2006). Ten different surface electrode placements were investigated using maximum tolerated stimulation. The National Institutes of Health Swallowing Safety Scale (NIH-SSS) and specific biomechanical measures of the larynx and hyoid at rest and during swallowing were made by raters blind to the swallowing conditions of stimulation and no stimulation. Results of this study raise concerns for biomechanical safety of NMES. Significant HLC descent occurred with stimulation at rest, and reduced HLC elevation occurred during swallowing; both movements are antagonistic to functional swallowing. Stimulated swallows were also judged to be "less safe" than non-stimulated swallows.

Studies of individuals with unimpaired physiology have documented an absence of change or potential worsening of biomechanical function. It could be argued that similar effects may not be evident in patients with impaired physiology. In response, the effectiveness of the VitalStim protocol in a population of patients with chronic pharyngeal phase dysphagia was evaluated by Ludlow and colleagues (2007). Time post-onset of dysphagia was 6 months or more. Blinded measurements were made of HLC movement and subglottic air column position on VFSS during no stimulation (no current induced), low stimulation (lowest intensity level, at which a participant felt a "tingling" sensation), and high stimulation (highest tolerable intensity without discomfort). Significant hyoid depression of up to 5 to 10 mm was observed during stimulation of the muscles at rest. Hyoid descent occurred, as targeted muscles for anterior and superior HLC elevation, mylohyoid and thyrohyoid, are too deep to stimulation. More superficial muscles such as the sternohyoid and sternothyroid, which lower the HLC, were stimulated. Low levels of stimulation resulted in improvement on the NIH-SSS but no improvement in airway invasion. Higher levels of stimulation, which would facilitate muscle contraction, had no effect on the NIH-SSS scores. An inverse relationship, however, was identified in which individuals with the greatest hyoid descent demonstrated the greatest reduction in airway invasion. Because of interference with HLC excursion, the authors conclude that "before such a tool is used in therapy, improved understanding of its immediate effects should be gained in the presence of specific types of swallowing difficulties before it is applied widely" (p. 9). The authors suggest that VitalStim may be used as a resistance exercise to facilitate HLC elevation. However, they caution that for this to be successful, patients must be able to overcome HLC depression; otherwise, increased risk of aspiration may occur. It is suggested that, for patients with reduced HLC elevation for whom VitalStim is considered as a therapy option, the effect of the stimulation be tested in VFSS. Only those patients who can overcome the downward pull of the HLC should be considered as candidates for the intervention.

This was echoed by more recent research evaluating response to treatment in younger (*n* = 20) versus older (*n* = 14) adults (Berretin-Felix, Sia, Barikroo, Carnaby, & Crary, 2016). Immediate effects following low-amplitude sensory stimulation (2 mA below motor response), high-amplitude motor stimulation (2 mA below maximum tolerance), or no stimulation (with electrodes in place) with lingual pressure and pharyngeal manometry were evaluated. Although there were no significant differences in sensory or motor stimulation amplitudes between the age groups, results indicated variable findings across groups and conditions. For example, elderly participants demonstrated increased BOT pressure following sensory stimulation, but decreased BOT pressure in young adults. Conversely, young adults demonstrated higher anterior lingual pressure than older adults across stimulation conditions. Further, both age groups demonstrated increased hypopharyngeal pressure following motor stimulation. The authors concluded by stating, "the collective results of this study suggest that a one-size-fits-all approach to [NMES] as an adjunctive modality in dysphagia rehabilitation may be misdirected" (p. 353).

Conflicting results were identified in a study by Blumenfeld, Hahn, LePage, Leonard, and Belafsky (2006), who undertook a retrospective study of 40 consecutive patients who underwent traditional dysphagia therapy (a combination of therapeutic exercise, diet texture modifications, and compensatory maneuvers) compared with 40 prospective patients who underwent NMES according to the VitalStim treatment paradigm. Patients were assigned a functional swallowing score based on the non-validated scale used by Freed and colleagues (2001); no control was provided for rater bias. Not surprisingly given the research design, those patients who were evaluated retrospectively using standard treatment (for that time period) did not demonstrate gains in swallowing treatment to the degree of those prospectively studied patients who underwent NMES. Twenty-two patients with swallowing disorders were evaluated by Kiger, Brown, and Watkins (2006) in another retrospective to prospective comparison of treatment. Participants were divided into two groups: the retrospective group received traditional dysphagia therapy, whereas the prospective group received VitalStim therapy. VFSS or videoendoscopy was used to evaluate swallowing function pre- and post-treatment based on a seven-point ordinal rating scale that described the patients' biomechanical swallowing functions as well as their ability to swallow different food consistencies. The traditional treatment group improved more in the oral phase than the VitalStim group. No significant differences in post-treatment outcomes for the pharyngeal phase, diet consistency tolerated, and oral intake measures were identified between the two groups.

According to Carnaby-Mann and Crary (2007), a meta-analysis of NMES research revealed a small but significant effect. In this analysis, seven articles met their inclusion criteria, which consisted of experimental studies with a quantifiable outcome measure, application of the intervention any time after the onset of dysphagia, and use of transcutaneous NMES. Their conclusion of significance, albeit small, should be viewed with substantial caution, as they used extremely lax inclusion criteria. For example, two of the studies were published in only abstract form and have never undergone peer-reviewed publication, and one of the studies (Freed et al., 2001) has been discussed earlier in terms of its poor design. As such, results are weak, thus without generalization to clinical practice. A subsequent meta-analysis was completed with eight studies of NMES; results indicated that "evidence was insufficient to indicate that neuromuscular electrical stimulation is superior to swallow therapy" (Chen, Chang, et al., 2016, p. 32).

Studies in patients with chronic dysphagia have been completed (Bülow, Speyer, Baijens, Woisard, & Ekberg, 2008; Carnaby-Mann & Crary, 2008; Kim, Park, & Nam, 2017; Nam, Beom, Oh, & Han, 2013). Inclusion criteria for the study by Carnaby-Mann and Crary were dysphagia for longer than 6 months, specific swallowing impairments of reduced HLC elevation, pharyngeal contraction and/or UES opening, and significantly reduced oral intake. Individuals completed 3 weeks of therapy (1 hour sessions/5 days a week) using VitalStim. This treatment was combined with the McNeill Dysphagia Treatment Program (MDTP) (Carnaby Mann & Crary, 2010; Crary, Carnaby, LaGoria, & Carvajal, 2012), in which patients used a "hard and fast swallow" to progress through a food hierarchy. Results revealed significantly improved clinical swallowing ability, functional oral intake, and patient perception. Decreased HLC elevation post-treatment was evident for thin liquids, but increased elevation was evident for thick liquids. Functional gains were maintained at a 6-month follow-up session. Bülow and associates completed a randomized clinical trial in which 25 patients with dysphagia following stroke of 3 months or longer were randomized to either VitalStim or traditional therapy. As with the Carnaby-Mann and Crary (2008) study, the experimental group completed 3 weeks of therapy (1-hour sessions 5 days a week) using NMES paired with instructions to "swallow hard and fast." The control group completed traditional therapy as determined by the patients' clinician. Therapy sessions were of the same length and duration as for the experimental group. Patient satisfaction and oral intake significantly improved with both groups; however, no changes on VFSS were evident following either treatment. Of importance, there was a poor correlation between outcome measures. That is, 2 patients reported subjective improvement in swallowing following NMES even though no objective VFSS gains were evident. These 2 patients advanced their own diets with resulting pneumonia.

Nam et al. (2013) provided stimulation to patients with dysphagia following stroke and brain injury (n = 50). Patients were randomly assigned to one of two groups, one receiving stimulation in the suprahyoid region and the other receiving simultaneous suprahyoid and infrahyoid stimulation. There was no control group or sham condition. Stimulation was provided in 10 to 15 sessions across 3 weeks, with pre- and post-treatment VFSS. The authors reported suprahyoid stimulation increased anterior hyoid excursion while combined supra and infrahyoid increased superior HLC excursion. Importantly, however, comparison of the groups revealed no significant differences in anterior hyoid excursion or superior laryngeal elevation across stimulation locations. Further, as all patients included were in the subacute phase, the authors state they could not rule out spontaneous recovery to account for at least some component of the results. Kim et al. (2017) provided NMES as a form of resistance training in conjunction with effortful swallowing to patients with dysphagia following stroke (n = 19). This training was implemented for 20 treatment sessions across 4 weeks, with stimulation provided to the infrahyoid region. Although there was no control group, results indicated significant improvements in hyoid excursion and a decrease in pharyngeal constriction ratio following training. Replication in a larger group with randomization and use of a sham condition is indicated, along with longer-term follow-up to analyze the maintenance of evidenced gains.

Similarly, the astute reader will note that with the VitalStim protocol, patients are instructed to swallow "hard," which is synonymous with an effortful swallow. Moreover, an additional therapy approach, MDTP, was used in conjunction with NMES in the study by Carnaby-Mann and Crary (2008). Participants receive intense swallowing therapy for 1 hour, resulting in numerous swallows; Carnaby-Mann and Crary reported a mean of 45 ± 27 swallows per session. Most patients do not receive traditional therapy of this intensity. Thus, was it the mass practice, the "effortful swallow," the food hierarchy and swallowing protocol of MDTP, or NMES that produced the results? Future studies must tease out the effects of these variables before the effects of NMES can be fully determined.

In summary, substantial excitement has been generated regarding the potential application of NMES in the treatment of swallowing impairment. Preliminary data are encouraging. However, clinical enthusiasm should be well balanced by a careful and intelligent evaluation of the presented data. Published meta-analyses have been conducted to analyze findings across the diverse patient groups and publications in this area. Tan, Liu, Li, Liu, and Chen (2013) state that NMES may be least effective in patients with stroke; coupled with documented adverse effects urges the clinician to respect the potential risks associated with NMES and be a smart clinical consumer. In a chapter on NMES, Alon (1991) comments: "The present disarray, and the natural tendency to accept nonscientific, subjective and commercially motivated claims . . . may threaten the substantive potential that electrical stimulation can offer as an objective clinical modality"

(p. 56). This comment was offered in reference to NMES applications in physical therapy but should serve as a warning to swallowing clinical practitioners. In our endeavor to provide optimal and innovative rehabilitative services to our patients with swallowing impairment, our best intentions need to be balanced with judiciousness and a critical eye.

Pharyngeal Electrical Stimulation

PES is applied to the pharyngeal mucosa via surface electrodes mounted on an intraluminal catheter, passed through the nose into the pharynx (Fraser et al., 2002). In a number of studies, researchers have demonstrated that PES primarily affects swallowing function through changes in the excitability of the pharyngeal representation in the primary motor cortex through this peripheral sensory stimulation. For example, PES using certain stimulus parameters can increase corticobulbar excitability in healthy research subjects and patients with dysphagia and, importantly, improve dysphagic symptoms, including aspiration score and pharyngeal transit times (Jayasekeran et al., 2010).

Power and colleagues (2004) demonstrated that PES applied to the muscles underlying the faucial pillar mucosa had frequency-specific inhibitory or facilitatory effects on corticobulbar motor excitability in healthy research participants. Interestingly, inhibitory faucial pillar PES resulted in a lengthened swallow response time, whereas facilitatory faucial pillar PES did not affect swallowing function. Similarly, a subsequent sham-controlled study of 16 patients following acute stroke (Power et al., 2006) showed no changes in swallowing function after facilitatory faucial pillar PES. In a meta-analysis of randomized controlled trials, Scutt, Lee, Hamdy, and Bath (2015) report an overall positive effect of PES in patients with dysphagia following stroke in terms of swallowing safety and function compared with a matched cohort who received sham or less-intensive stimulation. However, Vasant and colleagues (2016) investigated longer-term impacts of PES in a group of patients following acute stroke ($n = 36$). Participants were randomized to receive either PES or sham; researchers were blinded to their condition during analysis. Follow-up 2 weeks and 3 months after stimulation revealed no significant differences between PES and sham groups.

Bath and colleagues (2016) completed a multi-center randomized controlled trial investigating PES in patients with dysphagia following stroke (n = 162). Using PES or sham treatment on 3 consecutive days, consistent with prior studies, the researchers investigated safety of the PES procedure and dysphagia severity, including P-A Scale scores and swallowing-related quality of life. While no significant adverse effects were documented in this study, there were similarly no significant differences in swallowing-related outcomes as a result of PES. The authors speculated that operator characteristics may have impacted the outcomes. Optimal stimulation is recommended to be 10 minutes of PES at 75% of maximum tolerated intensity, yet when working with a patient, "maximum tolerated intensity" can be variable depending on clinician experience and comfort with applying PES. In the present study, Bath and colleagues found that up to 58.4% (n = 45) of patients potentially received "under-treatment" with less than optimal intensity of stimulation compared with prior data. While this may have affected results, further multi-center, randomized trials are indicated to clarify this point.

PES has been investigated in randomized studies to determine its efficacy in promoting decannulation in patients with tracheostomy as a result of a stroke. Suntrup, Marian, and colleagues (2015) investigated a randomized controlled trial in this population, providing either stimulation (n = 20) or sham stimulation (n = 10) across 3 days. Results indicated 75% of the PES stimulation group was able to be decannulated, compared with 20% decannulation in the sham group. Participants in the control group were subsequently crossed over to receive PES. Following this, a further five of seven patients were able to be decannulated. Importantly, this study was limited by a lack of blinding, which may have impacted decisions to decannulate. In a follow-up study of their original work by Suntrup, Marian, et al., Muhle and associates (2017) investigated the presence of "Substance P" in the saliva of PES participants. Substance P is a neuropeptide that is believed to enhance functions of swallowing and cough responses; reductions in Substance P are associated with dysphagia and aspiration. In patients with stroke who were decannulated following PES, 79% had an increase in Substance P in their saliva, with limited Substance P in the saliva of 89% of the individuals who were unable to be decannulated following PES. Whether the increase in Substance P was a result of PES, spontaneous recovery, or other mechanisms remains to be clarified. Importantly, Dziewas and colleagues (2017) are completing a larger follow-up study using a multiple baseline and single-blinded design to overcome limitations in prior work. Outcomes from this study are anticipated. In the interim, while PES appears to be a safe peripheral sensory stimulation technique that can be performed at bedside, further research is needed to help control for parameters such as stimulation intensity (Restivo & Hamdy, 2018). Pending ongoing research, this may be a promising future peripheral sensory stimulation modality.

21 Central Rehabilitation for Oropharyngeal Dysphagia

Extrinsic Modulation

CENTRAL STIMULATION TECHNIQUES

With increasing recognition of the role of the cortex in modulating the pharyngeal response, rehabilitation approaches have expanded to include mechanisms for eliciting central, rather than peripheral, change. Underlying this shift to central modulation is the assumption that if we can modify the underlying neurological substrates of swallowing, changes in swallowing biomechanics will be more robust and longer-lasting than those produced through peripheral muscle exercise alone. Non-behavioral and behavioral techniques for neural modulation are currently under development and provide promise for improved outcomes from rehabilitation of swallowing impairment. Among the non-behavioral approaches, non-invasive brain stimulation techniques induce changes in neural excitability using external (non-invasive) magnetic or electrical stimuli and are being actively evaluated in almost all areas of rehabilitation medicine.

The most frequently investigated techniques of this type are repetitive transcranial magnetic stimulation (rTMS) and transcranial direct current stimulation (tDCS), both of which stimulate neuronal networks within the brain through the intact skull with little or no discomfort, albeit through different mechanisms. These techniques have been investigated as a modality for neurorehabilitation following stroke, with subsequent facilitation of neuroplastic changes and motor recovery (Hummel & Cohen, 2006; Liew, Santarnecchi, Buch, & Cohen, 2014; Sandrini & Cohen, 2013).

Repetitive Transcranial Magnetic Stimulation

Initial reports of transcranial magnetic stimulation (TMS) were published by Barker, Jalinous, & Freeston (1985). Single pulse TMS generates a short-lasting magnetic field through a coil of wires placed over the head. This magnetic field passes through the scalp and skull and activates interneurons that project onto descending motor output neurons. The resulting descending current—the motor evoked potential—can be measured in the target muscle using surface electromyography. This technique has been used extensively to evaluate neural function (Griškova, Höppner, Rukšenas, & Dapsyš, 2006; Kobayashi & Pascual-Leone, 2003).

TMS application of low-intensity *repetitive* stimuli (e.g., rTMS) modulates transmembrane neural potentials and can be considered therapeutic as it produces long-term potentiation in the targeted neurons. The consequent effects on the stimulated neuronal networks are documented to outlast the stimulation period by 30 to 60 minutes (Esser et al., 2006; Goss, Hoffman, & Clark, 2012; Rossini & Rossi, 2007). Differential therapeutic effects are dependent on the nature of the stimulation protocol. Literature from corticospinal rehabilitation suggests that frequencies of <1 Hz inhibit cortical excitability; however, enhanced excitability is produced at frequencies >5 Hz (Klomjai, Katz, & Lackmy-Vallée, 2015). This stimulation to outcome pattern occurs also in the corticobulbar system. For example, 1 Hz rTMS has been shown to reduce excitability of corticobulbar motor projections to pharyngeal musculature when applied to healthy research participants (Mistry et al., 2007). This effect was accompanied by a reduction in swallowing reaction time of normal and fast swallows, as assessed by a swallowing reaction time task. Of note, the reaction time task was described as the time lag between a cue to swallow and onset of swallowing behavior. In an associated experiment, the inhibitory effects induced by 1 Hz rTMS were reversed by high-frequency 5 Hz rTMS applied to the contralateral hemisphere, which was associated with a restoration of swallowing function (Jefferson, Mistry, Michou, et al., 2009). It is unclear how this swallowing reaction time task functionally relates to pathophysiologic function in dysphagia. However, this early work rightly motivated investigation of rTMS as an approach for a recovery of swallowing function following stroke (Khedr, Abo-Elfetoh, & Rothwell, 2009; Mistry, Michou, Rothwell, & Hamdy, 2012).

The application of rTMS to patients with swallowing impairment was initially investigated in a series of research projects by Khedr and colleagues (Khedr & Abo-Elfetoh, 2010; Khedr et al., 2010). Both projects randomly assigned patients with general ischemic stroke (Khedr et al., 2010) and with lateral medullary infarct (Khedr & Abo-Elfetoh, 2010) to receive either a sham treatment or rTMS protocol. In both studies, patients who received rTMS demonstrated significantly improved swallowing over those receiving the sham treatment. A limitation of this work, however, was that dysphagia was not physiologically defined and assessments were all based on clinical observation rather than instrumental assessment. Thus, it is difficult to know the actual effect of the treatment on underlying biomechanics or pathophysiology.

This limitation persisted in subsequent studies. A more recent randomized, sham-controlled, double-blind study by Du et al. (2016) evaluated the effects of high-frequency versus low-frequency rTMS on patients with early post-stroke dysphagia. Forty-five patients were randomized between three groups (low frequency, high frequency, and sham conditions). Following five daily sessions, greater improvement in swallowing function as well as reduced functional disability were observed after real rTMS compared with sham rTMS; these changes persisted up to 3 months after the end of the treatment sessions. Low-frequency rTMS of 1 Hz increased cortical excitability of the affected hemisphere and decreased that of the non-affected hemisphere; however, 3 Hz rTMS only increased cortical excitability of the affected hemisphere. Although the study design was well developed, it is unfortunate that functional outcomes were based solely on clinical observational assessments, rather than instrumental measures.

Other research has provided greater specificity of outcomes. Park, Oh, Lee, Yeo, and Ryu (2013) randomized 18 patients to receive either 5 Hz rTMS over the contralesional hemisphere or sham 10 minutes daily for 2 weeks. Videofluoroscopic swallowing studies (VFSS) were performed prior to treatment, at the completion of treatment cessation, and 2 weeks afterward, with outcomes documented using the Videofluoroscopic Dysphagia Scale (VDS) (Kim et al., 2014) and the Penetration-Aspiration (P-A) Scale (Rosenbek, Robbins, Roecker, Coyle, & Wood, 1996). After rTMS, the prevalence of aspiration and pharyngeal residue was reduced significantly; however, no significant change was documented for delayed onset of pharyngeal swallowing or pharyngeal transit time. A subsequent study also documented mixed effects

(Lee, Kim, Lee, Lee, & Lee, 2015). Twenty-four patients were matched by age and site of lesion to two groups: one receiving rTMS overlying the pharyngeal motor cortex and the other receiving rTMS over a non-related muscle, serving as a control. Treatment was provided for 10 minutes per day for 10 days with outcomes measured immediately after and at 4 weeks following termination of treatment. Dysphagia status was measured with VFSS using the Functional Dysphagia Scale (FDS) (Paik, Kim, Kim, Oh, & Han, 2005), the P-A Scale, and the Dysphagia Outcome and Severity Scale (DOSS) (O'Neil, Purdy, Falk, & Gallo, 1999). Patients who received the active treatment improved significantly in their overall DOSS scores immediately and at 4 weeks after treatment compared with the control condition. However, there were no significant improvements in the FDS or PA-Scale for either group.

A recent study by Park, Kim, and colleagues (2017) evaluated three stimulation conditions: bilateral stimulation, unilateral stimulation of the ipsilesional cortex, and control stimulation of the bilateral motor cortices (although not well differentiated in the publication). Outcomes were measured immediately and 3 weeks post-intervention using clinical metrics and VFSS using a Clinical Dysphagia Scale (CDS) (Jung, Lee, Hong, & Han, 2005), the DOSS, the PA-Scale, and the VDS. Following 2 weeks of daily treatment at 10 Hz, patients in the bilateral stimulation group demonstrated greater gains as measured by the CDS than the other groups both immediately and 3 weeks after treatment. Greater gains were also appreciated in the DOSS, PA-Scale, and VDS, but only immediately post-treatment.

Positive outcomes have not been documented in all studies. Cheng et al. (2017) evaluated the outcomes of 5 Hz rTMS in patients with chronic dysphagia. Patients (n = 15) were assigned to an active or sham group, for 2 weeks of daily intervention. Outcomes were measured by a VFSS, swallowing-related quality-of-life questionnaire, and Iowa Oral Performance Instrument at 2, 6, and 12 months post stimulation. A broad range of biomechanical measures were evaluated, including oral transit time, stage transit time, pharyngeal transit time, pharyngeal constriction ratio, and normalized measures of pharyngeal residual. Although a small pilot study reported positive effects (Cheng, Chan, Wong, & Cheung, 2015), these findings were not confirmed in this larger trial. No significant changes were identified in any measure. This may suggest that rTMS holds less promise for those patients beyond the acute and subacute phases, in that by the 2-month post-treatment assessment period, any initial improvements were not retained. Rarely do we see published research that reports no significant treatment effect—there is a strong bias to publish on positive outcome. Thus, the results of this study warrant considerable regard.

Several systematic reviews have critically evaluated the literature related to rTMS or attempted to consolidate the data into meta-analyses (Gadenz, Moreira, Capobianco, & Cassol, 2015; Michou, Raginis-Zborowska, Watanabe, Lodhi, & Hamdy, 2016; Pisegna, Kaneoka, Pearson, Kumar, & Langmore, 2016; Yang, Pyun, Kim, Ahn, & Rhyu, 2015). The review by Michou et al. deserves particular note for their comparative critical appraisal of methods.

As the data accumulate to suggest possible clinical application of rTMS in routine dysphagia practice, it is important to consider the potential for adverse effects. Keeping in mind that the intent of rTMS is to alter neural function, it behooves clinicians to proceed with caution and appreciate the responsibility incumbent with provision of this treatment. For rTMS applications, minor and transient adverse effects have been reported to include headache, scalp discomfort, neck stiffness, twitching, or fatigue (Krishnan, Santos, Peterson, & Ehinger, 2015). Major side effects are reported infrequently, but any report suggests the need for care. Two reports of seizure induction (Chiramberro, Lindberg, Isometsä, Kähkönen, & Appelberg, 2013; Hu et al., 2011), particularly at higher frequency rTMS (>5 Hz) (Ebmeier & Lappin, 2001), and two reports of syncope (Kirton et al., 2008; Kirton, deVeber, Gunraj, & Chen, 2010) are documented in the literature. Safety guidelines have been recommended, which include avoiding TMS applications in those with a history of epilepsy or metal implants, including brain stimulators and cochlear implants (Krishnan et al., 2015; Rossi, Hallett, Rossini, & Pascual-Leone, 2009; Wassermann,1998).

Although rTMS offers potential for recovery of dysphagia secondary to stroke by stimulating central neural substrates, this technique is disadvantaged for routine clinical translation not only by potential adverse effects, as discussed in the preceding paragraph, but also by high cost and limited accessibility. There is slim likelihood that this technique will transition to usual clinical practice, within the domain of allied health. It is feasible that it may eventually move from the research domain to specialized clinics as a viable treatment option. However, alternative non-invasive brain stimulation approaches, which may be more accessible to allied health, are under evaluation, the most common of which is tDCS.

Transcranial Direct Current Stimulation

Transcranial DCS modifies neuronal activation in stimulated brain areas through application of low-intensity electrical direct currents. Similar to rTMS, the nature of how the stimulation is applied dictates the physiologic outcome; however, tDCS also influences outcomes through the direction of current flow between electrodes rather than stimulation frequency. Anodal stimulation of the motor cortex generally produces facilitation of motor cortical excitability, whereas cathodal stimulation reduces it. Application of tDCS protocols in stroke operates on the premise that stimulation corrects an imbalance in hemispheric activation caused by the stroke (Feng, Bowden, & Kautz, 2013). Anodal stimulation can be applied to upregulate excitability of the lesioned hemisphere. Cathodal stimulation can be applied over the contralesional hemisphere to downregulate excitability. Or bilateral stimulation that combines approaches may be used to inhibit activity in the lesioned hemisphere and optimize activity in the contralesional hemisphere to encourage task reorganization (Edwardson, Lucas, Carey, & Fetz, 2013; Feng et al., 2013).

Application for swallowing rehabilitation following stroke is emerging rapidly. As a first step to translation, it is important to determine if the directional characteristics of stimulation observed in the corticospinal system translate to the corticobulbar system. Functionally, when tDCS was applied to the region of pharyngeal motor representation for 10 min with an intensity of 1.5 mA and a cathodal current direction, reduced corticobulbar excitability was measured (Jefferson, Mistry, Singh, Rothwell, & Hamdy, 2009). In contrast, 10 min of 1.5 mA and 20 min of 1 mA anodal stimulation increased corticobulbar excitability. The finding of anodal facilitation was confirmed by Cosentino et al. (2014) in a double-blind randomized trial of effects in healthy volunteers. Anodal tDCS over the right M1 (20 min at 1.5 mA) enhanced oral sucking and swallowing-related EMG measures compared with the sham group, whereas cathodal tDCS did not.

Jefferson, Mistry, Singh, and colleagues (2009) also evaluated frequency effects in healthy participants, by comparing low-intensity (1 mA for 10 min) and high-intensity (1.5 mA for 10 min or 1 mA for 20 min) tDCS. Low-intensity anodal or cathodal tDCS did not alter pharyngeal motor evoked potentials, a measure of neural change. This is in contrast to findings from the corticospinal literature (Nitsche & Paulus, 2001). However, corticobulbar excitability following anodal and cathodal tDCS was increased or decreased, respectively, in response to increases in duration and intensity of the applied current (Jefferson, Mistry, Singh, et al., 2009). These findings were largely confirmed in subsequent studies (Suntrup et al., 2013; Vasant et al., 2014) verifying that compared with the corticospinal system, changes in swallowing will require extended duration of treatment and higher stimulation intensities.

The research by Suntrup and colleagues (2013) also sought to evaluate the physiologic effect of tDCS on cortical networks using a crossover design. In this study, tDCS and a sham condition were applied over pharyngeal regions of the left and right motor cortices during performance of a swallowing reaction time task. Data from this study suggest that interhemispheric connections for swallowing are synergistic, with stimulation in either hemisphere producing increased bilateral activation.

Application of tDCS to patients with dysphagia following stroke is slowly accumulating. Kumar and colleagues (2011) investigated the functional correlates of tDCS-induced plasticity in a small study of 14 subacute stroke patients assigned to receive either anodal tDCS over the non-lesioned hemisphere or a sham condition. All participants received one session of 60 effortful swallows (one swallow every 30 s, while sucking on a flavored lollipop), with or without tDCS, on 5 consecutive days. The DOSS was used to measure outcomes and identified that those receiving tDCS demonstrated significantly greater improvement than a sham group. A significant limitation of the study, however, was the absence of blinding in assessing outcomes and a scale that might be considered susceptible to examiner bias.

Two additional studies have taken the approach of applying 1 mA tDCS (or sham) not to the contralesional hemisphere but to the lesioned hemisphere, using similar protocols consisting of 10 treatments of 20 min paired with swallowing training (Shigematsu, Fujishima, & Ohno, 2013; Yang et al., 2012). In both studies, there were no significant treatment effects measured with the FDS for either group. However, by 3 months post-treatment, significant gains were demonstrated in the tDCS group compared with the sham in the Yang et al. study.

The final approach of bi-hemispheric anodal tDCS was recently explored by Ahn et al. (2017). Patients were assigned to either an anodal or sham condition with anodal electrodes placed over M1 and cathodal electrodes over the supraorbital regions of the contralateral hemisphere. All participants received 10 sessions of 20 min at 1 mA current intensity. Outcomes were measured using the DOSS immediately before and after the intervention. Although there was no significant difference between the tDCS and the sham group, the anodal tDCS group demonstrated significant improvement on DOSS scores as a function of treatment. Unlike the prior study by Kumar et al. (2011), who also used the DOSS, a double-blind design was incorporated in this study to control for assessment bias. However, for this study and others, the choice of generalized scales as a primary outcome measure does not provide specific information about the nature of physiologic change and may lack sensitivity for identifying subtle improvements.

TRANSLATING rTMS AND tDCS INTO CLINICAL DYSPHAGIA REHABILITATION

These early studies of neuromodulation in patients with stroke-related dysphagia suggest promise for increasing options for rehabilitation in this group. By providing controlled stimulation to neuronal networks underlying swallowing, there appears to be preliminary, but not consistent, evidence of improved biomechanics and functional swallowing. The mechanisms engaged with these techniques suggest that stimulation should be provided as a component of a clustered therapy protocol. Again, the assumption is that experimental brain stimulation can "repair" imbalanced brain function caused by insult or disease (Ridding & Rothwell, 2007). However, most stimulation protocols have limited duration of effects: 60 min for rTMS, 20 min for tDCS. Thus, modulatory treatments in and of themselves do not result in long-term, functionally relevant neural changes. The most effective strategy may therefore be to promote the brain's intrinsic, neural repair mechanisms using neuromodulatory techniques, then provide conventional rehabilitative training during a period of experimentally enhanced cortical excitability. In this case, the generation of a one hour "therapeutic window" induced through neuromodulatory techniques would be sufficient for most training protocols. Use of a paired treatment approach then provides a functional target for the neural enhancement. There is evidence in the corticospinal motor system for the efficacy of such an approach in both healthy subjects and stroke patients (Conforto et al., 2010; McDonnell, Hillier, Miles, Thompson, & Ridding, 2007).

A recent meta-analysis addressed both techniques and reported moderate overall effect size for four randomized controlled trials utilizing rTMS in dysphagia rehabilitation post-stroke (Pisegna et al., 2016; Figure 21–1). When evaluating the most influential protocol, this meta-analysis found a greater effect of rTMS over the unaffected hemisphere with a significant combined effect size of 0.65 compared with an effect size of 0.46 for rTMS over the affected hemisphere. Despite this overall positive effect based on a small number of studies, entry of this technique into practice would be premature. Details of treatment protocol, outcome measurement, and patient characteristics require significant refinement.

The Pisegna et al. (2016) study also evaluated the limited number of studies using tDCS. Although the overall effect is not significant, there is the strong suggestion of a positive effect; with a larger number of studies, this outcome may likely change. In contrast to rTMS, tDCS has most effectively been used when applied in combination with various types of behavioral rehabilitation for limb function (Hummel & Cohen, 2006; Schlaug, Renga, & Nair, 2008). The use of paired protocols may compound the measurement of independent treatment outcomes of tDCS, since outcome data for our other rehabilitation approaches are inadequate. Thus, if treatment effect is not significant, is that a reflection of tDCS or the accompanying behavioral treatment approach? Transcranial DCS has several advantages over rTMS applications, such as cost-efficiency and fewer side effects (Simons & Hamdy, 2017), thus further research in this area is warranted.

THE NEED FOR INTELLIGENT ENTHUSIASM

As our specificity in diagnosis improves and our depth of rehabilitative understanding deepens, we can eagerly anticipate new developments in swallowing rehabilitation. It is an exciting time in the profession. But as our existing data would indicate, it is also a time that we need to carefully consider emerging options and base our developing treatments on theory and outcome. Although rTMS is perhaps unlikely to achieve uptake in clinical dysphagia rehabilitation delivery by allied

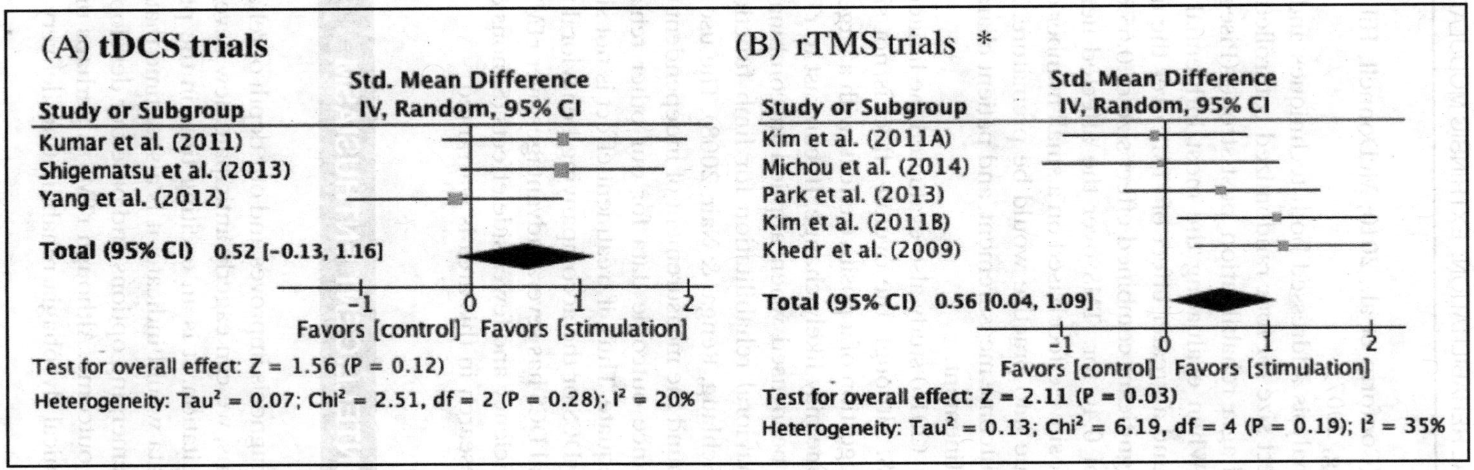

Figure 21–1. **A**. Effect sizes of tDCS trials on post-stroke dysphagia. **B**. Effect sizes of rTMS trials on post-stroke dysphagia. Source: J. M. Pisegna, A. Kaneoka, W. G. Pearson, S. Kumar, and S. E. Langmore, "Effects of non-invasive brain stimulation on post-stroke dysphagia: A systematic review and meta-analysis of randomized controlled trials." *Clinical Neurophysiology, 127*(1), 956–968. Copyright @ 2016, by permission of Elsevier.

health, tDCS is much more accessible. With a much lower price tag, this instrumentation can be on a clinician's desk following a very quick and inexpensive purchase online. This availability, however, does not abdicate responsibility to ensure that the treatment is efficacious and appropriate and that the clinician is knowledgeable in clinical delivery. Modulation of neural function is as potentially promising as it is potentially problematic. These approaches open the door for considerable issues regarding boundaries of professional practice and expansion of professional preparation. Doeltgen and Huckabee (2012) prepared a summary of emerging modalities, which at the time did not include tDCS, and offered caution and suggestions for how we might proceed in addressing newer and more invasive technologies. This is suggested reading for those wishing to pursue these rehabilitation options.

A substantial limitation of all externally applied neuromodulatory techniques is the lack of specificity they provide. Stimulation of "brain," even somewhat targeted regions, is assumed and indeed proven to effect a change in behavior. But what behavior? To date, research that is focused on exploring neuromodulatory approaches has not hypothesized its intent to address any specific biomechanical impairment. Clinicians thus have no guidance on which presentation of dysphagia would be an appropriate therapeutic target. To further the confusion, research has utilized mostly very global measures of swallowing function to assess outcomes of neuromodulatory approaches. These may document some change in "dysphagia." But dysphagia has many presentations and a non-specific outcome measure provides little guidance on how to target this intervention approach. After decades of research, it behooves us to advance well beyond generalities and target more physiologically specific treatment approaches.

22 Central Rehabilitation for Oropharyngeal Dysphagia

Behavioral Adaptation[1]

Behavioral interventions for swallowing impairment have traditionally focused on restoring safe and effective swallowing through functional modification of biomechanics in the peripheral structures—the muscles (Chapter 20). Most literature suggests that this approach changes muscle, with little effect on central mechanisms. As we are learning, swallowing may not require maximal muscle contraction; in some patients, strengthening may be the wrong approach. Neuromodulatory approaches (Chapter 21) have gone a long way to encourage a rethinking of our rehabilitation targets. These techniques focus on changes not at the periphery through muscle strengthening, but through lasting modulation of the neuronal circuitries involved in swallowing motor control. They change the brain first, with the intent of altered functional swallowing as a consequence. However, they are non-specific to swallowing biomechanics. This leads to a question: Can we develop approaches that first target specific swallowing biomechanics, but then encode those changes in the brain?

This chapter addresses the advent of behavioral adaptation to change the neural swallowing system in dysphagia rehabilitation. Skill-based training represents a category of emerging approaches to specifically target cortical modulation of swallowing in a task-specific manner. These approaches are considered to maintain the biomechanical specificity of muscle strengthening by focusing on specific features of impaired swallowing, while also capturing the longer-lasting change associated with neural adaptation.

[1]Portions of this section have been reprinted with permission of RightsLink/Springer Nature: Huckabee, M. L., and Lamvik-Gozdzikowska, K. (2018). Reconsidering rehabilitation for neurogenic dysphagia: Strengthening skill in swallowing. *Current Physical Medicine and Rehabilitation Reports*, *6*(3), 186–191.

SKILL-BASED TRAINING PARADIGMS: DYSPHAGIA AS A MOTOR PLANNING DISORDER

A central theme in this text has been the need for diagnostic specificity and how our current techniques allow us clear evaluation of biomechanics but little insight into the underlying pathophysiology that causes impaired movement. This leaves us to base our intervention, quite inadequately, on assumptions. Whereas strengthening approaches appear to be predicated on an assumption of weakness underlying swallowing impairment, it could be argued that skill-based training is predicated on an assumption of impaired motor planning and execution.

In one of the very first publications on management of dysphagia nearly 40 years ago, George Larsen recognized that "rehabilitation of this disorder depends on careful assessment of spared and damaged processes responsible for swallowing" (Larsen, 1972, p. 189). When commenting on rehabilitation, he proffered that rehabilitation should maximize "use of assets, capitalizing on intelligence to support reflex behavior" (p. 191). This theme was reflected again nearly 20 years later by Stevenson and Allaire (1991). In an article on development of swallowing in pediatrics, they commented that swallowing is reflexive at birth; however, the ability to modify developmental swallowing behavior is linked to a process of encephalization. This suggests that the "skill" component of ingestive swallowing is acquired through cortical expansion and modulation of the primitive brainstem-driven swallowing response. In the face of injury or disease, relearning or modifying the complex sequence of events involved in swallowing poses a much greater challenge. However, skill-based paradigms essentially are targeted toward recruiting cortical control mechanisms to alter the impaired response—an essential expansion of cortical modulation of swallowing that is well documented in the literature.

Skill-based training may be simply defined as the acquisition of skill through functional repetition and refinement of movement patterns (Huckabee & Macrae, 2014; Plautz, Milliken, & Nudo, 2000). As with most rehabilitation approaches, we have bolstered our development of skill-based training paradigms from research in other areas of rehabilitation medicine. And as with other approaches, translation to swallowing cannot necessarily be assured due to the differences in composition and neural processes (Chhabra & Sapienza, 2007). In the physical therapy domain, skill-based training has been shown to induce cortical reorganization of motor networks (Lefebvre et al., 2015) and has been investigated as an approach for motor recovery (Kitago & Krakauer, 2013; Krakauer, 2006; Matthews, Johansen-Berg, & Reddy, 2004). The principles of neural plasticity (Kleim & Jones, 2008) outlined in Chapter 19 are critically relevant in discussions of skill-based training, particularly the concepts of specificity of practice (plasticity is experience specific), task challenge (use it and improve it), and feedback (salience).

Barnett, Ross, Schmidt, and Todd (1973) proposed that specific motor skills are developed and stored through practice, and that these motor skills do not generalize across tasks. Thus, specificity of practice is crucial to encouraging skill acquisition. There is evidence of this in the literature relative to corticobulbar function. A series of studies have reported that a tongue protrusion exercise resulted in increased size of cortical representation of the tongue (Sessle et al., 2007, 2005; Svensson, Romaniello, Arendt-Nielsen, & Sessle, 2003; Svensson, Romaniello, Wang, Arendt-Nielsen, & Sessle, 2006) and increased excitability (Svensson et al., 2003, 2006) of corticobulbar projections (see Sessle et al., 2007, for review). Despite these increases in the tongue motor cortex, the authors report that no increase was seen in representation of the "cortical masticatory area/swallow cortex" (Sessle et al., 2005, pp. 111–112), suggesting a lack of generalization from one repetitive task to a structurally related function. This research emphasizes the importance of task specificity, the need for exercise that replicates the desired task—that of swallowing—in skill-based training. Historically, strategies such as effortful swallowing, Mendelsohn maneuver, or Masako maneuver have been applied using maximal contraction in a strength-training approach. However, by adapting functional swallowing for recruitment of greater strength or duration, there is a suggestion that some strengthening exercises may have a skill-based training component that would not be apparent in exercises that are not executed within a functional context, such as the head lift. Interestingly, limb-based skill training has been documented to influence strength gains to a greater extent than strength training alone, despite training at submaximal levels of muscle contraction (Liu-Ambrose, Taunton, MacIntyre, McConkey, & Khan, 2003). This phenomenon has been attributed to improved movement coordination and neural adaptation due to proprioceptive facilitation in skill-based training. Task-oriented training programs inherently incorporate proprioceptive facilitation (Borsa, Sauers, & Lephart, 1999). Adler, Beckers, and Buck (2008), therefore, suggest that skill-based paradigms are recommended for motor deficits with underlying impairments in both coordination and muscle strength. The importance of task-oriented exercise training has been documented in many physical therapy research studies and is considered crucial to foster optimal motor learning (see Rensink, Schuurmans, Lindeman, & Hafsteinsdottir, 2009 for an in-depth review).

However, repetition of motor activity alone is not thought to result in functional recovery, particularly in the context of rehabilitation where impaired motor performance is then repeated. Another key component of skill-based training, and a principle of neural plasticity, is that of task challenge, the "use it and improve it" principle. Encouraging "practice" of dysphagic swallowing with no adaptation or adjustment, although preventing against disuse, is unlikely to produce a more functional swallowing response and may encourage maladaptive behaviors. Skill-based training involves the introduction of a challenge component, requiring an individual to evaluate and adjust the movement with each repetition, rather than memorizing and replaying the same sequence of muscle contractions (Krakauer, 2006). Task challenge extends neural activation to different brain circuits than those associated with previously acquired movements (Luft & Buitrago, 2005). This extension induces neural and behavioral changes associated with learning. Motor learning, rather than motor repetition, is required for functional cortical reorganization (Plautz et al., 2000). Translated to clinical routines, ingestion of a safely tolerated diet may facilitate pulmonary safety but may also be considered "practicing" impaired swallowing unless ongoing feedback and adjustments are made to swallowing behavior. Eating may be important to maintain existing neural pathways but is unlikely to have therapeutic benefits. However, systematically challenging the system in a controlled therapeutic environment may facilitate recovery. This appears to be one of the tenets of the McNeill Dysphagia Therapy Program (MDTP) (Crary, Carnaby, LaGorio, & Carvajal, 2012), constituting a type of skill-based training.

The final key element in motor learning is the necessity for feedback regarding task performance, related to the principle of neural plasticity of "salience" (Rose & Robert, 2006; Schmidt & Lee, 1999). Execution of motor tasks requires movement awareness to be paired with kinesthetic intrinsic feedback from joint receptors, muscle spindles, and Golgi tendon organs and consequently transferred to the central nervous system (Schmidt & Lee, 1999). If a mismatch between the projected motor plan and the actual performance occurs, correction of the motor plan ensues during subsequent trials. Guidance and integrated feedback are critical for improved performance (Salmoni, Schmidt, & Walter, 1984). Rehabilitation of swallowing poses significantly greater challenges than the limb in this regard. No clear external movement patterns are observed in swallowing, and intrinsic feedback systems are likely to be impaired in neurological disorders. Thus, learning through repetition is less likely to occur. Particularly in swallowing skill-based training, exteroceptive feedback is likely necessary to provide a salient means for conveying cues regarding movement accuracy, thus allowing improvement in swallowing motor function.

Development of Skill-Based Training Paradigms for Swallowing

The ultimate goal in swallowing skill-based training, very simply put, is for a patient to return to oral ingestive swallowing that is safe, pleasurable, and sufficient for sustaining nutrition and hydration. In a higher-level therapeutic sense, one might define the goal of skill-based training as to acquire skill in execution of specific aspects of swallowing biomechanics that are encoded at a central level. Several approaches for translating the construct of skill-based training to the practice of dysphagia rehabilitation have emerged. The MDTP is a systematic exercise framework that is predicated on components of strength training (Crary et al., 2012). An additional key component of this approach appears to be the systematic and hierarchical presentation of oral intake. This emphasizes task specificity in that the treatment is focused on swallowing repetition, although it is not specific to individual pathophysiologic features of swallowing. Task challenge is met through the hierarchical presentation of food, with the purveyors of this approach advocating that assessment of task performance for advancement on the hierarchy is based on clinical presentation of bolus tolerance. The researchers have documented positive outcomes of the MDTP in subsequent studies (Crary et al., 2012; Lan, Ohkubo, Berretin-Felix, Carnaby-Mann, & Crary, 2012; Sia, Carvajal,

Lacy, Carnaby, & Crary, 2015). However, as the approach fundamentally is focused on repetition of a type of effortful swallowing task, the "active treatment" is unclear.

Stepp, Britton, Chang, Merati, and Matsuoka (2014) evaluated the feasibility of skill-based therapy for dysphagia rehabilitation by utilizing surface electromyography (sEMG) biofeedback. Electrodes were placed bilaterally on the anterior neck, overlying the thyrohyoid, sternohyoid, and omohyoid muscles. Six healthy participants and one patient with severe oropharyngeal dysphagia following brainstem stroke received real-time visual feedback of muscle activity on a computer screen placed in front of them. Surface EMG data were presented in video-game format, with the leading edge of the waveform represented as a large fish that moves vertically on the screen based on the magnitude of sEMG output. The game involved using the muscles in an organized manner such that the larger fish "caught" a smaller fish (target) that moved at a constant speed across the horizontal (time) axis but with a variable amplitude across the vertical axis. In the baseline session, healthy volunteers "caught" significantly more fish than the single patient participant. Throughout five subsequent sessions, the patient significantly increased target accuracy and reported improved secretion management. As is evident, this study utilized biofeedback to increase task performance and provided significant challenge to facilitate motor learning. However, physiologic swallowing was not required to complete the task, thus task specificity was not optimized.

Athukorala, Jones, Sella, and Huckabee (2014) addressed the limitation in task specificity in the above study with a similar approach. Using submental electrode placement to detect timing and magnitude of the anterior belly of the digastric, mylohyoid, and geniohyoid muscles, 10 patients with dysphagia secondary to Parkinson's disease completed a 2-week, daily treatment protocol. The task, executed with specialized software, required the patient to control the timing and degree of muscle activation during swallowing such that the peak of the time-by-amplitude waveform "hit" a target box that was placed randomly on the visualized computer screen. All targets were calibrated to fall within 2 and 25 sec of a 30-sec screen sweep and between 20% and 80% of maximal sEMG amplitude during five effortful swallows, thus avoiding the confound of effortful-type swallowing. Task challenge was provided by a decrease in the size of the target by 10% following three successive "hits," and, conversely, an increase of 10%

in target size in the event of three successive misses. One hundred repetitions of the task were executed in blocks of 10, with 30 sec between trials and 90 sec between blocks. Outcomes were measured using the Timed Water Swallowing Test (Hughes & Wiles, 1996), the Test of Masticating and Swallowing Solids (TOMASS) (Huckabee et al., 2018), and sEMG timing measures of pre-motor, pre-swallow, and total swallowing duration times. The Swallowing Quality of Life (Swal-QOL) (McHorney et al., 2002) was also derived. In this within-subject ABA design, patients demonstrated stable performance across a 2-week baseline period. They demonstrated significant improvement on all measures, with the exception of those from the TOMASS, following 2 weeks of treatment, with no decline in performance at 2 weeks following discontinuation of treatment. The absence of change on TOMASS measures likely reflected an absence of impairment in solid bolus swallowing, as described by participants and demonstrated through pre-treatment TOMASS scores. Although improvement was demonstrated and maintained in functional swallowing measures following this treatment that was swallowing-task specific, skill-based training in this context did not target a specific physiologic abnormality (e.g., reduced hyoid movement). Rather, this approach monitored floor of mouth muscle condition as a mechanism to increase cortical modulation of swallowing strength and timing in a more general sense.

Steele et al. (2013) reported results from a tongue-pressure strength and accuracy training intervention in six individuals following acquired brain injury. The aim of this study was to determine if a mixed strength and skill-based (e.g., accuracy) training would increase tongue strength for maximum isometric pressures, as well as improve swallowing safety and efficiency. Participants completed 24 twice-weekly sessions in which the target was to complete a lingual strength and accuracy task using the Iowa Oral Performance Instrument (IOPI). While the strength task was to complete maximum isometric pressures with the anterior and posterior tongue, the skill-based task was accomplished only using 20% to 90% of maximum isometric pressure. Participants were asked to generate a randomly selected target pressure as accurately as possible within that submaximal pressure band. Feedback was provided through IOPI pressure amplitudes, and an equal number of trials between the strength and skill tasks were completed within a session. In addition to lingual pressure measures, pre- and post-treatment videofluoroscopic swallowing studies (VFSS) were undertaken to investigate differences in swallowing biomechanics.

Results indicated increases in anterior and posterior tongue strength; however, VFSS data revealed no improvements in bolus clearance, with worsening pharyngeal residual in the majority of participants (n = 5) in the absence of any (unrelated) worsening in disease state or dysphagia severity. This result is consistent with findings from studies of other strength-based exercises, such as the effortful swallow (Molfenter, Hsu, Lu, & Lazarus, 2018), which have documented increased pharyngeal residual following the intervention, as discussed in Chapter 20. Further assessment of lingual accuracy tasks, trained independently from maximal isometric tasks, is indicated.

Huckabee, Lamvik, and Jones (2014) reported results from a group of patients (n = 16) with atypical pathophysiologic features of dysphagia. On VFSS, this patient cohort presented with decreased pharyngeal motility, diffuse pharyngeal residue, and frequent nasal redirection. Subsequent assessment with pharyngeal manometry revealed a mis-sequenced pattern of pharyngeal pressure, with simultaneous pressure in the proximal and distal pharynx, respectively. All participants were seen for intensive, skill-based training 5 days per week for a period of 2 weeks (10 days), for a total of 10 one-hour sessions. Previous research has documented that pressure and duration of brainstem-generated pharyngeal swallowing can be cortically modulated (Bülow, Olsson, & Ekberg, 2001, 2002; Ertekin, 2011; Wheeler-Hegland, Rosenbek, Sapienza, 2008); thus, participants were instructed to volitionally increase the temporal separation between the proximal and distal pharyngeal pressure waveforms when swallowing using pharyngeal manometry as a visual biofeedback modality. Following this intervention, the mean latency between peak pressures at the proximal and distal pharynx increased from a pre-treatment average of 15 ms (95% CI = −2 to 33 ms) to a post-treatment mean of 137 ms (95% CI = 86–187 ms). This correlated to subjective improvements in oral intake and led to a subsequent experiment evaluating the capacity for skill-based adaptation of pharyngeal swallowing in healthy adults (Lamvik, Jones, Sauer, Erfmann, & Huckabee, 2015).

In a more recent publication, Martin-Harris and colleagues (2016) evaluated performance of a skill-based respiration-swallow training intervention in participants (n = 30) with head and neck cancer. The aims of this study were to: (i) determine whether the use of a respiratory-related feedback protocol was effective in training desired respiratory-swallowing coordinative patterns, measured with respect to expiration preceding and following deglutitive apnea, and

(ii) investigate the stability of the training 1 month post-treatment. Participants completed a 1 hour session twice weekly for a duration of 4 weeks. During these sessions, respiratory-swallowing coordination was trained with visual biofeedback from a KayPENTAX Digital Swallowing Workstation on a motor skill acquisition hierarchy in which participants were first taught to identify the target, perform the desired response with a minimum of 80% accuracy, and finally master the production in at least 90% of trials. Using this approach, patients were able to learn and implement an optimal respiratory-swallowing pattern after treatment ($p < 0.001$); in fact, all study participants mastered the optimal pattern within 8 sessions, with carryover effects seen at 1 month follow-up. These gains in motor skill were associated with improvements in VFSS measures, including improved laryngeal vestibule closure ($p < 0.001$), improved tongue-base retraction ($p < 0.001$), and a reduction in pharyngeal residual ($p = 0.01$).

Development of skill-based training paradigms may hold promise for rehabilitation above and beyond traditional strength-based methods. While the abovementioned studies provide favorable proof-of-concept and positive indicators that skill-based intervention may circumvent some limitations with existing strength-based intervention modalities, it is clear that further research is needed. These studies are limited by small sample sizes and heterogeneous etiologies, including Parkinson's disease, acquired brain injury, and head and neck cancer. It is simply too early to make wider inferences and generalization without additional research.

There is, however, a rapidly progressing field of research regarding skill training in the limb literature, with researchers documenting superior outcomes for task-oriented skill training over strength-training programs (Hogan et al., 2006; Liu-Ambrose et al., 2003; Nelles, Jentzen, Jueptner, Müller, & Diener, 2001; Rensink et al., 2009; Risberg, Holm, Myklebust, & Engebretsen, 2007). Further, skill-based training in the limb literature has been linked with an increase in corticomotor excitability (Jensen, Marstrang, & Nielsen, 2005), increase in plasticity of the motor cortex, and greater functional movement improvements (Remple, Bruneau, Vandenberg, Goertzen, & Kleim, 2001). The critical component appears to be optimization of motor learning, rather than motor repetition, to stimulate functional cortical reorganization (Plautz et al., 2000).

As discussed in Chapter 19, our current diagnostic methods have a great impact on subsequent rehabilitation decisions. This begs the question, how does a clinician determine if residual on VFSS is secondary to a reduction of muscular strength or deficits in swallowing motor programming? Weakness can really only reliably and objectively be assessed through specific muscle function tests; current work is pursuing development of a clinical test of this differentiation. Despite this, further research is also warranted directly comparing skill-based training to strength-based treatment. The studies evaluating only skill-based intervention documented favorable outcomes (Athukorala et al., 2014; Huckabee et al., 2014; Stepp et al., 2011). The two studies where skill training and strength training were combined produced dissimilar results (Crary et al., 2012; Steele et al., 2013). Steele and colleagues produced the sole study to document a worsening of pharyngeal residual following their mixed strength and skill-based rehabilitation paradigm. This fits with emerging evidence regarding negative sequelae following use of a similar strength-based exercise, namely, effortful swallowing (Molfenter et al., 2018). Whether it be a strength-based or skill-based rehabilitation approach, it is wise to remember that if an intervention is powerful enough to effect a positive change, then it is inherently powerful enough to effect a negative change. Until further data are accrued and the picture becomes clearer, practicing clinicians should always question their rehabilitation decisions.

BIOFEEDBACK

Outcomes of skill-based swallowing rehabilitation, and truly all behavioral intervention, may be limited by several factors:

- We are dealing with a largely abstract concept. Rehabilitation of impaired swallowing frequently requires neuromuscular adaptation of a pseudo-reflexive process that most individuals typically perform without conscious thought or manipulation. In the event of dysphagia subsequent to stroke, clinicians ask individuals not only to engage an impaired system but to modulate that system in a manner that is quite unlike anything they have ever done. Although execution of effortful swallowing may appear relatively simple, other techniques, such as interventions targeting pharyngeal sequencing (Huckabee et al., 2014), will challenge even the patient with minor impairment and can sometimes present an overwhelming obstacle for those with cognitive impairment.

- There are limited reliable means to assess whether exercises are done correctly. Asking a patient to swallow with effort or sustain hyolaryngeal excursion may produce visible effort on the part of the patient, but it is unclear exactly where that effort lies. Swallowing produces very few externally observable cues on performance. Thus, it challenges the clinician to provide feedback to the patient for adaptation of behavior if the clinician has little insight into how that behavior is executed. This may be even more challenging in skill-based tasks where patients are asked to finely modulate a select component of their swallowing at precise levels of timing or intensity.
- There is little objective measurement of change; thus, meaningful goal delineation is difficult at best. Research has unquestionably documented poor validity in the clinical assessment for evaluating swallowing biomechanics. This impacts our initial diagnostic formulation but also heavily influences our rehabilitation approaches. If we cannot see within the pharynx, how do we know pharyngeal improvement is occurring? How do we maintain motivation for treatment when external evidence of treatment is obscure? How do we document small increments of change?
- Finally, as a consequence of the hurdles we face in rehabilitation, it is likely that treatment is discontinued prematurely due to frustration with the therapeutic process.

Clinicians facilitating swallowing rehabilitation need to be creative and inventive, and possess a bit of dogged determination to make identified rehabilitation techniques accessible to individuals with neurologic impairment. Mere instruction will rarely be sufficient. As discussed above, the process of consolidating skill acquisition at the neural level first requires sufficient specificity of practice (Rensink et al., 2009), sufficient task challenge (Krakauer, 2006) as well as the use of some form of biofeedback (Rose & Christina, 2006; Schmidt & Lee, 1999). It is notable that, in the studies reviewed above, biofeedback was implemented to enhance skill-based training in all but a single study (Crary et al., 2012).

Although the studies used different modalities, biofeedback enables online modification of performance and may be particularly critical in deglutition, improving the saliency of rehabilitation (Humbert & Joel, 2012). Biofeedback has been defined as:

> [t]he technique of using equipment (usually electronic) to reveal to human beings some of their internal physiological events, normal and abnormal, in the form of visual and auditory signals in order to teach them to *manipulate these otherwise involuntary or unfelt events by manipulating the displayed signals.* (Basmajian & DeLuca, 1985, p. 132)

This final italicized point is an important one. In the event of cognitive impairment that hinders manipulation of swallowing physiology, manipulation of a waveform may present a much easier, more accessible task. Kasman (1996) extends this definition by commenting that biofeedback modalities represent "instantaneous performance-contingent feedback . . . and provide an extension of the patients' or clinicians' senses" (p. 4). Because clinical measurement in swallowing presents such a challenge, our estimations of treatment response in the short term rely heavily on our "clinical sense." Many of our available biofeedback modalities are able to provide some quantification of swallowing behavior. This can be either through direct measurement of the targeted task, as in the case of manometric feedback of upper esophageal sphincter (UES) opening, or through a less firmly validated proxy measure, such as sEMG of floor of mouth muscles. The addition of quantitative information offered through instrumentation may provide encouragement for the patient and clinician alike to persevere with treatment when progress has not yet begun to manifest clinically.

Modalities for Biofeedback

Archer, Wellwood, Smith, and Newham (2013) surveyed 138 speech pathologists working in stroke rehabilitation across a variety of settings; 84% ($n = 101$) of respondents reported not using any method of biofeedback during swallowing exercises. Of these, 94.1% ($n = 80$) reported limited access to necessary equipment and 75.3% ($n = 64$) reported insufficient training or experience to use biofeedback. While these findings may be discouraging, it is important for the clinician to remember that biofeedback modalities for dysphagia rehabilitation may take many forms, many able to be adapted online for use. Logemann and Kahrilas (1990) published a case report of a patient for whom the VFSS was used as a biofeedback modality to impress on a patient the concept of pharyngeal residual and clearance. Although clearly fluoroscopy has its limitations as biofeedback—the invasiveness and expense of the technique render it challenging—these authors provide a good lesson. Do not miss an opportunity when it presents itself to enhance insight into pathophysiology and recovery. Allowing the patient observation of the monitor during VFSS may add very little time and exposure to the study, but the online feedback of pharyngeal swallowing may provide a valuable baseline for extending patients' perception of swallowing behavior.

Other modalities have been reported. Denk and Kaider (1997) employed videoendoscopy as an ongoing biofeedback modality in a group of head and neck cancer patients. Those who received biofeedback recovered more rapidly than those in a control group without feedback. Additionally, in the earlier rehabilitation section discussing oral lingual exercises, the use of the IOPI was described as a biofeedback modality (Nicosia et al., 2000; Robbins et al., 2005; Robbins, Levine, Wood, Roecker, & Luschei, 1995). Kahrilas, Logemann, Krugler, and Flanagan (1991) used tactile biofeedback in conjunction with changes in swallowing maneuvers to alter UES opening in healthy participants (n = 7) as evaluated by manofluoroscopy. Macrae, Anderson, Taylor-Kamara, and Humbert (2014) trained healthy participants (n = 16) to perform a volitional laryngeal vestibule closure maneuver during swallowing either with or without visual biofeedback. Results indicated participants in the biofeedback group made significant improvement in duration of laryngeal vestibule closure, while there was no difference from baseline in the no feedback group. Intensive manometric biofeedback training enabled healthy adults and patients following neurologic impairment to substantially reduce the temporal separation between proximal and distal pharyngeal pressure during volitional swallowing (Huckabee et al., 2014; Lamvik et al., 2015). This has been expanded with the advent of high-resolution manometry, which has a well-documented history of use as a biofeedback modality in other fields, such as anorectal biofeedback, and recently in a strength-based rehabilitation paradigm for oropharyngeal swallowing (O'Rourke & Humphries, 2017). Essentially, any tool that allows for a visual, tactile, or auditory representation of some aspect of swallowing that can be immediately fed back to the patient to provide information about performance can be used as a biofeedback modality. Using this definition, ultrasound, oxygen saturation, nasal air flow, endoscopy, and other clinical or diagnostic tools can be employed.

Biofeedback using sEMG is historically the most well-recognized feedback type for swallowing rehabilitation. This requires surface measurement of electrical activity in underlying musculature, which is displayed as a time-by-amplitude waveform, which provides a visual representation of relative strength and timing of muscle contraction. Through online monitoring of muscle activity, this modality supplies an alternative feedback system of proprioception, thus attenuating the patient's or clinician's awareness of one aspect of swallowing behavior. By yielding a visible representation of even the smallest motor response, rehabilitative efforts are maximized, allowing the patient and clinician a means of confronting automatic physiologic behaviors and enhancing access to volitional motor control. Incorporated into swallowing treatment, the technique appears to be most useful for monitoring execution of rehabilitative techniques related to pharyngeal phase dysphagia; however, it may also be used to monitor activity associated with orolingual movement. As sEMG biofeedback has been most predominantly reported in the swallowing rehabilitation literature, several publications reporting applications have emerged and will be discussed in a separate section below. Of interest when reflecting on prior discussions of skill-based training is that many of the studies using sEMG biofeedback used this modality as a means to provide feedback during muscle strengthening tasks. Although the presumed "active treatment" was strengthening, it would appear possible, if not probable, that many of the positive outcomes were a reflection not of the strengthening exercises themselves, but of the skill acquired through adjusting performance using biofeedback.

Importantly, recent research has highlighted the importance of specificity in biofeedback modality selection. In a study of healthy adults ($n = 30$), Azola, Sunday, and Humbert (2017) evaluated response to training of a volitional laryngeal vestibule closure maneuver with either submental sEMG, VFSS, or a combination of modalities. Interestingly, their results revealed that sEMG biofeedback was the least reliable, with an accuracy of 67% compared with a task-performance accuracy of 92% using VFSS biofeedback. Of concern, clinicians provided cues about accuracy of task performance correctly only 61% of the time when using sEMG as biofeedback compared with 83% during VFSS. The researchers postulate that the reduced accuracy with sEMG likely relates to a lack of relevant kinematic data to perform the laryngeal vestibule closure task, which is logical considering sEMG measured activation of submental musculature in this instance.

Two interesting neuroimaging studies provide indirect support that some of the treatment effects may have been secondary to the biofeedback modality itself. Kawai and colleagues (2009) evaluated the influence of swallowing sounds and videos on brain activation during swallowing. The supplementary motor area was activated during swallowing with auditory feedback only. When only visual stimuli were presented, the premotor and primary motor areas of both hemispheres and the left prefrontal area were activated. When audiovisual stimuli were presented, bilateral prefrontal and premotor areas were activated, providing strong support for the enhancing effects of feedback. Humbert and Joel (2012) followed this research with a study of signal responses dependent on blood-oxygen level during swallowing when modulated using three types of sensory input (taste, cutaneous electrical stimulation, and visual biofeedback) compared with a control condition of ingestion in healthy adults. The visual biofeedback task activated primarily frontal regions with less activation in S1 than water or other sensory modalities, suggesting a potential role of visual feedback in motor planning.

In the discussion of biofeedback modalities, it is impossible to determine from existing studies whether the positive outcomes were due to the intensity of treatment or the use of exteroceptive feedback. A recent meta-analysis evaluated 23 studies investigating whether biofeedback improves functional swallowing outcomes compared with treatment without biofeedback modalities (Benfield, Everton, Bath, & England, 2018). Results indicated that the three most common types of biofeedback in dysphagia rehabilitation were sEMG (36.6%), accelerometry (33.4%), and tongue manometry (14.9%). Dose appeared highly variable with a range of input from 4 to 72 sessions occurring at an intensity of twice daily to less than one session per week. At present, there are no randomized controlled trials to evaluate the efficacy of biofeedback; however, pooled study results reveal sEMG may enhance hyoid displacement (Benfield et al., 2018). The authors cautioned that existing studies were at risk of bias, with limited control and use of predominantly non-validated outcome measures to document improvement. Stated clearly, sEMG "can be a powerful tool that enhances motor learning and motivates patients during the therapy sessions when paired with movements that the signal directly represents (as shown in the limbs). Nevertheless, its proper use and limitations need to be clearly understood by clinicians involved in swallowing rehabilitation" (Azola et al., 2017, p. 122). Ongoing research is needed to demonstrate specific application of the various modalities of biofeedback to support increased specificity, engagement, and understanding of dysphagia rehabilitation.

Specific Research of the Use of sEMG Biofeedback

Clinical sEMG biofeedback has been extensively evaluated in other realms of physical medicine and rehabilitation, with numerous studies demonstrating clinical efficacy for a variety of neuromuscular disorders. Many of these studies have evaluated the use of sEMG in patients with intact cognition. However, a key study by Balliet, Levy, and Blood (1986) describes the use of sEMG as an adjunct to upper extremity retraining in patients with cognitive impairment. In this study, five patients with chronic upper extremity paresis, all of whom had aphasia and notably impaired comprehension, regained upper extremity function after 50 sessions using EMG biofeedback of the weakened limb. This study documents the benefits of this technology in assisting patients who may otherwise not be treatment candidates based on the severity of cognitive/communication deficits. Indeed, patients with unimpaired cognition may benefit from dysphagia rehabilitation without biofeedback; it is the patients with cognitive decline who will require the additional information from the external feedback. Although not an assessment of the application of biofeedback to dysphagia rehabilitation, the study carries significant implications, as many patients with dysphagia present with concomitant cognitive and/or communication deficits. These data, paired with research on motor learning theory, provide a foundation for the application of biofeedback in physical rehabilitation (Rubow, 1984; Wolf, 1994).

The discipline of speech pathology has yet to extensively evaluate this modality. The application of sEMG biofeedback in dysarthria rehabilitation, despite the neuromuscular nature of this type of disorder, has been grossly under-evaluated. A string of case studies documents consistently both the short-term and long-term benefits of this treatment modality in facilitating primarily facial muscle control in patients with both acute and chronic deficits. As documented in some, but not all, of the studies, this increased control subsequently resulted in improved appearance and speech production skills through greater volitional use of primarily the labial articulators (Brown, Nahai, & Basmajian, 1991; Brudny, Hammerschlag, Cohen, & Ransohoff, 1988; Daniel-Whitney, 1989; Draizar, 1984; Jankel, 1978; Netsell & Cleeland, 1973). However, there are no experimentally controlled studies that compare this modality with more traditional treatment.

A similar string of case studies has begun to emerge regarding the use of sEMG biofeedback in swallowing treatment. The first such paper was presented by Draizar (1984), who outlined the use of biofeedback in the treatment of dysarthria and dysphagia; however, little detail is provided regarding specific treatment methods or evaluation of progress. A more detailed account was provided by Bryant (1991), who presented a description of the use of sEMG biofeedback in the treatment of a patient with oral pharyngeal carcinoma. This patient, a 40-year-old female with severe dysphagia secondary to resection and radiation, was able to discontinue tube feedings and return to a near normal diet after 10 weeks of treatment.

Relevant to stroke, Crary (1995) described the treatment course of 6 patients with chronic dysphagia secondary to brainstem infarct treated with sEMG biofeedback. All 6 patients, with a mean time since onset of 18.8 months (range, 5–54 months), were able to return to oral feedings with discontinuation of tube feedings. Huckabee and Cannito (1999) extended this work by offering a report of 10 additional patients with dysphagia secondary to brainstem injury who participated in a 1-week accelerated swallowing treatment program with sEMG monitoring. Of these 10 patients, with a mean time post-onset of 26 months, 8 returned to full oral feeding with removal of feeding tube on average of 5.3 months after treatment initiation. All maintained oral feeding with the exception of 2, both of whom suffered further neurologic injury unrelated to their swallowing disorder. Crary, Carnaby-Mann, Groher, and Helseth (2004) completed an additional retrospective analysis of 45 patients, 25 of whom were dysphagic subsequent to stroke, using a therapy approach with sEMG biofeedback. Of the patients with stroke in this study, 92% demonstrated gains in functional oral intake, with a return to full oral diet in 65% after an average of 12.32 sessions (range, 4–28 sessions). A further, very similar study was completed on a small sample of 11 patients with dysphagia following stroke with an average time post-onset of 31 months (Bogaardt, Grolman, & Fokkens, 2009). Following an average of 7 sessions, scores on the Functional Oral Intake Scale (Crary, Mann, & Groher, 2004) increased from 2.6 (SD ±2.3) to 5.6 (SD ±1.6). Six of 8 patients who were initially fed via feeding tube were able to discontinue tube feedings. These studies document positive outcomes in patients who are not within the acute phase of recovery. These are promising findings. What must be remembered, however, is that these outcome data suggest improvement subsequent to swallowing rehabilitation exercises. Although sEMG was used as an adjunct, no control groups were utilized to differentiate the effect of biofeedback over and above traditional treatment approaches.

TAKE-HOME POINTS

The adverse effects reported with peripheral strengthening exercises, such as effortful swallowing (Chapter 20) as well as limitations in non-invasive brain stimulation modalities (Chapter 21), have inspired current research based on the use of behavioral adaptation to change the central swallowing system. However, despite the rehabilitation paradigm used, biofeedback likely plays a critical role in the ability to maximize cortical capacity to modulate aspects of pharyngeal swallowing (Humbert & Joel, 2012). Individualization of training targets could be expanded in future studies by providing increasingly specific goal-oriented, skill-based criteria to delineate performance outcomes and effect of biofeedback. Patients could continue to practice the adapted pharyngeal motor plan following the end of formal biofeedback training and hence further increase, rather than lose, their newly acquired and highly beneficial skill. This may reflect increases in neural plasticity, but much research is needed to elucidate this theory (Kleim & Jones, 2008; Robbins, Butler, et al., 2008).

23 Medical and Surgical Management

Randomized controlled clinical trials have not been conducted to determine the effectiveness of medical or surgical interventions on the management of dysphagia following stroke. Although not exclusive to stroke, medical and surgical interventions proposed to target specific physiologic problems are addressed in this chapter. A referral for medical and/or surgical management of dysphagia following stroke should only occur following detailed assessment of oropharyngeal swallowing function. As medical and surgical procedures are invasive, often irreversible and provide additional risks, a clear understanding of impairments at the biomechanical level is indicated to optimize outcomes and results. As stated by Martino and McCulloch (2016), "applying the same surgical management approach to [an] entire patient group is not appropriate and predicting the added value of a surgical intervention is very difficult" (p. 671). For example, when considering surgical options for upper esophageal sphincter (UES) dysfunction, the clinician must remember that in some patients, the primary cause for reduced UES opening is attributable to decreased anterior hyolaryngeal complex (HLC) movement rather than failed neural relaxation of the cricopharyngeus muscle. Hence, medical or surgical intervention would not facilitate UES opening in patients for whom impaired HLC movement was the underlying problem of decreased UES opening. Thus, the onus is on the astute clinician to pursue an accurate differential diagnosis.

MEDICAL MANAGEMENT

Botulinum Toxin

Botulinum toxin (Botox) has been used since 2000 to treat UES dysfunction. It is produced by the bacteria *Clostridium botulinum* and is the neurotoxin in botulism, which is a deadly, paralyzing disease that occurs when food contaminated with the toxin is swallowed. There are seven types of botulinum toxin; however, Botox type A is most commonly used in patients with UES dysfunction (Regan et al., 2014). For therapeutic purposes, Botox is injected into target muscles to yield paralysis and atrophy. The duration of the Botox effect is limited as nerve endings regenerate, which may be beneficial in acute patients who are spontaneously recovering or as a differential diagnosis tool to assess candidacy prior to performing invasive surgical procedures, such as cricopharyngeal myotomy (Martino & McCulloch, 2016). However, the temporary nature of Botox requires repeated reinjections in chronic patients (Ravich, 2001). As with all medical and surgical procedures for the UES, patients under consideration for this procedure should present with adequate pharyngeal motility and HLC excursion, indicating the root cause of the dysphagia is insufficient neural relaxation at the level of the cricopharyngeus muscle. As discussed in Chapter 13, preliminary assessment with a procedure such as pharyngeal manometry can be a valuable first step to clarify a diagnosis of UES dysfunction.

Individuals can have highly variable responses to Botox injections due to numerous factors, including the dose administered, needle gauge, injection site and injection method (Alfonsi et al., 2017). Further, administration is dependent on practitioner experience and preference. Medical professionals typically administer Botox under videoendoscopic guidance or transcutaneously with electromyography (Regan et al., 2014). Importantly, inappropriately placed Botox can affect functioning of laryngeal and pharyngeal musculature, leading to increased risk of dysphagia and reduced airway protection (Martino & McCulloch, 2016). A recent Cochrane Systematic Review highlighted that although Botox continues to be widely used internationally, there is insufficient evidence regarding its use (Regan et al., 2014). Non-randomized studies report improved swallowing as evidenced by instrumental examination and/or patient report, with efficacy reported anywhere between 43% and 100% (Alberty, Oelerich, Ludwig, Hartmann, & Stoll, 2000; Haapaniemi, Laurikainen, Pulkkinen, & Marttila, 2001; Parameswaran & Soliman, 2002; Regan et al., 2014; Shaw & Searl, 2001), with results lasting from 1 to 14 months post-injection (Shaw & Searl, 2001). However, most of these studies are retrospective and use heterogeneous populations, with no placebo control. More recently, in a prospective research study of Botox injections in patients with stroke (n = 24), Alfonsi and colleagues (2017) reported that 62.5% ($n = 15$) of the patients with stroke benefited from Botox for greater than 4 months post-injection. Short-term negative outcomes included worsening of dysphagia ($n = 3$) for up to 3 weeks following injection and increased dysphonia and breathiness ($n = 1$) for the first week following injection. As with other medical and surgical techniques, randomized controlled clinical trials have not been conducted to determine the effectiveness of Botox in dysphagia following stroke. Ongoing research is critical to further clarify patient candidacy, dose, administration, and other important methodological considerations for this medical procedure.

Dilation

Dilation may also be used to treat cricopharyngeal dysfunction; however, no study has specifically focused on this procedure in dysphagia following stroke. Medical dilation differs from the behavioral intervention termed "modified catheter balloon dilatation"; the reader is referred to a discussion of this rehabilitation approach in Chapter 20. The purpose of medical dilation is to stretch the UES tissues to increase compliance. This has been historically done in patients with post-radiation fibrotic changes or esophageal strictures; the theoretical basis for administration of dilation in dysphagia following stroke remains unclear. Stretching and tearing the muscle fibers to create a manual increase in opening may increase the risk of scar-tissue formation without attending to the primary failure to provide neural relaxation of the tonically contracted cricopharyngeus muscle. Nevertheless, dilation may be completed with a bougienage, a rigid dilator pushed through to a prescribed circumference, or a balloon, which can be inflated to specific dimensions. Historically, medical professionals have utilized round dilators that were designed for dilation in the esophagus; however, pilot research has provided preliminary data that the ovoid-shaped UES may benefit from a customized approach, such as twin dilators that replicate a kidney-like shape (Belafsky et al., 2013).

Generally, efficacy for dilation has been reported to be anywhere between 58% and 100% (Kocdor, Siegel, & Tulunay-Ugur, 2016), with the risk of treatment failure as high as 16%. Importantly, benefits of dilation are usually short term, with up to 58% of patients requiring multiple dilation procedures (Belafsky et al., 2013). Response to cricopharyngeal intervention with either dilation or myotomy was studied in a heterogeneous group of subjects, including two confirmed patients with stroke (Ali, Wallace, et al., 1997). Results suggested that 58% of subjects who underwent dilation had a subjective improvement in swallowing at 6 weeks following the procedure. Long-term response was not assessed.

SURGICAL INTERVENTION

Cricopharyngeal Myotomy

Cricopharyngeal myotomy is the most commonly performed surgery to alleviate oropharyngeal dysphagia (Cook & Kahrilas, 1999). In review of efficacy of myotomy in neurogenic dysphagia, Cook and Kahrilas report a 63% rate of improved response. However, this surgical procedure has the highest rate of complication (up to 39%) as compared with Botox (up to 20%) and dilation (up to 25%) (Kocdor et al., 2016). Although no controlled clinical trial has been completed to evaluate the effectiveness of cricopharyngeal myotomy in dysphagia following stroke, such a trial has been completed following surgery for head and neck cancer (Jacobs et al., 1999). Results revealed no significant differences in swallowing between those patients who underwent myotomy and those who did not.

Studies completed to date in neurogenic populations are frequently retrospective, use subjective versus objective outcome measures, and are limited by small sample sizes (e.g., Berg, Jacobs, Persky, & Cohen, 1985; Gilheaney, Kerr, Béchet, & Walshe, 2016; Kos, David, Klinkenberg-Knol, & Mahieu, 2010; Poirier et al., 1997). In a review of population-specific response to myotomy, patients presenting with idiopathic dysphagia showed complete improvement, while outcomes in patients with neurologic impairment or head and neck cancers had reduced success rates of less than 25% (Kos et al., 2010). As discussed earlier, the exact nature of UES dysfunction must be understood before proceeding with surgical or medical intervention in dysphagia following stroke. It appears that "myotomy is less reliable in patients after stroke and with myopathic disease, which can not only impact UES relaxation but also affect opening due to weakened hyolaryngeal elevation and pharyngeal bolus propulsion" (Martino & McCulloch, 2016, p. 672).

Thus, specific criteria have been suggested before considering a patient with neurogenic dysphagia for myotomy: (a) normal voluntary swallowing, (b) adequate tongue movement, (c) intact laryngeal functioning and phonation, and (d) no dysarthria (Duranceau, 1997). As discussed above, a manometric evaluation of the UES could also aid in facilitating identification of patients who will respond favorably to myotomy. Further, a trial with an appropriately placed Botox injection may serve as a beneficial screening to determine patients who may benefit from a further myotomy procedure. It has been suggested that in patients with non-progressive diseases, such as stroke, a myotomy should not be completed until 6 months post-injury, as many patients may spontaneously recover function within that time frame (Logemann, 1998). These same criteria should also be applied when deciding on other medical interventions for UES dysfunction.

Diverticulum Resection

Zenker's diverticulum is believed to be produced following prolonged pressure to a triangular region of anatomic weakness, termed Killian's dehiscence, between the pharyngeal constrictor muscles and cricopharyngeus muscle (Beard & Swanstrom, 2017). The pressure generated during pharyngeal swallowing in patients with reduced opening of the UES is believed to lead to this sac-like outpouching (Bizzotto, Iacopini, Landi, & Costamagna, 2013). While there is a limited understanding of the incidence of Zenker's diverticulum following stroke, Walters, Battle, Portera, Blizzard, and Browder (1998) reported that 66.7% of elderly patients (n = 12) presented with a diverticulum followed by brainstem or basilar lesions.

Symptoms of a Zenker's diverticulum include regurgitation, halitosis, globus, and odynophagia. Over time, this "pouch" can progressively increase in size, leading to an increased risk of aspiration, malnutrition, weight loss, and worsened overall health. The evidence regarding surgical methods for diverticulum resection is limited by a lack of randomized controlled studies comparing efficacy and outcomes (Bizzotto et al., 2013). However, usual treatment generally consists of a surgical procedure to eliminate the resistance at the level of the UES (e.g., myotomy) combined with resection of the diverticulum. The difficulty of this procedure increases with increased size of the pouch; thus, early identification and prevention are key. The reader is directed to Chapter 15, in which a case study involving a diverticulum is discussed.

Laryngeal Procedures

Vocal fold medialization is the procedure generally performed to treat aspiration due to an incompetent larynx. As discussed in earlier chapters, the clinician will recall that unilateral true vocal fold (TVF) paralysis is not uncommon in patients with a lateral medullary stroke. If recovery of function is anticipated (e.g., following stroke), augmentation of the TVF with an absorbable material, such as collagen, is recommended (Ergun & Kahrilas, 1997). Restoring laryngeal competence can also be accomplished through a thyroplasty, where a small implant is placed lateral to the TVF to aid in medialization. In a study of a heterogeneous population, including patients post-stroke, who underwent videofluoroscopic swallowing studies pre- and post-TVF medialization, the incidence of airway invasion did not significantly decrease following surgery (Bhattacharyya, Kotz, & Shapiro, 2002). However, evidence in populations with iatrogenic and idiopathic unilateral TVF paralysis indicate improved swallowing-related quality of life after TVF medialization (Cates, Venkatesan, Strong, Kuhn, & Belafsky, 2016); replication of these studies in populations with neurologic impairment, including stroke, is indicated.

A tracheotomy may be performed for patients following stroke with chronic aspiration. Although it will not improve swallowing, it will facilitate pulmonary toileting. Tracheotomy generally is performed only on the most severe patients with stroke. Laryngotracheal separation is a more radical attempt at preventing chronic aspiration, although allowing for oral intake. Whereas patients may return to oral diets, the ability to phonate is eliminated. If physiologic aspects of swallowing improve sufficiently, this procedure can be reversed, as the glottis is not removed (Eisele, 1991). Case reports have documented successful use of this procedure with the neurogenic population; however, only limited specification of outcome measures have been provided (Butcher, 1982; Krespi, Quatela, Sisson, & Som, 1984). Lastly, in severe, palliative cases, a total laryngectomy may be considered; however, this eliminates the ability for laryngeal phonation and requires a highly invasive, irreversible surgical procedure.

24 Lagniappe[1]

MANAGEMENT EFFECTIVENESS FOR PATIENTS WITH STROKE

It is important that swallowing management be proven effective. To do this, large-scale randomized controlled trials are warranted. Data from such studies can be used to support provision of services, staffing, and reimbursement from third-party payers for the evaluation and treatment of swallowing disorders. Prior chapters in this text have systematically reviewed existing literature on specific intervention techniques. A few additional studies have addressed rehabilitation programs, in which comprehensive management outcomes were evaluated. A clinical trial on swallowing intervention was completed in patients with stroke-related dysphagia and revealed positive results on the effects of treatment (Carnaby, Hankey, & Pizzi, 2006). In this study, 306 patients with acute stroke and a clinical diagnosis of dysphagia were randomly assigned to one of three treatment groups: (1) usual care as prescribed by the physician (n = 102), (2) low-intensity treatment (n = 102), and (3) high-intensity treatment (n = 102). The usual care (control) group was managed by the physician in the routine manner and may have consisted of referral to speech pathology in which patients were primarily supervised for feedings and given precautions for safe swallowing. The low-intensity group received directed intervention composed of compensatory strategies and precautions for safe swallowing. The high-intensity group received direct swallowing exercises. Treatment for the two experimental groups was based on results from the clinical swallowing examination and the videofluoroscopic swallowing study (VFSS).

---

[1]Lagniappe (lan yap) is a Creole word derived from American Spanish meaning "a little something extra" and is a favorite expression and treat in New Orleans.

Results revealed that the proportion of surviving patients who returned to a normal diet at 6 months was significantly greater for the high-intensity treatment group (70%) compared with the low-intensity treatment group (64%), which was greater than the usual care group (56%). Return to functional swallowing was significantly greater in the active treatment groups, and chest infection and complications related to dysphagia were significantly less in these two treatment groups compared with the control group. The number of sessions and duration of sessions were significantly greater for the experimental treatment groups compared with the control group. Not unexpectedly, the control group returned to a normal diet quicker than the treatment groups. It was noted that participants in the usual care group frequently received a regular diet prior to assessment.

Although not as rigorous as the randomized controlled clinical trial from Carnaby and colleagues (2006), other studies in the past two decades have provided evidence of treatment effects of swallowing intervention using large cohorts of patients with non-progressive neurologic disease, including stroke (Bartolome, Prosiegel, & Yassouridis, 1997; Neumann, 1993; Neumann, Bartolome, Buchholz, & Prosiegel, 1995). In the study by Neumann and colleagues, 58 consecutive patients were referred for swallowing therapy. Eleven patients were greater than 6 months following onset of deficits; the remaining 47 were less than 6 months. No patient was receiving exclusive oral intake, with 86% receiving only tube feeding. Patients received either indirect (e.g., rehabilitative exercises, thermal-tactile application) swallowing treatment or combined indirect and direct management (e.g., compensatory postures, swallowing maneuvers). Treatment lasted a median of 15 weeks. Results revealed that 67% of patients progressed to exclusive oral feeding at the end of treatment, with only 14% receiving only tube feeding. Time from onset of deficit (greater than 6 months, less than 6 months) was not associated with outcome, as both groups demonstrated a similar success rate in returning to oral intake. Patients greater than 6 months post-deficit tended to require a longer duration of treatment. These results support earlier outcomes from Neumann and are supported by later findings from Bartolome and colleagues. Of interest, Neumann identified decreased attention to be associated with negative outcomes. This was not confirmed by Neumann et al.; however, attentional deficits were associated with longer treatment durations.

Evidence suggests that the influence of rehabilitative recovery is markedly less than that of spontaneous recovery (Drulia & Ludlow, 2013); however, several case series are presented in Chapter 22 that suggest positive outcomes in treatment of individuals averaging 1.5 years post-stroke (Crary, 1995; Crary, Carnaby-Mann, Groher, & Helseth, 2004; Huckabee & Cannito, 1999; Huckabee, Lamvik & Jones, 2016). From these findings, clinicians may have greater confidence in the benefits of swallowing therapy as an active treatment, by excluding the significant influence of spontaneous recovery. Nevertheless, continued research is needed to replicate findings, determine response to specific types of treatment programs, and identify specific dose requirements.

While we acknowledge the growing list of rehabilitation publications since the first edition of this book, we also acknowledge that stronger evidence is needed. In this book, we noted the absence of evidence to support thermal-tactile application as a rehabilitation technique for delayed onset of the pharyngeal swallow. Yet, evidence is limited for many of our compensatory and rehabilitation techniques. For example, we discuss 3-second prep as a compensatory technique for pre-swallow pooling; however, there is **no** empirical evidence to support its use, nor is there evidence to support the use of chin tuck to decrease vallecular residue. Other examples of limited evidence include the Masako maneuver, for which long-term effects have never been evaluated in a patient population. Like the Masako maneuver, lingual strengthening exercises are included in our rehabilitation armament to increase base of tongue (BOT) to posterior pharyngeal wall (PPW) contact, thereby decreasing vallecular residue. However, most studies do not report any evidence demonstrating that it improves BOT-PPW contact or reduces valleculae residue (e.g., Robbins et al., 2007; Rogus-Pulia et al., 2016). At best, weak evidence is available in the form of a single case study in which decreased vallecular residue for semisolids and increased BOT to PPW pressure were reported (Juan et al., 2013). Even our management strategies with stronger evidence such as expiratory muscle strength training need to be further studied in patients with dysphagia following stroke, as well as replicated by investigators not associated with the lab where the treatment was first studied. While it is difficult to obtain funding for replication studies, this type of research is crucial in demonstrating that treatments work without negative effects.

Foley, Teasall, Salter, Kruger, and Martino (2008) provided a systematic review of randomized controlled trials in swallowing rehabilitation. A mere 15 articles met their inclusion criteria for evaluation; only 2 of these evaluated programmatic changes (Carnaby et al., 2006;

DePippo, Holas, Reding, Mandel, & Lesser, 1994). The authors of this review concluded that although evidence is lacking to support our current practices, they "do not suggest that they be discontinued, since current treatments have their roots in clinical experience and approaches that are physiologically based" (p. 263). Clearly, a fitting proverb is: "Absence of proof is not proof of absence." As researchers, however, we must do better in providing strong research to support evidence-based clinical practice. We need to: (1) have focused outcomes, (2) ensure that research participants have the underlying impairments targeted, not just signs such as Penetration-Aspiration Scale score 3 (penetration with laryngeal residue) or vallecular residue, and (3) use measurement techniques that target the outcome. This is particularly critical if we truly think rehabilitation must target specific physiological or biomechanical impairments. For example, if we want to use lingual exercises to increase BOT retraction and decrease vallecular residue with or without post-swallow airway invasion and have the evidence to support its use for this, researchers need to: (1) ensure that participants have the problem of vallecular residue with or without post-swallow residue due to decreased BOT retraction, and (2) employ measures that assess vallecular residue, airway invasion, and BOT retraction and/or BOT-PPW contact pressure. Only in this manner will we be able to determine whether lingual strengthening exercises can address this underlying biomechanic deficit and the associated signs.

In reading the above paragraphs, one might argue that we would be best to pack up shop and go home. Although our lack of empirical support is a harsh reality, it should also be our strong motivation to move forward in conscientious clinical practice using the best available evidence to target our patients' goals and conduct continued systematic empirical research. Doing nothing is not an option.

REASSESSMENT

Instrumental reassessment of swallowing must be considered on an individual basis in patients with stroke and is influenced by changes in the patient's medical status, cognition, and response to swallowing treatment. Studies have suggested that significant improvement in swallowing occurs in the first month following stroke in those patients with supratentorial stroke (Barer, 1989; Logemann, 1998); however, continued dysphagia also has been documented at 6 months post-stroke (Mann, Hankey, & Cameron, 1999).

Certain external factors may help the clinician determine response to treatment. A gross estimate of onset of the laryngeal elevation, duration, and distance of laryngeal movement may be achieved by palpating the larynx. Reduction in expectoration may indicate a more efficient swallow. Surface electromyography or ultrasound may facilitate objective quantification of treatment results. Before compensatory strategies are removed, however, instrumental reevaluation is recommended. This will allow objective documentation of changes in biomechanical functioning, as well as assessment of safety of swallowing with less restricted consistencies or without the use of postural compensation. The reassessment will also indicate whether further treatment is warranted and guide the direction of continued rehabilitation.

If clinical improvement is not evident, outcome measures should be reviewed for appropriateness and modified as needed. Improvement cannot be properly determined if outcome measures are poorly selected. Outcome measures should include both functional and objective swallowing measures. If outcome measures are appropriate but progress is not apparent, then modification of the treatment should be considered. For example, if effortful swallowing is used to target reduced BOT to PPW contact and little progress is evident, the clinician may want to consider adding visual feedback such as surface electromyography or manometry (see Chapters 20 and 22). Additionally, as addressed in Chapter 19, an absence of treatment effect may indicate that the treatment dose was insufficient to produce the desired effect, and modifications in service delivery would be indicated. Finally, poor treatment outcomes may also suggest that the wrong rehabilitation approach was selected.

If after considerable readjustment of the treatment plan improvement in swallowing is still not evident, discontinuation of treatment must be considered. Reassessment of swallowing with an instrumental examination should be considered prior to termination of treatment to document lack of progress.

As the patient with stroke is complex and behaviors in addition to swallowing are impaired, specific factors such as decreased cognition and attention may impede progress, particularly initially. In patients with acute stroke, cognitive behaviors may need to be addressed before swallowing rehabilitation is undertaken. As cognition improves, the response to swallowing treatment may increase. Reassessment of swallowing should also be considered when a change in swallowing functioning is reported in those patients previously discharged from therapy. Reevaluation by speech pathology may reveal changes in swallowing pathophysiology that are more amenable to rehabilitation. In addition, new treatment techniques may be available that may improve swallowing.

Optimal times when swallowing rehabilitation should be initiated or is most effective have not been established. It is frequently assumed that rehabilitation is best implemented in the acute phase post-stroke; however, empiric research is not available to confirm this. Several case-series studies of rehabilitation of dysphagia have focused on treatment composed of effortful swallowing and the Mendelsohn maneuver and have documented functional and physiologic improvement in patients well beyond the post-acute period (Crary, 1995; Crary et al., 2004; Huckabee & Cannito, 1999). The average time post-onset reported by Huckabee and Cannito was 26.9 months (range, 8–84 months). Although the number of participants was limited ($n = 10$), time post-onset was not a significant variable in recovery. One of the two patients with a time post-onset of less than 1 year was the slowest to have tube feeding discontinued. As a result, reassessment and potential reestablishment of treatment should be considered when the clinician is reconsulted for previously treated patients.

LAST THOUGHTS

Writing a book is hard work . . . perhaps even more so the third time around. It is time-consuming, tedious, and at times just plain boring. But, in balance, it also offers the rare opportunity for academics, who live in a world of evidence and science, to offer opinion and perspective and to reveal bias. We present these last ideas as food for thought: challenges to clinicians to be considered in shaping their clinical routines, warnings about potential speed bumps we see on the horizon, and finally, enthusiasm for the great potential that we have to offer patients with swallowing impairment.

1. *Reactive or proactive?* Our research tells us that dysphagia following stroke resolves quickly in many patients in the acute phase.

As clinicians, we have listened to this research and, therefore, have frequently adopted a practice of compulsive reevaluation. An initial assessment is completed and some decision made regarding immediate diet management (to feed or not to feed, that is the question!), but we hesitate, perhaps quite intelligently, to refer for instrumental assessment, even in the presence of subtle clinical signs. Perhaps the problem will resolve? So we return 2 days later and reassess. Given the lack of sensitivity in clinical assessment, the patient looks much the same. So we wait again and return 2 days later for reassessment. And again. And again, waiting for something to change or for the confidence that nothing will change. Sadly, the development of pneumonia is sometimes the "change" that prompts the instrumental assessment. A recent randomized controlled trial evaluating the inclusion of cough reflex testing by Miles, Zeng, McLauchlan, and Huckabee (2013) identified that in a control group of patients who ultimately received VFSS, *all* had developed pneumonia before referral for this assessment. Although the sample size was extremely small, even in a very few patients this would suggest a problematic clinical practice. The research by Wilson (2012) and Wilson and Howe (2012), summarized in Chapter 15, strongly supports the cost-effectiveness of early execution of instrumental assessment. Einstein defined insanity as doing the same thing over and over again and expecting different results. Are you a proactive or reactive clinician in managing dysphagia following stroke?

2. *Consultative or rehabilitative service?* The wait-and-see trap extends to management as well. It is imperative that clinicians not just evaluate swallowing with an instrumental examination, identify the presence of dysphagia, prescribe a diet with or without the inclusion of a compensatory technique, and then monitor the patient. If this scenario is followed, we become a consultative service, not a rehabilitative service. We are consulted to evaluate and *rehabilitate*, that is, to assist the patient in recovery. A diagnosis of dysphagia without subsequent rehabilitation does little for the patient and demeans our profession.

Our definition of management has changed. As discussed in Chapter 19, we are expanding our focus more heavily into rehabilitation research. Bolstered by the emergence of data that support these efforts, clinicians can strengthen their confidence in the application of rehabilitation programs. Rehabilitation will finally surpass compensation. It would never be considered acceptable for a physician to treat a urinary tract infection by advising bed rest and aspirin. Antibiotics would be expected. Likewise, except in cases of severe cognitive impairment where rehabilitation is not accessible to the patient, recommending a diet change and chin tuck is not an acceptable approach for swallowing impairment. Rehabilitation is expected. Intensive efforts are vital for success, and our research has documented preliminary evidence of substantial improvement even in patients with chronic and severe swallowing disability. We have not yet identified clear parameters for rehabilitation candidacy. Until these data emerge, every patient with stroke-related dysphagia should be considered a rehabilitation candidate until he or she proves not to be. Bottom line: Once the clinician decides the patient will not benefit from treatment, he or she will not benefit from treatment. Until that decision is made, there is potential for improvement. The responsibility for rehabilitation should not be taken lightly given the social and health ramifications of non-oral status; disuse and lack of stimulation of the swallowing sensorimotor system may have further negative effects on neural plasticity (Chapter 19). Moreover, if speech pathology wants to continue to be the preferred profession consulted for the evaluation and treatment of oropharyngeal dysphagia, we must remember that rehabilitation is part of this responsibility.

3. *New challenges: Will we be ready?* In the first edition of this text, we included a chapter on "Emerging Modalities in Dysphagia Rehabilitation." In the ensuing years, these described techniques fully merged into clinical consideration, thus shifting to Chapter 21 of this third edition. Progress continues in rehabilitation research, with the emergence of techniques that can be classified as "neuromodulatory" rapidly approaching. These techniques, including repetitive transcranial magnetic stimulation (TMS) and transcranial direct current stimulation, represent a significant shift away from manipulation of peripheral swallowing biomechanics to extrinsic manipulation of the underlying neural systems that support swallowing. By exciting or inhibiting neural activity, there is early evidence that biomechanical changes will follow, with improved swallowing efficiency and decreased adverse signs of dysphagia. At this point, we consider these techniques to still be highly experimental in nature. The interested reader is referred to more thorough review of techniques and potential application

in dysphagia rehabilitation provided by Doeltgen and Huckabee (2012). However, we wanted to confront clinicians with the professional challenges that will accompany the techniques, more than with the techniques themselves.

The use of neuromodulation in other areas of physical medicine has well preceded our ventures into swallowing recovery. As with most procedures in health care delivery, these techniques are not performed without potential risk to the patient population. As they have moved into experimental and clinical research, the International Federation of Clinical Neurophysiology formed a consensus panel to develop guidelines for use of TMS in particular (Rossi, Hallett, Rossini, & Pascual-Leone, 2009). These guidelines classify the relative risk of application of TMS in several classes, with recommendations for professionals, training, and supervision at each level. Protection of patient safety is paramount in these guidelines.

Currently, neuromodulatory techniques for the purpose of swallowing rehabilitation are currently only used by trained researchers conducting carefully monitored experimental protocols in a few research centers across the world. With very promising early results, it is very likely that the push to translate this work into clinical regimes will follow in fairly short time. This will bring significant professional challenges. The emergence of every new "medical" modality into speech-language pathology practices has required a redefinition of scope of practice. Our techniques in swallowing diagnosis and management, by necessity, are ever more invasive, to the point that we are now moving toward direct manipulation of the central nervous system. Once again, we need to redefine our scope of practice. Who will provide these neuromodulatory treatments? How can we ensure adequate training to safeguard patient safety? Under what conditions and in what contexts should the treatments be done? The professional responsibilities associated with this type of invasive treatment are remarkable and bear careful consideration *prior to* the techniques landing on the doorstep of clinical practice. We encourage clinicians to begin these discussions now, with their peers, their multidisciplinary health care teams, and, very importantly, with their professional organizations.

4. *Commercialization of knowledge.* The foundation for our work in swallowing diagnosis and management was laid through the

innovative thinking, exploratory research, and widespread clinical education offered by Jeri Logemann. Imagine what our practices would be like if she had commercialized her intellectual property. Where would the field be if she did not publish the techniques of how to conduct a VFSS or how to implement specific treatment techniques?

Open availability of specific details of evaluation and treatment methods allows clinicians to implement these techniques and researchers to replicate findings. This is true for all areas of our profession, not just dysphagia, and extends as well to all areas of health care. Open-source use of techniques, however, brings with it a host of issues with improper implementation and misuse. A benefit of commercialization of intellectual property is that "certification" provides some assurance that, at one point in time, users of the technique or instrumentation demonstrated some cursory level of competence. As evaluation and management techniques become more invasive—for instance, neuromodulation with TMS—assurance of competency is a must.

With open-source availability comes the responsibility to clinicians to ensure that the most up-to-date knowledge is obtained prior to implementation and that continued review of the literature is maintained. Thirty-five years ago, could a clinician read Logemann's groundbreaking text (1983) and then successfully complete a VFSS? No. At that time, training in swallowing and swallowing disorders was not part of the curriculum, but continuing educational conferences by Logemann and other experts allowed clinicians to obtain the necessary knowledge to successfully implement VFSS in clinical practice. Just because materials are freely available does not make the clinician any less responsible for obtaining the most up-to-date knowledge possible.

Commercialization of intellectual property provides challenges to the peer-review process. In the interest of protecting intellectual property, peer-reviewed research is submitted without full disclosure of research methods. It is difficult to fairly evaluate a technique, recommend for publication, and replicate findings if only cursory details of the methods are provided.

The applicability of a technique may be limited by commercialization. What is a potentially very positive advancement toward the improvement or resolution of dysphagia is limited to patients who are served by health care systems affluent enough to purchase the protocol. Free market may be all well and good when buying a car, but not when coping with the effects of illness.

With all of this said, our ultimate goal is to provide evidence-based evaluation and treatment for our clients with dysphagia. At the 2007 meeting of the Dysphagia Research Society, a presentation was given by Deborah Batjer, a very determined woman who recovered swallowing function after 2.5 years of nonoral feeding secondary to neurologic injury. She commented, "As you already know, dysphagia is a package deal. It is not just the dysfunctional synchronization of nerves and muscles. It also involves a complex matrix of emotions." In her talk, she also provided great insights into the possibility of recovery. "I will never forget the clinician's words after she saw my dismal test results. Without offering any promise of success (and, more importantly, of not predicting failure), she simply said, 'Let's try.' This was all I needed to hear—a hopeful message with effort to back it up."

References

Aagaard, P., Andersen, J. L., Dyhre-Poulsen, P., Leffers, A. M., Wagner, A., Magnusson, S. P., . . . Simonsen, E. B. (2001). A mechanism for increased contractile strength of human pennate muscle in response to strength training: Changes in muscle architecture. *Journal of Physiology*, *534*(2), 613–623.

Abdala, A. P. L., Rybak, I. A., Smith, J. C., Zoccal, D. B., Machado, B. H., St-John, W. M., & Paton, J. F. R. (2009). Multiple pontomedullary mechanisms of respiratory rhythmogenesis. *Respiratory Physiology & Neurobiology*, *168*(1–2), 19–25.

Abdul Wahab, N., Jones, R. D., & Huckabee, M. L. (2010). Effects of olfactory and gustatory stimuli on neural excitability for swallowing. *Physiology & Behavior*, *101*, 568–575.

Abdul Wahab, N., Jones, R. D., & Huckabee, M. L. (2011). Effects of olfactory and gustatory stimuli on the biomechanics of swallowing. *Physiology & Behavior*, *102*, 485–490.

Abernethy, P. J., Jürimäe, J., Logan, P. A., Taylor, A. W., & Thayer, R. E. (1994). Acute and chronic response of skeletal muscle to resistance exercise. *Sports Medicine*, *17*(1), 22–38.

Adams, V., Mathisen, B., Baines, S., Lazarus, C., & Callister, R. (2013). A systematic review and meta-analysis of measurements of tongue and hand strength and endurance using the Iowa Oral Performance Instrument (IOPI). *Dysphagia*, *28*(3), 350–369.

Adams, V., Mathisen, B., Baines, S., Lazarus, C., & Callister, R. (2015). Reliability of measurements of tongue and hand strength and endurance using the Iowa Oral Performance Instrument with elderly adults. *Disability and Rehabilitation*, *37*(5), 389–395.

Addington, W. R., Stephens, R. E., & Gilliland, K. A. (1999). Assessing the laryngeal cough reflex and the risk of developing pneumonia after stroke: An interhospital comparison. *Stroke*, *30*(6), 1203–1207.

Addington, W. R., Stephens, R. E., & Goulding, R. E. (1999). Anesthesia for the superior laryngeal nerves and tartaric acid-induced cough. *Archives of Physical Medicine and Rehabilitation*, *80*(12), 1584–1586.

Addington, W. R., Stephens, R. E., Phelipa, M. M., Widdicombe, J., & Ockey, R. R. (2008). Intra-abdominal pressures during voluntary and reflex cough. *Cough*, *4*(1), 2. https://doi.org/10.1186/1745-9974-4-2

Adler, S. S., Beckers, D., & Buck, M. (2008). *PNF in practice: An illustrated guide*. Heidelberg, Germany: Springer.

Adnerhill, I., Ekberg, O., & Groher, M. E. (1989). Determining normal bolus size for thin liquids. *Dysphagia*, *4*(1), 1–3.

Ahn, Y. H., Sohn, H. J., Park, J. S., Ahn, T. G., Shin, Y. B., Park, M., . . . Shin, Y. I. (2017). Effect of bihemispheric anodal transcranial direct current stimulation for dysphagia in chronic stroke patients: A randomized clinical trial. *Journal of Rehabilitation Medicine*, *49*(1), 30–35.

Aithal, G. P., Nylander, D., Dwarakanath, A. D., & Tanner, A. R. (1999). Subclinical esophageal peristaltic dysfunction during the early phase following a stroke. *Digestive Diseases and Sciences*, *44*(2), 274–278.

Alberts, M. J., Horner, J., Gray, L., & Brazer, S. R. (1992). Aspiration after stroke: Lesion analysis by brain MRI. *Dysphagia*, *7*(3), 170–173.

Alberty, J., Oelerich, M., Ludwig, K., Hartmann, S., & Stoll, W. (2000). Efficacy of botulinum toxin A for treatment of upper esophageal sphincter dysfunction. *Laryngoscope*, *110*(7), 1151–1156.

Alfonsi, E., Restivo, D. A., Cosentino, G., De Icco, R., Bertino, G., Schindler, A., . . . Tassorelli, C. (2017). Botulinum toxin is effective in the management of neurogenic dysphagia: Clinical-electrophysiological findings and tips on safety in different neurological disorders. *Frontiers in Pharmacology*, *8*, 80. https://doi.org/10.3389/fphar.2017.00080

Alfonso, M., Ferdjallah, M., Shaker, R., & Wertsch, J. J. (1998). Electrophysiologic validation of deglutitive UES opening head lift exercise [Abstract]. *Gastroenterology*, *114*(4), G2942.

Ali, G. N., Cook, I. J., Laundl, T. M., Wallace, K. L., & De Carle, D. J. (1997). Influence of altered tongue contour and position on deglutitive pharyngeal and UES function. *American Journal of Physiology–Gastrointestinal and Liver Physiology*, *273*(5), G1071–G1076.

Ali, G. N., Laundl, T. M., Wallace, K. L., deCarle, D. J., & Cook, I. J. (1996). Influence of cold stimulation on the normal pharyngeal swallow response. *Dysphagia*, *11*(1), 2–8.

Ali, G. N., Wallace, K. L., Laundl, T. M., Hunt, D. R., deCarle, D. J., & Cook, I. J. (1997). Predictors of outcome following cricopharyngeal disruption for pharyngeal dysphagia. *Dysphagia*, *12*(3), 133–139.

Allen, J. E., White, C., Leonard, R., & Belafsky, P. C. (2012). Comparison of esophageal screen findings on videofluoroscopy with full esophagram results. *Head & Neck*, *34*(2), 264–269.

Allen, J. E., White, C. J., Leonard, R. J., & Belafsky, P. C. (2010). Prevalence of penetration and aspiration on videofluoroscopy in normal individuals without dysphagia. *Otolaryngology–Head and Neck Surgery*, *142*(2), 208–213.

Alon, G. (1991). Principles of electrical stimulation. In R. M. Nelson & D. P. Currier (Eds.), *Clinical electrotherapy* (2nd ed., pp. 35–101). Norwalk, CT: Appleton & Lange.

Al-Toubi, A. K., Doeltgen, S. H., Daniels, S. K., Corey, D. M., & Huckabee, M. L. (2015). Pharyngeal pressure differences between four types of swallowing in healthy participants. *Physiology & Behavior*, *140*, 132–138.

American Speech-Language-Hearing Association. (1992, March). Instrumental diagnostic procedures for swallowing. *Asha, 34*(Suppl. 7), 25–33.

American Speech-Language-Hearing Association (2004). *Preferred practice patterns for the profession of speech-language pathology* [Preferred Practice Patterns]. Available from http://www.asha.org/policy

American Speech-Language-Hearing Association (2007). *Graduate curriculum on swallowing and swallowing disorders (adult and pediatric dysphagia)* [Technical report]. Available from http://www.asha.org/policy

American Speech-Language-Hearing Association (2009). *Frequently asked questions (FAQ) on swallowing screening: Special emphasis on patients with acute stroke.* Available from https://www.asha.org/uploadedFiles/FAQs-on-Swallowing-Screening.pdf

Amri, M., & Car, A. (1988). Projections from the medullary swallowing center to the hypoglossal motor nucleus: A neuroanatomical and electrophysiological study in sheep. *Brain Research, 441*(1–2), 119–126.

Amri, M., Car, A., & Jean, A. (1984). Medullary control of the pontine swallowing neurones in sheep. *Experimental Brain Research, 55*(1), 105–110.

Amri, M., Car, A., & Roman, C. (1990). Axonal branching of medullary swallowing neurons projecting on the trigeminal and hypoglossal motor nuclei: Demonstration by electrophysiological and fluorescent double labeling techniques. *Experimental Brain Research, 81*(2), 384–390.

Anderson, J. A., Pathak, S., Rosenbek, J. C., Morgan, R. O., & Daniels, S. K. (2016). Rapid aspiration screening for suspected stroke: Part 2: Initial and sustained nurse accuracy and reliability. *Archives of Physical Medicine and Rehabilitation, 97*(9), 1449–1455.

Anis, M. K., Abid, S., Jafri, W., Abbas, Z., Shah, H. A., Hamid, S., & Wasaya, R. (2006). Acceptability and outcomes of the percutaneous endoscopic gastrostomy (PEG) tube placement-patients' and care givers' perspectives. *BMC Gastroenterology, 6*(1), 37. https://doi.org/10.1186/1471-230X-6-37

Antonios, N., Carnaby-Mann, G., Crary, M., Miller, L., Hubbard, H., Hood, K., . . . Sillman, S. (2010). Analysis of a physician tool for evaluating dysphagia on an inpatient stroke unit: The Modified Mann Assessment of Swallowing Ability. *Journal of Stroke and Cerebrovascular Disease, 19*(1), 49–57.

Archer, S. K., Wellwood, I., Smith, C. H., & Newham, D. J. (2013). Dysphagia therapy in stroke: A survey of speech and language therapists. *International Journal of Language & Communication Disorders, 48*(3), 283–296.

Athukorala, R. P., Jones, R. D., Sella, O., & Huckabee, M. L. (2014). Skill training for swallowing rehabilitation in patients with Parkinson's disease. *Archives Physical Medicine and Rehabilitation, 95*(7), 1374–1382.

Aviv, J. E. (1997). Effects of aging on sensitivity of the pharyngeal and supraglottic areas. *American Journal of Medicine, 103*(5A), 74S–76S.

Aviv, J. E., Martin, J. H., Jones, M. E., Wee, T. A., Diamond, B., Keen, M. S., & Blitzer, A. (1994). Age-related changes in pharyngeal and supraglottic sensation. *Annals of Otology, Rhinology & Laryngology, 103*(10), 749–752.

Aydogdu, I., Ertekin, C., Tarlaci, S., Turman, B., Kiylioglu, N., & Secil, Y. (2001). Dysphagia in lateral medullary infarction (Wallenberg's syndrome): An acute disconnection syndrome in premotor neurons related to swallowing activity. *Stroke, 32*(9), 2081–2087.

Azola, A. M., Greene, L. R., Taylor-Kamara, I., Macrae, P., Anderson, C., & Humbert, I. A. (2015). The relationship between submental surface electromyography and hyo-laryngeal kinematic measures of Mendelsohn maneuver duration. *Journal of Speech, Language, and Hearing Research, 58*(6), 1627–1636.

Azola, A. M., Sunday, K. L., & Humbert, I. A. (2017). Kinematic visual biofeedback improves accuracy of learning a swallowing maneuver and accuracy of clinician cues during training. *Dysphagia, 32*(1), 115–122.

Babaei, A., Lin, E. C., Szabo, A., & Massey, B. T. (2015). Determinants of pressure drift in Manoscan™ esophageal high-resolution manometry system. *Neurogastroenterology & Motility, 27*(2), 277–284.

Babaei, A., Szabo, A., Yorio, S. D., & Massey, B. T. (2018). Pressure exposure and catheter impingement affect the recorded pressure in the Manoscan 360™ system. *Neurogastroenterology & Motility*, e13329. https://doi.org/10.1111/nmo.13329

Baker, L. L., McNeal, D. R., Benton, L. A., Bowman, B. R., & Waters, R. L. (1993). *Neuromuscular electrical stimulation: A practical guide.* Downey, CA: Los Amigos Research and Education Institute.

Balliet, R., Levy, B., & Blood, K. M. (1986). Upper extremity sensory feedback therapy in chronic cerebrovascular accident patients with impaired expressive aphasia and auditory comprehension. *Archives of Physical Medicine and Rehabilitation, 67*(5), 304–310.

Balou, M., McCullough, G. H., Aduli, F., Brown, D., Stack, B. C., Snoddy, P., & Guidry, T. (2014). Manometric measures of head rotation and chin tuck in healthy participants. *Dysphagia, 29*(1), 25–32.

Barbiera, F., Condello, S., De Palo, A., Todaro, D., Mandracchia, C., & De Cicco, D. (2006). Role of videofluorography swallow study in management of dysphagia in neurologically compromised patients. *La Radiologia Medica, 111*(6), 818–827.

Barer, D. H. (1989). The natural history and functional consequences of dysphagia after hemispheric stroke. *Journal of Neurology, Neurosurgery, and Psychiatry, 52*(2), 236–241.

Barker, A. T., Jalinous, R., & Freeston, I. L. (1985). Non-invasive magnetic stimulation of human motor cortex. *Lancet, 325*(8437), 1106–1107.

Barnett, M. L., Ross, D., Schmidt, R. A., & Todd, B. (1973). Motor skills learning and the specificity of training principle. *Research Quarterly. American Association for Health, Physical Education and Recreation, 44*(4), 440–447.

Bartolome, G., & Neumann, S. (1993). Swallowing therapy in patients with neurological disorders causing cricopharyngeal dysfunction. *Dysphagia, 8*(2), 146–149.

Bartolome, G., Prosiegel, M., & Yassouridis, A. (1997). Long-term functional outcome in patients with neurogenic dysphagia. *NeuroRehabilitation*, *9*(3), 195–204.

Basmajian, J. V., & DeLuca, C. J. (1985). *Muscles alive: Their functions revealed by electromyography* (5th ed.). Baltimore, MD: Williams and Wilkins.

Bassim, C. W., Gibson, G., Ward, T., Paphides, B. M., & DeNucci, D. J. (2008). Modification of the risk of mortality from pneumonia with oral hygiene care. *Journal of the American Geriatrics Society*, *56*(9), 1601–1607.

Bath, P. M., Scutt, P., Love, J., Clavé, P., Cohen, D., Dziewas, R., . . . Hamdy, S. (2016). Pharyngeal electrical stimulation for treatment of dysphagia in subacute stroke: A randomized controlled trial. *Stroke*, *47*(6), 1562–1570.

Bath, P. M., Bath, F. J., & Smithard, D. G. (2000). Interventions for dysphagia in acute stroke. *Cochrane Database System Review*, *2*.

Bautista, T. G., & Dutschmann, M. (2014). Pontomedullary nuclei involved in the generation of sequential pharyngeal swallowing and concomitant protective laryngeal adduction in situ. *Journal of Physiology*, *592*(12), 2605–2623.

Baylow, H. E., Goldfarb, R., Taveira, C. H., & Steinberg, R. S. (2009). Accuracy of clinical judgment of the chin-down posture for dysphagia during the clinical/bedside assessment as corroborated by videofluoroscopy in adults with acute stroke. *Dysphagia*, *24*(4), 423–433.

Beard, K., & Swanström, L. L. (2017). Zenker's diverticulum: Flexible versus rigid repair. *Journal of Thoracic Disease*, *9*(Suppl 2), S154–S162.

Beckstead, R. M., Morse, J. R., & Norgren, R. (1980). The nucleus of the solitary tract in the monkey: Projections to the thalamus and brain stem nuclei. *Journal of Comparative Neurology*, *190*(2), 259–282.

Belafsky, P. C., Mouadeb, D. A., Rees, C. J., Pryor, J. C., Postma, G. N., Allen, J., & Leonard, R. J. (2008). Validity and reliability of the Eating Assessment Tool (EAT-10). *Annals of Otology, Rhinology & Laryngology*, *117*(12), 919–924.

Belafsky, P. C., Plowman, E. K., Mehdizadeh, O., Cates, D., Domer, A., & Yen, K. (2013). The upper esophageal sphincter is not round: A pilot study evaluating a novel, physiology-based approach to upper esophageal sphincter dilation. *Annals of Otology, Rhinology & Laryngology*, *122*(4), 217–221.

Benfield, J. K., Everton, L. F., Bath, P. M., & England, T. J. (2018). Does therapy with biofeedback improve swallowing in adults with dysphagia? A systematic review and meta-analysis. *Archives of Physical Medicine and Rehabilitation*. https://doi.org/10.1016/j.apmr.2018.04.031

Benjamin, R. M., & Burton, H. (1968). Projection of taste nerve afferents to anterior opercular-insular cortex in squirrel monkey (Saimiri sciureus). *Brain Research*, *7*(2), 221–231.

Bennett, J. W., Van Lieshout, P. H. H. M., Pelletier, C. A., & Steele, C. M. (2009). Sip-sizing behaviors in natural drinking conditions compared to instructed experimental conditions. *Dysphagia*, *24*(2), 152–158.

Berg, H. M., Jacobs, J. B., Persky, M. S., & Cohen, N. L. (1985). Cricopharyngeal myotomy: A review of surgical results in patients with cricopharyngeal achalasia of neurogenic origin. *Laryngoscope*, *95*(11), 1337–1340.

Bernard, S., Loeslie, V., & Rabatin, J. (2016). Use of a modified Frazier Water Protocol in critical illness survivors with pulmonary compromise and dysphagia: A pilot study. *American Journal of Occupational Therapy*, *70*(1), 1–5. https://doi.org/10.5014/ajot.2016.016857

Berntson, G. G., Potolicchio, S. J., & Miller, N. E. (1973). Evidence for higher functions of the cerebellum: Eating and grooming elicited by cerebellar stimulation in cats. *Proceedings of the National Academy of Sciences*, *70*(9), 2497–2499.

Berretin-Felix, G., Sia, I., Barikroo, A., Carnaby, G. D., & Crary, M. A. (2016). Immediate effects of transcutaneous electrical stimulation on physiological swallowing effort in older versus young adults. *Gerodontology*, *33*(3), 348–355.

Bhattacharyya, N., Kotz, T., & Shapiro, J. (2002). Dysphagia and aspiration with unilateral vocal cord immobility: Incidence, characterization, and response to surgical treatment. *Annals of Otology, Rhinology & Laryngology*, *111*(8), 672–679.

Bickerman, H. A., & Barach, A. L. (1954). The experimental production of cough in human subjects induced by citric acid aerosols: Preliminary studies on the evaluation of antitussive agents. *American Journal of the Medical Sciences*, *228*(2), 156–163.

Bickerman, H. A., Cohen, B. M., & German, E. (1956). The cough response of normal human subjects stimulated experimentally by citric acid aerosol: Alterations produced by antitussive agents. I. Methology. *American Journal of the Medical Sciences*, *232*(1), 57–66.

Bisch, E. M., Logemann, J. A., Rademaker, A. W., Kahrilas, P. J., & Lazarus, C. L. (1994). Pharyngeal effects of bolus volume, viscosity, and temperature in patients with dysphagia resulting from neurologic impairment and in normal subjects. *Journal of Speech and Hearing Research*, *37*(5), 1041–1059.

Bizzotto, A., Iacopini, F., Landi, R., & Costamagna, G. (2013). Zenker's diverticulum: Exploring treatment options. *ACTA Otorhinolaryngologica Italica*, *33*(4), 219–229.

Blumenfeld, L., Hahn, Y., Lepage, A., Leonard, R., & Belafsky, P. C. (2006). Transcutaneous electrical stimulation versus traditional dysphagia therapy: A nonconcurrent cohort study. *Otolaryngology–Head and Neck Surgery*, *135*(5), 754–757.

Blumenstein, I., Shastri, Y., & Stein, J. (2014). Gastroenteric tube feeding: Techniques, problems and solutions. *World Journal of Gastroenterology*, *20*(26), 8505–8524.

Bodén, K., Hallgren, A., & Witt Hedstrom, H. (2006). Effects of three different swallow maneuvers analyzed by videomanometry. *Acta Radiologica*, *47*(7), 628–633.

Bogaardt, H. C., Grolman, W., & Fokkens, W. J. (2009). The use of biofeedback in the treatment of chronic dysphagia in stroke patients. *Folia Phoniatrica et Logopaedica*, *61*(4), 200–205.

Bolser, D. C., Gestreau, C., Morris, K. F., Davenport, P. W., & Pitts, T. E. (2013). Central neural circuits for coordination of swallowing, breathing, and coughing: Predictions from computational modeling and simulation. *Otolaryngologic Clinics of North America, 46*(6), 957–964.

Bolser, D. C., Pitts, T. E., Davenport, P. W., & Morris, K. F. (2015). Role of the dorsal medulla in the neurogenesis of airway protection. *Pulmonary Pharmacology & Therapeutics, 35*, 105–110.

Bonilha, H. S., Blair, J., Carnes, B., Huda, W., Humphries, K., McGrattan, K., . . . Martin-Harris, B. (2013). Preliminary investigation of the effect of pulse rate on judgments of swallowing impairment and treatment recommendations. *Dysphagia, 28*(4), 528–538.

Borr, C., Hielscher-Fastabend, M., & Lucking, A. (2007). Reliability and validity of cervical auscultation. *Dysphagia, 22*(3), 225–234.

Borsa, P. A., Sauers, E. L., & Lephart, S. M. (1999). Functional training for the restoration of dynamic stability in the PCL-injured knee. *Journal of Sport Rehabilitation, 8*(4), 362–378.

Bourne, M. (2002). *Food texture and viscosity: Concept and measurement* (2nd ed.). New York, NY: Academic Press.

Bours, G. J. J. W., Speyer, R., Lemmens, J., Limburg, M., & deWit, R. (2009). Bedside screening tests vs. videofluoroscopy or fiberoptic endoscopic evaluation of swallowing to detect dysphagia in patients with neurological disorders: Systematic review. *Journal of Advanced Nursing, 65*(3), 477–493.

Bove, M., Mansson, I., & Eliasson, I. (1998). Thermal oral-pharyngeal stimulation and elicitation of swallowing. *Acta Oto-Laryngologica, 118*(5), 728–731.

Brandimore, A. E., Hegland, K. W., Okun, M. S., Davenport, P. W., & Troche, M. S. (2017). Voluntary upregulation of reflex cough is possible in healthy older adults and Parkinson's disease. *Journal of Applied Physiology, 123*(1), 19–26.

Britton, D., Roeske, A., Ennis, S. K., Benditt, J. O., Quinn, C., & Graville, D. (2018). Utility of pulse oximetry to detect aspiration: An evidence-based systematic review. *Dysphagia, 33*(3), 282–292.

Brodal, P., & Bjaalie, J. G. (1992). Organization of the pontine nuclei. *Neuroscience Research, 13*(2), 83–118.

Brodal, P., & Bjaalie, J. G. (1997). Salient anatomic features of the cortico-ponto-cerebellar pathway. In *Progress in brain research* (Vol. 114, pp. 227–249). Cambridge, MA: Elsevier.

Brodsky, M. B., Suiter, D. M., Gonzalez-Fernandez, M., Michtalik, H. J., Frymark, T. B., Venediktov, R., & Schooling, T. (2016). Screening accuracy for aspiration using bedside water swallow tests. *Chest, 150*(1), 148–163.

Brogan, E., Langdon, C., Brookes, K., Budgeon, C., & Blacker, D. (2014). Respiratory infections in acute stroke: Nasogastric tubes and immobility are stronger predictors than dysphagia. *Dysphagia, 29*(3), 340–345

Broussard, D. L., & Altschuler, S. M. (2000). Central integration of swallow and airway-protective reflexes. *American Journal of Medicine, 108*(Suppl. 4a), 62S–67S.

Brown, D. M., Nahai, F., & Basmajian, J. V. (1991). Electromyographic biofeedback in the reeducation of facial palsy. *Americal Journal of Physical Medicine, 57*, 183–190.

Brudny, J., Hammerschlag, P. E., Cohen, N. L., & Ransohoff, J. (1988). Electromyographic rehabilitation of facial function and introduction of a facial paralysis grading scale for hypoglossal-facial nerve anastomosis. *Laryngoscope, 98*(4), 405–410.

Bryant, M. (1991). Biofeedback in the treatment of a selected dysphagic patient. *Dysphagia, 6*(3), 140–144.

Bülow, M., Olsson, R., & Ekberg, O. (1999). Videomanometric analysis of supraglottic swallow, effortful swallow, and chin tuck in healthy volunteers. *Dysphagia, 14*(2), 67–72.

Bülow, M., Olsson, R., & Ekberg, O. (2001). Videomanometric analysis of supraglottic swallow, effortful swallow, and chin tuck in patients with pharyngeal dysfunction. *Dysphagia, 16*(3), 190–195.

Bülow, M., Olsson, R., & Ekberg, O. (2002). Supraglottic swallow, effortful swallow, and chin tuck did not alter hypopharyngeal intrabolus pressure in patients with pharyngeal dysfunction. *Dysphagia, 17*(3), 197–201.

Bülow, M., Olsson, R., & Ekberg, O. (2003). Videoradiographic analysis of how carbonated thin liquids and thickened liquids affect the physiology of swallowing in subjects with aspiration on thin liquids. *Acta Radiologica, 44*(4), 366–372.

Bülow, M., Speyer, R., Baijens, L, Woisard, V., & Ekberg, O. (2008). Neuromuscular electrical stimulation (NMES) in stroke patients with oral and pharyngeal dysfunction. *Dysphagia, 23*(3), 203–209.

Burkhead, L. M., Sapienza, C. M., & Rosenbek, J. C. (2007). Strength-training exercise in dysphagia rehabilitation: Principles, procedures, and directions for future research. *Dysphagia, 22*(3), 251–265.

Burnett, T. A., Mann, E. A., Stoklosa, J. B., & Ludlow, C. L. (2005). Self-triggered functional electrical stimulation during swallowing. *Journal of Neurophysiology, 94*(6), 4011–4018.

Bussell, S. A., & Gonzalez-Fernandez, M. (2011). Racial disparities in the development of dysphagia after stroke: Further evidence from the Medicare database. *Archives of Physical Medicine and Rehabilitation, 92*(5), 737–742.

Butcher, R. B. (1982). Treatment of chronic aspiration as a complication of cerebrovascular accident. *Laryngoscope, 92*(6 Pt. 1), 681–685.

Butler, S. G. (2006). *The SLP's clinical use of pharyngeal and upper esophageal sphincter manometry*. Lincoln Park, NJ: KayPentax.

Butler, S. G., Markley, L., Sanders, B., & Stuart, A. (2015). Reliability of the penetration aspiration scale with flexible endoscopic evaluation of swallowing. *Annals of Otology, Rhinology & Laryngology, 124*(6), 480–483.

Butler, S. G., Postma, G. N., & Fischer, E. (2004). Effects of viscosity, taste, and bolus volume on swallowing apnea duration of normal adults. *Otolaryngology–Head and Neck Surgery, 131*(6), 860–863.

Butler, S. G., Stuart, A., Castell, D., Russell, G. B., Koch, K., & Kemp, S. (2009). Effects of age, gender, bolus condition, viscosity, and volume on pharyngeal and upper esophageal sphincter pressure and temporal measurements during swallowing. *Journal of Speech, Language, and Hearing Research*, *52*(1), 240–253.

Butler, S. G., Stuart, A., Leng, X., Rees, C., Williamson, J., & Kritchevsky, S. B. (2010). Factors influencing aspiration during swallowing in healthy older adults. *Laryngoscope*, *120*(11), 2147–2152.

Butler, S. G., Stuart, A., Markley, L., Feng, X., & Kritchevsky, S. B. (2018). Aspiration as a function of age, sex, liquid type, bolus volume, and bolus delivery across the healthy adult life span. *Annals of Otology, Rhinology & Laryngology*, *127*(1), 21–32.

Butler, S. G., Stuart, A., Markley, L., & Rees, C. (2009). Penetration and aspiration in healthy older adults as assessed during endoscopic evaluation of swallowing. *Annals of Otology, Rhinology, & Larnygology*, *118*(3), 190–198.

Butler, S. G., Stuart, A., Pressman, H., Poage, G., & Roche, W. J. (2007). Preliminary investigation of swallowing apnea duration and swallow/respiratory phase relationships in individuals with cerebral vascular accident. *Dysphagia*, *22*(3), 215–224.

Callahan, C. M., Haag, K. M., Buchanan, N. N., & Nisi, R. (1999). Decision making for percutaneous endoscopic gastrostomy among older adults in a community setting. *Journal of the American Geriatrics Society*, *47*(9), 1105–1109.

Campion, M. B., Haynos, J., & Palmer, J. B. (2007). An individualized approach to the videofluoroscopic swallowing study. *Perspectives on Swallowing and Swallowing Disorders*, *16*(1), 7–11.

Capra, N. F. (1995). Mechanisms of oral sensation. *Dysphagia*, *10*(4), 235–247.

Car, A. (1970). Cortical control of the bulbar swallowing center [in French]. *Journal of Physiology (Paris)*, *62*(4), 361–386.

Car, A. (1973). Cortical control of deglutition. 2. Medullary impact of corticofugal swallowing pathways [in French]. *Journal of Physiology (Paris)*, *66*(5), 553–575.

Car, A., & Amri, M. (1982). Pontine deglutition neurons in sheep. I. Activity and localization [in French]. *Experimental Brain Research*, *48*(3), 345–354.

Car, A., Jean, A., & Roman, C. (1975). A pontine primary relay for ascending projections of the superior laryngeal nerve. *Experimental Brain Research*, *22*(2), 197–210.

Carey, T. S., Hanson, L., Garrett, J. M., Lewis, C., Phifer, N., Cox, C. E., & Jackman, A. (2006). Expectations and outcomes of gastric feeding tubes. *American Journal of Medicine*, *119*(6), 527, e11–e16. https://doi.org/10.1016/j.amjmed.2005.11.021

Carl, L. R., & Johnson, P. R. (2006). *Drugs and dysphagia: How medications can affect eating and swallowing*. Austin, TX: Pro-Ed.

Carlaw, C., Finlayson, H., Beggs, K., Visser, T., Marcoux, C., Coney, D., & Steele, C. M. (2012). Outcomes of a pilot water protocol project in a rehabilitation setting. *Dysphagia*, *27*(3), 297–306.

Carnaby, G., Hankey, G. J., & Pizzi, J. (2006). Behavioural intervention for dysphagia in acute stroke: A randomised controlled trial. *Lancet Neurology*, *5*(1), 31–37.

Carnaby, G. D., & Harenberg, L. (2013). What is "usual care" in dysphagia rehabilitation: A survey of USA dysphagia practice patterns. *Dysphagia*, *28*(4), 567–574.

Carnaby-Mann, G. D., & Crary, M. A. (2007). Examining the evidence for neuromuscular electrical stimulation: A meta-analysis. *Archives of Otolaryngology–Head & Neck Surgery*, *133*(5), 743–749.

Carnaby-Mann, G. D., & Crary, M. A. (2008). Adjunctive neuromuscular electrical stimulation for treatment-refractory dysphagia. *Annals of Otology, Rhinology & Laryngology*, *117*(6), 564–571.

Carnaby-Mann, G. D., & Crary, M. A. (2010). McNeil Dysphagia Therapy Program: A case-control study. *Archives of Physical Medicine and Rehabilitation*, *91*(5), 743–749.

Carpenter, M. B. (1978). *Core text of neuroanatomy* (1st ed.). Baltimore, MD: Williams and Wilkins.

Carter, G., Lee, M., McKelvey, V., Sourial, A., Halliwell, R., & Livingston, M. (2004). Oral health status and oral treatment needs of dependent elderly people in Christchurch. *New Zealand Medical Journal (Online)*, *117*(1194).

Castell, J. A., & Castell, D. O. (1993). Modern solid state computerized manometry of the pharyngoesophageal segment. *Dysphagia*, *8(3)*, 270–275.

Castell, J. A., Dalton, C. B., & Castell, D. O. (1990). Pharyngeal and upper esophageal sphincter manometry in humans. *American Journal of Physiology*, *258*(2 Pt. 1), G173–G178.

Casaubon, L. K., Boulanger, J. M., Blacquiere, D., Boucher, S., Brown, K., Goddard, T., . . . Lindsay, P. (2015). Canadian stroke best practice recommendations: Hyperacute stroke care guidelines, update 2015. *International Journal of Stroke*, *10*(6), 924–940.

Cates, D. J., Venkatesan, N. N., Strong, B., Kuhn, M. A., & Belafsky, P. C. (2016). Effect of vocal fold medialization on dysphagia in patients with unilateral vocal fold immobility. *Otolaryngology–Head and Neck Surgery*, *155*(3), 454–457.

Cerenko, D., McConnel, F. M., & Jackson, R. T. (1989). Quantitative assessment of pharyngeal bolus driving forces. *Otolaryngology–Head and Neck Surgery*, *100*(1), 57–63.

Chang, A. B., Phelan, P. D., Roberts, R. G., & Robertson, C. F. (1996). Capsaicin cough receptor sensitivity test in children. *European Respiratory Journal*, *9*(11), 2220–2223.

Chang, A. B., Phelan, P. D., & Robertson, C. F. (1997). Cough receptor sensitivity in children with acute and non-acute asthma. *Thorax*, *52*(9), 770–774.

Chaudhuri, G., Hildner, C. D., Brady, S., Hutchins, B., Aliga, N., & Abadilla, E. (2002). Cardiovascular effects of the supraglottic and super-supraglottic swallowing maneuvers in stroke patients with dysphagia. *Dysphagia*, *17*(1), 19–23.

Chee, C., Arshad, S., Singh, S., Mistry, S., & Hamdy, S. (2005). The influence of chemical gustatory stimuli and oral anesthesia on healthy human pharyngeal swallowing. *Chemical Senses, 30*(5), 393–400.

Chen, M. Y., Ott, D. J., Peele, V. N., & Gelfand, D. W. (1990). Oropharynx in patients with cerebrovascular disease: Evaluation with videofluoroscopy. *Radiology, 176*(3), 641–643.

Chen, P. C., Chuang, C. H., Leong, C. P., Guo, S. E., & Hsin, Y. J. (2016). Systematic review and meta-analysis of the diagnostic accuracy of the water swallow test for screening aspiration in stroke patients. *Journal of Advanced Nursing, 72*(11), 2575–2586.

Chen, Y. W., Chang, K. H., Chen, H. C., Liang, W. M., Wang, Y. H., & Lin, Y. N. (2016). The effects of surface neuromuscular electrical stimulation on post-stroke dysphagia: A systemic review and meta-analysis. *Clinical Rehabilitation, 30*(1), 24–35.

Cheng, I. K., Chan, K. M., Wong, C. S., & Cheung, R. T. (2015). Preliminary evidence of the effects of high-frequency repetitive transcranial magnetic stimulation (rTMS) on swallowing functions in post-stroke individuals with chronic dysphagia. *International Journal of Language & Communication Disorders, 50*(3), 389–396.

Cheng, I. K., Chan, K. M., Wong, C. S., Li, L. S., Chiu, K. M., Cheung, R. T., & Yiu, E. M. (2017). Neuronavigated high-frequency repetitive transcranial magnetic stimulation for chronic post-stroke dysphagia: A randomized controlled study. *Journal of Rehabilitation Medicine, 49*(6), 475–481.

Chhabra, A., & Sapienza, C. (2007). A review of neurogenic and myogenic adaptations associated with specific exercise. *Communicative Disorders Review, 1*(3–4), 175–194.

Chhetri, D. K., & Berke, G. S. (1997). Ansa cervicalis nerve: Review of the topographic anatomy and morphology. *Laryngoscope, 107*(10), 1366–1372.

Chi-Fishman, G. (2005). Quantitative lingual, pharyngeal and laryngeal ultrasonography in swallowing research: A technical review. *Clinical Linguistics & Phonetics, 19*(6-7), 589–604.

Chi-Fishman, G., & Sonies, B. C. (2000). Motor strategy in rapid sequential swallowing: New insights. *Journal of Speech, Language, and Hearing Research, 43*(6), 1481–1492.

Chi-Fishman, G., & Sonies, B. C. (2002a). Effects of systematic bolus viscosity and volume changes on hyoid movement kinematics. *Dysphagia, 17*(4), 278–287.

Chi-Fishman, G., & Sonies, B. C. (2002b). Kinematic strategies for hyoid movement in rapid sequential swallowing. *Journal of Speech, Language, and Hearing Research, 45*(3), 457–468.

Chiara, T., Martin, A. D., Davenport, P. W., & Bolser, D. C. (2006). Expiratory muscle strength training in persons with multiple sclerosis having mild to moderate disability: Effect on maximal expiratory pressure, pulmonary function, and maximal voluntary cough. *Archives of Physical Medicine and Rehabilitation, 87*(4), 468–473.

Chiara, T., Martin, D., & Sapienza, C. (2007). Expiratory muscle strength training: Speech production outcomes in patients with multiple sclerosis. *Neurorehabilitation and Neural Repair, 21*(3), 239–249.

Chiramberro, M., Lindberg, N., Isometsä, E., Kähkönen, S., & Appelberg, B. (2013). Repetitive transcranial magnetic stimulation induced seizures in an adolescent patient with major depression: A case report. *Brain Stimulation, 6*(5), 830–831.

Chong, M. S., Lieu, P. K., Sitoh, Y. Y., Meng, Y. Y., & Leow, L. P. (2003). Bedside clinical methods useful as screening test for aspiration in elderly patients with recent and previous strokes. *Annals of the Academy of Medicine, Singapore, 32*(6), 790–794.

Cichero, J. A., Hay, G., Murdoch, B. E., & Halley, P. J. (1997). Videofluoroscopic fluids versus mealtime fluids: Differences in viscosity and density made clear. *Journal of Medical Speech-Language Pathology, 5*(3), 203–215.

Cichero, J. A., Jackson, O., Halley, P. J., & Murdoch, B. E. (2000). How thick is thick? Multicenter study of the rheological and material property characteristics of mealtime fluids and videofluoroscopy fluids. *Dysphagia, 15*(4), 188–200.

Cichero, J. A., Lam, P., Steele, C. M., Hanson, B., Chen, J., Dantas, R. O., . . . Stanschus, S. (2017). Development of international terminology and definitions for texture-modified foods and thickened fluids used in dysphagia management: The IDDSI framework. *Dysphagia, 32*(2), 293–314.

Cichero, J. A., & Murdoch, B. E. (2002). Detection of swallowing sounds: Methodology revisited. *Dysphagia, 17*(1), 40–49.

Ciocon, J. O., Silverstone, F. A., Graver, L. M., & Foley, C. J. (1988). Tube feedings in elderly patients. Indications, benefits, and complications. *Archives of Internal Medicine, 148*(2), 429–433.

Clark, H. M., Henson, P. A., Barber, W. D., Stierwalt, J. A., & Sherrill, M. (2003). Relationships among subjective and objective measures of tongue strength and oral phase swallowing impairments. *American Journal of Speech-Language Pathology, 12*(1), 40–50.

Clark, H. M., O'Brien, K., Calleja, A., & Corrie, S. N. (2009). Effects of directional exercise on lingual strength. *Journal of Speech, Language, and Hearing Research, 52*(4), 1034–1047.

Clavé, P., Arreola, V., Romea, M., Medina, L., Palomear, E., & Serra-Prat, M. (2008). Accuracy of the volume-viscosity swallow test for clinical screening of oropharyngeal dysphagia and aspiration. *Clinical Nutrition, 27*(6), 806–815.

Clavé, P., de Kraa, M., Arreola, V., Girvent, M., Farre, R., Palomera, E., & Serra-Prat, M. (2006). The effect of bolus viscosity on swallowing function in neurogenic dysphagia. *Alimentary Pharmacology and Therapeutics, 24*(9), 1385–1394.

Cock, C., Jones, C. A., Hammer, M. J., Omari, T. I., & McCulloch, T. M. (2017). Modulation of upper esophageal sphincter (UES) relaxation and opening during volume swallowing. *Dysphagia, 32*(2), 216–224.

Cock, C., & Omari, T. (2017). Diagnosis of swallowing disorders: How we interpret pharyngeal manometry. *Current Gastroenterology Reports, 19*(3), 11. https://doi.org/10.1007/s11894-017-0552-2

Cohen, M. D. (2009). Can we use pulsed fluoroscopy to decrease the radiation dose during video fluoroscopic feeding studies in children? *Clinical Radiology, 64*(1), 70–73.

Cola, M. G., Daniels, S. K., Corey, D. M., Lemen, L. C., McClain, M., & Foundas, A. L. (2010). Relevance of subcortical stroke in dysphagia. *Stroke, 41*(3), 482–486.

Cola, P. C., Gatto, A. R., Silva, R. G. D., Spadotto, A. A., Ribeiro, P. W., Schelp, A. O., . . . Henry, M. A. (2012). Taste and temperature in swallow transit time after stroke. *Cerebrovascular Diseases Extra, 2*(1), 45–51

Cola, P. C., Gatto, A. R., Silva, R. G. D., Spadotto, A. A., Schelp, A. O., & Henry, M. A. (2010). The influence of sour taste and cold temperature in pharyngeal transit duration in patients with stroke. *Arquivos de Gastroenterologia, 47*(1), 18–21.

Collins, M. J., & Bakheit, A. M. (1997). Does pulse oximetry reliably detect aspiration in dysphagic stroke patients? *Stroke, 28*(9), 1773–1775.

Colodny, N. (2000). Comparison of dysphagics and nondysphagics on pulse oximetry during oral feeding. *Dysphagia, 15*(2), 68–73.

Colodny, N. (2002). Interjudge and intrajudge reliabilities in fiberoptic endoscopic evaluation of swallowing (FEES) using the Penetration-Aspiration Scale: A replication study. *Dysphagia, 17*(4), 308–315.

Colodny, N. (2005). Dysphagic independent feeders' justifications for noncompliance with recommendations by a speech-language pathologist. *American Journal of Speech-Language Pathology, 14*(1), 61–70.

Conforto, A. B., Ferreiro, K. N., Tomasi, C., dos Santos, R. L., Moreira, V., Marie, S. K., . . . Cohen, L. G. (2010). Effects of somatosensory stimulation on motor function after subacute stroke. *Neurorehabilitation and Neural Repair, 24*(3), 263–272.

Cook, I. J. (1993). Cricopharyngeal function and dysfunction. *Dysphagia, 8*(3), 244–251.

Cook, I. J., Dodds, W. J., Dantas, R. O., Kern, M. K., Massey, B. T., Shaker, R., & Hogan, W. J. (1989). Timing of videofluoroscopic, manometric events, and bolus transit during the oral and pharyngeal phases of swallowing. *Dysphagia, 4*(1), 8–15.

Cook, I. J., Dodds, W. J., Dantas, R. O., Massey, B., Kern, M. K., Lang, I. M., . . . Hogan, W. J. (1989). Opening mechanisms of the human upper esophageal sphincter. *American Journal of Physiology-Gastrointestinal and Liver Physiology, 257*(5), G748–G759.

Cook, I. J., & Kahrilas, P. J. (1999). AGA technical review on management of oropharyngeal dysphagia. *Gastroenterology, 116*(2), 455–478.

Cook, I. J., Weltman, M. D., Wallace, K., Shaw, D. W., McKay, E., Smart, R. C., & Butler, S. P. (1994). Influence of aging on oral-pharyngeal bolus transit and clearance during swallowing: Scintigraphic study. *American Journal of Physiology–Gastrointestinal and Liver Physiology, 266*(6), G972–G977.

Cosentino, G., Alfonsi, E., Brighina, F., Fresia, M., Fierro, B., Sandrini, G., . . . Priori, A. (2014). Transcranial direct current stimulation enhances sucking of a liquid bolus in healthy humans. *Brain Stimulation*, *7*(6), 817–822.

Crary, M. A. (1995). A direct intervention program for chronic neurogenic dysphagia secondary to brainstem stroke. *Dysphagia*, *10*(1), 6–18.

Crary, M. A., Carnaby, G. D., LaGoria, L. A., & Carvajal, P. J. (2012). Functional and physiological outcomes from an exercise-based dysphagia therapy: A pilot investigation of McNeil Dysphagia Therapy Program. *Archives of Physical Medicine and Rehabilitation*, *93*(7), 1173–1178.

Crary, M. A., Carnaby, G. D., & Sia, I. (2014). Spontaneous swallow frequency compared with clinical screening in the identification of dysphagia in acute stroke. *Journal of Stroke and Cerebrovascular Diseases*, *23*(8), 2047–2053.

Crary, M. A., Carnaby, G. D., Sia, I., Khanna, A., & Waters, M. F. (2013). Spontaneous swallowing frequency has potential to identify dysphagia in acute stroke. *Stroke*, *44*(12), 3452–3457.

Crary, M. A., Carnaby-Mann, G. D., Groher, M. E., & Helseth, E. (2004). Functional benefits of dysphagia therapy using adjunctive sEMG biofeedback. *Dysphagia*, *19*(3), 160–164.

Crary, M. A., Mann, G. D., & Groher, M. E. (2005). Initial psychometric assessment of a functional oral intake scale for dysphagia in stroke patients. *Archives of Physical Medicine and Rehabilitation*, *86*(8), 1516–1520.

Curtis, D. J., Braham, S. L., Karr, S., Holborow, G. S., & Worman, D. (1988). Identification of unopposed intact muscle pair actions affecting swallowing: Potential for rehabilitation. *Dysphagia*, *3*(2), 57–64.

Daggett, A., Logemann, J., Rademaker, A., & Pauloski, B. (2006). Laryngeal penetration during deglutition in normal subjects of various ages. *Dysphagia*, *21*(4), 270–274.

Daniel-Whitney, B. (1989). Severe spastic-ataxic dysarthria in a child with traumatic brain injury: Questions for management. In K. Yorkston & D. Beukelman (Eds.), *Recent advances in clinical dysarthria* (pp. 129–137). Boston, MA: College-Hill.

Daniels, S. K. (2000). Swallowing apraxia: A disorder of the praxis system? *Dysphagia*, *15*(3), 159–166.

Daniels, S. K., Anderson, J. A., & Petersen, N. J. (2013). Implementation of stroke dysphagia screening the emergency department. *Nursing Research and Practice*, article ID 304190. https://doi.org/10.1155/2013/304190

Daniels, S. K., Anderson, J. A., & Willson, P. C. (2012). Valid items for screening dysphagia risk in patients with stroke: A systematic review. *Stroke*, *43*(3), 892–897.

Daniels, S. K., Brailey, K., & Foundas, A. L. (1999). Lingual discoordination and dysphagia following acute stroke: Analyses of lesion localization. *Dysphagia*, *14*(2), 85–92.

Daniels, S. K., Brailey, K., Priestly, D. H., Herrington, L. R., Weisberg, L. A., & Foundas, A. L. (1998). Aspiration in patients with acute stroke. *Archives of Physical Medicine and Rehabilitation*, *79*(1), 14–19.

Daniels, S. K., Corey, D. M., Hadskey, L. D., Legendre, C., Priestly, D. H., Rosenbek, J. C., & Foundas, A. L. (2004). Mechanism of sequential swallowing during straw drinking in healthy young and older adults. *Journal of Speech, Language, and Hearing Research*, *47*(1), 33–45.

Daniels, S. K., Corey, D. M., Schulz, P. E., Foundas, A. L., & Rosenbek, J. C. (2007). Effects of evaluation variables on swallowing performance in mild Alzheimer's disease [Abstract]. *Dysphagia*, *22*(4), 386.

Daniels, S. K., & Foundas, A. L. (1997). The role of the insular cortex in dysphagia. *Dysphagia*, *12*(3), 146–156.

Daniels, S. K., & Foundas, A. L. (1999). Lesion localization in acute stroke patients with risk of aspiration. *Journal of Neuroimaging*, *9*(2), 91–98.

Daniels, S. K., & Foundas, A. L. (2001). Swallowing physiology of sequential straw drinking. *Dysphagia*, *16*(3), 176–182.

Daniels, S. K., Foundas, A. L., Iglesia, G. C., & Sullivan, M. A. (1996). Lesion site in unilateral stroke patients with dysphagia. *Journal of Stroke and Cerebrovascular Disease*, *6*(1), 30–34.

Daniels, S. K., McAdam, C. P., Brailey, K., & Foundas, A. L. (1997). Clinical assessment of swallowing and prediction of dysphagia severity. *American Journal of Speech-Language Pathology*, *6*(4), 17–24.

Daniels, S. K., Pathak, S., Mukhi, S. V., Stach, C. B., Morgan, R. O., & Anderson, J. A. (2017). The relationship between lesion localization and dysphagia in acute stroke. *Dysphagia*, *32*(6), 777–784.

Daniels, S. K., Pathak, S., Rosenbek, J. C., Morgan, R. O., & Anderson, J. A. (2016). Rapid aspiration screening for suspected stroke: Part 1: Development and validation. *Archives of Physical Medicine and Rehabilitation*, *97*(9), 1440–1448.

Daniels, S. K., Pathak, S., Stach, C. B., Mohr, T. M., Morgan, R. O., & Anderson, J. A. (2015). Speech pathology reliability for stroke swallowing screening items. *Dysphagia*, *30*(5), 565–570.

Daniels, S. K., Schroeder, M. F., DeGeorge, P. C., Corey, D. M., & Rosenbek, J. C. (2007). Effects of verbal cue on bolus flow during swallowing. *American Journal of Speech-Language Pathology*, *16*(2), 140–147.

Daniels, S. K., Schroeder, M. F., DeGeorge, P. C., Corey, D. M., Foundas, A. L., & Rosenbek, J. C. (2009). Defining and measuring dysphagia following stroke. *American Journal of Speech-Language Pathology*, *18*(1), 74–81.

Daniels, S. K., Schroeder, M. F., McClain, M., Corey, D. M., Rosenbek, J. C., & Foundas, A. L. (2006). Dysphagia in stroke: Development of a standard method to examine swallowing recovery. *Journal of Rehabilitation, Research, and Development*, *43*(3), 347–356.

Dantas, R. O., Kern, M. K., Massey, B. T., Dodds, W. J., Kahrilas, P. J., Brasseur, J. G., . . . Lang, I. M. (1990). Effect of swallowed bolus variables on oral and pharyngeal phases of swallowing. *American Journal of Physiology–Gastrointestinal and Liver Physiology*, *258*(5), G675–G681.

Davalos, A., Ricart, W., Gonzalez-Huix, F., Soler, S., Marrugat, J., Molins, A., . . . Genis, D. (1996). Effect of malnutrition after acute stroke on clinical outcome. *Stroke*, *27*(6), 1028–1032.

Davies, A. E., Kidd, D., Stone, S. P., & MacMahon, J. (1995). Pharyngeal sensation and gag reflex in healthy subjects. *Lancet*, *345*(8948), 487–488.

Dejaeger, E., & Pelemans, W. (1996). Swallowing and the duration of the hyoid movement in normal adults of different ages. *Aging Clinical and Experimental Research*, *8*(2), 130–134.

Denes, G., Perazzolog, C., & Piccione, F. (1996). Intensive versus regular speech therapy in global aphasia: A controlled study. *Aphasiology*, *10*(4), 385–394.

Denk, D. M., & Kaider, A. (1997). Videoendoscopic biofeedback: A simple method to improve the efficacy of swallowing rehabilitation of patients after head and neck surgery. *ORL*, *59*(2), 100–105.

Dennis, M., Lewis, S., Cranswick, G., & Forbes, J. (2006). FOOD: A multicentre randomised trial evaluating feeding policies in patients admitted to hospital with a recent stroke. *Health Technology Assessment*, *10*(2). https://doi.org/10.3310/hta10020

DePippo, K. L., Holas, M. A., & Reding, M. J. (1992). Validation of the 3-oz water swallow test for aspiration following stroke. *Archives of Neurology*, *49*(12), 1259–1261.

DePippo, K. L., Holas, M. A., Reding, M. J., Mandel, F. S., & Lesser, M. L. (1994). Dysphagia therapy following stroke: A controlled trial. *Neurology*, *44*(9), 1655–1660.

Dick, T. E., Oku, Y., Romaniuk, J. R., & Cherniack, N. S. (1993). Interaction between central pattern generators for breathing and swallowing in the cat. *Journal of Physiology*, *465*, 715–730.

Dicpinigaitis, P. V. (2003). Cough reflex sensitivity in cigarette smokers. *Chest*, *123*(3), 685–688.

Dicpinigaitis, P. V., & Rauf, K. (1998). The influence of gender on cough reflex sensitivity. *Chest*, *113*(5), 1319–1321.

Ding, R., Logemann, J. A., Larson, C. R., & Rademaker, A. W. (2003). The effects of taste and consistency on swallow physiology in younger and older healthy individuals: A surface electromyographic study. *Journal of Speech, Language, and Hearing Research*, *46*(4), 977–989.

Dodds, W. J., Hogan, W. J., Reid, D. P., Stewart, E. T., & Arndorfer, R. C. (1973). A comparison between primary esophageal peristalsis following wet and dry swallows. *Journal of Applied Physiology*, *35*(6), 851–857.

Dodds, W. J., Kahrilas, P. J., Dent, J., & Hogan, W. J. (1987). Considerations about pharyngeal manometry. *Dysphagia*, *1*(4), 209–214.

Dodds, W. J., Man, K. M., Cook, I. J., Kahrilas, P. J., Stewart, E. T., & Kern, M. K. (1988). Influence of bolus volume on swallow-induced hyoid movement in normal subjects. *AJR American Journal of Roentgenology*, *150*(6), 1307–1309.

Dodds, W. J., Stewart, E. T., & Logemann, J. A. (1990). Physiology and radiology of the normal oral and pharyngeal phases of swallowing. *AJR American Journal of Roentgenology*, *154*(5), 953–963.

Doeltgen, S. H., Hofmayer, A., Gumbley, F., Witte, U., Moran, C., Carroll, G., & Huckabee, M. L. (2007). Clinical measurement of pharyngeal surface electromyography: Exploratory research. *Neurorehabilitation and Neural Repair*, *21*(3), 250–262.

Doeltgen, S. H., & Huckabee, M. L. (2012). Swallowing neurorehabilitation: From the research laboratory to routine clinical application. *Archives of Physical Medicine and Rehabilitation*, *93*(2), 207–213.

Doeltgen, S. H., Ong, E., Scholten, I., Cock, C., & Omari, T. (2017). Biomechanical quantification of Mendelsohn maneuver and effortful swallowing on pharyngoesophageal function. *Otolaryngology–Head and Neck Surgery*, *157*(5), 816–823.

Doeltgen, S. H., Witte, U., Gumbley, F., & Huckabee, M. L. (2009). Evaluation of manometric measures during tongue hold swallows. *American Journal of Speech-Language Pathology*, *18*(1), 65–73.

Donovan, N. J., Daniels, S. K., Edmiaston, J., Weinhardt, J., Summers, D., & Mitchell, P. H. (2013). Dysphagia screening: State of the art: Invitational conference proceeding from the State-of-the-Art Nursing Symposium, International Stroke Conference 2012. *Stroke*, *44*(4), e24–e31.

Donzelli, J., & Brady, S. (2004). The effects of breath-holding on vocal fold adduction: Implications for safe swallowing. *Archives of Otolaryngology–Head and Neck Surgery*, *130*(2), 208–210.

Doty, R. W. (1968). Neural organization of deglutition. In C. F. Code (Ed.), *Handbook of physiology: Alimentary canal: Motility* (Sec. 6, Vol. 4, pp. 1861–1902). Washington, DC: American Physiology Society.

Doty, R. W., & Bosma, J. F. (1956). An electromyographic analysis of reflex deglutition. *Journal of Neurophysiology*, *19*(1), 44–60.

Doty, R. W., Richmond, W. H., & Storey, A. T. (1967). Effect of medullary lesions on coordination of deglutition. *Experimental Neurology*, *17*(1), 91–106.

Dou, Z., Zu, Y., Wen, H., Wan, G., Jiang, L., & Hu, Y. (2012). The effect of different catheter balloon dilatation modes on cricopharyngeal dysfunction in patients with dysphagia. *Dysphagia*, *27*(4), 514–520.

Dozier, T. S., Brodsky, M. B., Michel, Y., Walters, B. C., Jr., & Martin-Harris, B. (2006). Coordination of swallowing and respiration in normal sequential cup swallows. *Laryngoscope*, *116*(8), 1489–1493.

Draizar, A. (1984). Clinical EMG feedback in motor speech disorders. *Archives of Physical Medicine and Rehabilitation*, *65*(8), 481–484.

Drulia, T. C., & Ludlow, C. L. (2013). Relative efficacy of swallowing versus non-swallowing tasks in dysphagia rehabilitation: Current evidence and future directions. *Current Physical Medicine and Rehabilitation Reports*, *1*(4), 242–256.

Du, J., Yang, F., Liu, L., Hu, J., Cai, B., Liu, W., . . . Liu, X. (2016). Repetitive transcranial magnetic stimulation for rehabilitation of poststroke dysphagia: A randomized, double-blind clinical trial. *Clinical Neurophysiology*, *127*(3), 1907–1913.

Dua, K. S., Ren, J., Bardan, E., Xie, P., & Shaker, R. (1997). Coordination of deglutitive glottal function and pharyngeal bolus transit during normal eating. *Gastroenterology*, *112*(1), 73–83.

Dudik, J. M., Coyle, J. L., El-Jaroudi, A., Sun, M., & Sejdić, E. (2016). A matched dual-tree wavelet denoising for tri-axial swallowing vibrations. *Biomedical Signal Processing and Control*, *27*, 112–121.

Dudik, J. M., Coyle, J. L., & Sejdić, E. (2015). Dysphagia screening: Contributions of cervical auscultation signals and modern signal-processing techniques. *IEEE Transactions on Human-Machine Systems*, *45*(4), 465–477.

Dudik, J. M., Kurosu, A., Coyle, J. L., & Sejdić, E. (2016). A statistical analysis of cervical auscultation signals from adults with unsafe airway protection. *Journal of Neuroengineering and Rehabilitation*, *13*(1), 7. https://doi.org/10.1186/s12984-015-0110-9

Duranceau, A. (1997). Cricopharyngeal myotomy in the management of neurogenic and muscular dysphagia. *Neuromuscular Disorders*, *7*(Suppl. 1), S85–S89.

Dyer, J. C., Leslie, P., & Drinnan, M. J. (2008). Objective computer-based assessment of valleculae residue: Is it useful? *Dysphagia*, *23*(1), 7–15.

Dziewas, R., Mistry, S., Hamdy, S., Minnerup, J., Van Der Tweel, I., Schäbitz, W., . . . PHAST-TRAC Investigators. (2017). Design and implementation of PHAryngeal electrical STimulation for early de-cannulation in TRACheotomized (PHAST-TRAC) stroke patients with neurogenic dysphagia: A prospective randomized single-blinded interventional study. *International Journal of Stroke*, *12*(4), 430–437.

Dziewas, R., Ritter, M., Schilling, M., Konrad, C., Oelenberg, S., Nabavi, D. G., . . . Lüdemann, P. (2004). Pneumonia in acute stroke patients fed by nasogastric tube. *Journal of Neurology, Neurosurgery, and Psychiatry*, *75*(6), 852–856.

Dziewas, R., Sörös, P., Ishii, R., Chau, W., Henningsen, H., Ringelstein, E. B., . . . Pantev, C. (2003). Neuroimaging evidence for cortical involvement in the preparation and in the act of swallowing. *NeuroImage*, *20*(1), 135–144.

Dziewas, R., Warnecke, T., Hamacher, T., Oelenberg, S., Teismann, I., Kraemer, C., . . . Schaebitz, W. R. (2008). Do nasogastric tubes worsen dysphagia in patients with acute stroke? *BMC Neurology*, *8*, 28. https://doi.org/10.1186/1471-2377-8-28

Dziewas, R., Warnecke, T., Ölenberg, S., Teismann, I., Zimmermann, J., Krämer, C., . . . Schäbitz, W. R. (2008). Towards a basic endoscopic assessment of swallowing in acute stroke—development and evaluation of a simple dysphagia score. *Cerebrovascular Diseases*, *26*(1), 41–47.

Easterling, C., Grande, B., Kern, M., Sears, K., & Shaker, R. (2005). Attaining and maintaining isometric and isokinetic goals of the Shaker exercise. *Dysphagia*, *20*(2), 133–138.

Ebihara, T., Ebihara, S., Maruyama, M., Kobayashi, M., Itou, A., Arai, H., & Sasaki, H. (2006). A randomized trial of olfactory stimulation using black pepper oil in older people with swallowing dysfunction. *Journal of the American Geriatrics Society, 54*(9), 1401–1406.

Ebihara, T., Takahashi, H., Ebihara, S., Okazaki, T., Sasaki, T., Watando, A., . . . Sasaki, H. (2005). Capsaicin troche for swallowing dysfunction in older people. *Journal of American Geriatric Society, 53*(5), 824–828.

Ebmeier, K. P., & Lappin, J. M. (2001). Electromagnetic stimulation in psychiatry. *Advances in Psychiatric Treatment, 7*(3), 181–188.

Edmiaston, J., Connor, L. T., Loehr, L., & Nassief, A. (2010). Validation of a dysphagia screening tool in acute stroke patients. *American Journal of Critical Care, 19*(4), 357–364.

Edmiaston, J., Connor, L. T., Steger-May, K., & Ford, A. L. (2014). A simple bedside stroke dysphagia screen, validated against videofluoroscopy, detects dysphagia and aspiration with high sensitivity. *Journal of Stroke and Cerebrovascular Diseases, 23*(4), 712–716.

Edwardson, M. A., Lucas, T. H., Carey, J. R., & Fetz, E. E. (2013). New modalities of brain stimulation for stroke rehabilitation. *Experimental Brain Research, 224*(3), 335–358.

Eisele, D. W. (1991). Surgical approaches to aspiration. *Dysphagia, 6*(2), 71–78.

Eisenhuber, E., Schima, W., Schober, E., Pokieser, P., Stadler, A., Scharitzer, M., & Oschatz, E. (2002). Videofluoroscopic assessment of patients with dysphagia: Pharyngeal retention is a predictive factor for aspiration. *AJR American Journal of Roentgenology, 178*(2), 393–398.

Elshukri, O., Michou, E., Mentz, H., & Hamdy, S. (2016). Brain and behavioral effects of swallowing carbonated water on the human pharyngeal motor system. *Journal of Applied Physiology, 120*(4), 408–415.

Emshoff, R., Bertram, S., & Strobl, H. (1999). Ultrasonographic cross-sectional characteristics of muscles of the head and neck. *Oral Surgery, Oral Medicine, Oral Pathology, Oral Radiology and Endodontics, 87*(1), 93–106.

Engstrom, C. M., Loeb, G. E., Reid, J. G., Forrest, W. J., & Avruch, L. (1991). Morphometry of the human thigh muscles. A comparison between anatomical sections and computer tomographic and magnetic resonance images. *Journal of Anatomy, 176*, 139–156.

Eom, M. J., Chang, M. Y., Oh, D. H., Kim, H. D., Han, N. M., & Park, J. S. (2017). Effects of resistance expiratory muscle strength training in elderly patients with dysphagic stroke. *NeuroRehabilitation, 41*(4), 747–752.

Ergun, G. A., & Kahrilas, P. J. (1997). Medical and surgical treatment interventions in deglutitive dysfunction. In A. L. Perlman & K. Schulze-Delreiu (Eds.), *Deglutition and its disorders* (pp. 463–490). San Diego, CA: Singular.

Ergun, G. A., Kahrilas, P. J., & Logemann, J. A. (1993). Interpretation of pharyngeal manometric recordings: Limitations and variability. *Diseases of the Esophagus, 6*(3), 11–16.

Ertekin, C. (2011). Voluntary versus spontaneous swallowing in man. *Dysphagia, 26*(2), 183–192.

Esposito, F., Cè, E., Gobbo, M., Veicsteinas, A., & Orizio, C. (2005). Surface EMG and mechanomyogram disclose isokinetic training effects on quadriceps muscle in elderly people. *European Journal of Applied Physiology, 94*(5-6), 549–557.

Esser, S. K., Huber, R., Massimini, M., Peterson, M. J., Ferrarelli, F., & Tononi, G. (2006). A direct demonstration of cortical LTP in humans: A combined TMS/EEG study. *Brain Research Bulletin, 69*(1), 86–94.

Falsetti, P., Acciai, C., Palilla, R., Bosi, M., Carpinteri, F., Zingarelli, A., . . . Lenzi, L. (2009). Oropharyngeal dysphagia after stroke: Incidence, diagnosis, and clinical predictors in patients admitted to a neurorehabilitation unit. *Journal of Stroke and Cerebrovascular Diseases, 18*(5), 329–335.

Farneti, D., Fattori, B., & Bastiani, L. (2017). The endoscopic evaluation of the oral phase of swallowing (Oral-FEES, O-FEES): A pilot study of the clinical use of a new procedure. *Acta Otorhinolaryngologica Italica, 37*(3), 201–206.

Farneti, D., Fattori, B., Nacci, A., Mancini, V., Simonelli, M., Ruoppolo, G., & Genovese, E. (2014). The pooling-score (P-score): Inter- and intra-rater reliability in endoscopic assessment of the severity of dysphagia. *ACTA Otorhinolaryngologica Italica, 34*(2), 105–110.

Fattal, M., Suiter, D. M., Warner, H. L., & Leder, S. B. (2011). Effect of presence/absence of a nasogastric tube in the same person on incidence of aspiration. *Otolaryngology-Head and Neck Surgery, 145*(5), 796–800.

Feinberg, M. J. (1993). Radiographic techniques and interpretation of abnormal swallowing in adult and elderly patients. *Dysphagia, 8*(4), 356–358.

Feng, W., Bowden, M. G., & Kautz, S. (2013). Review of transcranial direct current stimulation in poststroke recovery. *Topics in Stroke Rehabilitation, 20*(1), 68–77.

Ferdjallah, M., Wertsch, J. J., & Shaker, R. (2000). Spectral analysis of surface electromyography (EMG) of upper esophageal spinchter-opening muscles during head lift exercise. *Journal of Rehabilitation Research and Development, 37*(3), 335–340.

Ferrari, M., Olivieri, M., Sembenini, C., Benini, L., Zuccali, V., Bardelli, E., . . . LoCascio, V. (1995). Tussive effect of capsaicin in patients with gastroesophageal reflux without cough. *American Journal of Respiratory and Critical Care Medicine, 151*(2 Pt. 1), 557–561.

Fife, T. A., Butler, S. G., Langmore, S. E., Lester, S., Wright Jr, S. C., Kemp, S., . . . Rees Lintzenich, C. (2015). Use of topical nasal anesthesia during flexible endoscopic evaluation of swallowing in dysphagic patients. *Annals of Otology, Rhinology & Laryngology, 124*(3), 206–211.

Finestone, H. M., Greene-Finestone, L. S., Wilson, E. S., & Teasell, R. W. (1996). Prolonged length of stay and reduced functional improvement rate in malnourished stroke rehabilitation patients. *Archives of Physical Medicine and Rehabilitation*, 77(4), 340–345.

Flowers, H. L., Al Harbi, M. A., Mikulis, D., Silver, F. L., Rochon, E., Streiner, D., & Martino, R. (2017). MRI-based neuroanatomical predictors of dysphagia, dysarthria, and aphasia in patients with first acute ischemic stroke. *Cerebrovascular Diseases Extra*, *7*(1), 21–34.

Flowers, H. L., Skoretz, S. A., Streiner, D. L., Silver, F. L., & Martino, R. (2011). MRI-based neuroanatomical predictors of dysphagia after acute ischemic stroke: A systematic review and meta-analysis. *Cerebrovascular Diseases*, *32*(1), 1–10.

Foley, N., Teasell, R., Salter, K., Kruger, E., & Martino, R. (2008). Dysphagia treatment post stroke: A systematic review of randomized controlled trials. *Age and Ageing*, *37*(3), 258–264.

Folland, J. P., & Williams, A. G. (2007). Morphological and neurological contributions to increased strength. *Sports Medicine*, *37*(2), 145–168.

Foundas, A. L., Macauley, B. L., Raymer, A. M., Maher, L. M., Heilman, K. M., & Gonzalez Rothi, L. J. (1995). Ecological implications of limb apraxia: Evidence from mealtime behavior. *Journal of the International Neuropsychological Society*, *1*(1), 62–66.

Frank, U., van den Engel-Hoek, L., Nogueira, D., Schindler, A., Adams, S., Curry, M., & Huckabee, M. L. (2018, in press). International standardization of the Test of Masticating and Swallowing Solids in Children (TOMASS-C). *Journal of Oral Rehabilitation*, https://doi.org/10.1111/joor.12728

Fraser, C., Power, M., Hamdy, S., Rothwell, J., Hobday, D., Hollander, I., . . . Thompson, D. (2002). Driving plasticity in human adult motor cortex is associated with improved motor function after brain injury. *Neuron*, *34*(5), 831–840.

Fraser, S., & Steele, C. M. (2012). The effect of chin down position on penetration-aspiration in adults with dysphagia. *Canadian Journal of Speech-Language Pathology and Audiology*, *36*(2), 142–148.

Freed, M. L., Freed, L., Chatburn, R. L., & Christian, M. (2001). Electrical stimulation for swallowing disorders caused by stroke. *Respiratory Care*, *46*(5), 466–474.

Freeland, T. R., Pathak, S., Garrett. R. R., Anderson, J. A., & Daniels, S. K. (2016). Using medical mannequins to train nurses in stroke swallowing screening. *Dysphagia*, *31*(1), 104–110.

Frey, K. L., & Ramsberger, G. (2011). Comparison of outcomes before and after implementation of a water protocol for patients with cerebrovascular accident and dysphagia. *Journal of Neuroscience Nursing*, *43*(3), 165–171.

Fritz, M., Cerrati, E., Fang, Y., Verma, A., Achlatis, S., Lazarus, C., . . . Amin, M. (2014). Magnetic resonance imaging of the effortful swallow. *Annals of Otology, Rhinology & Laryngology*, *123*(11), 786–790.

Fujii, N., Inamoto, Y., Saitoh, E., Baba, M., Okada, S., Yoshioka, S., . . . Palmer, J. B. (2011). Evaluation of swallowing using 320-detector-row multislice CT. Part I: Single-and multiphase volume scanning for three-dimensional morphological and kinematic analysis. *Dysphagia*, *26*(2), 99–107.

Fujiu, M., & Logemann, J. A. (1996). Effect of a tongue-holding maneuver on posterior pharyngeal wall movement during deglutition. *American Journal of Speech-Language Pathology*, *5*(1), 23–30.

Fujiu, M., Logemann, J. A., & Pauloski, B. (1995). Increased post-operative posterior pharyngeal wall movement in patients with anterior oral cancer: Preliminary findings and possible implications for treatment. *American Journal of Speech-Language Pathology*, *4*(1), 24–30.

Gabriel, D. A., Kamen, G., & Frost, G. (2006). Neural adaptations to resistive exercise: Mechanisms and recommendations for training practices. *Sports Medicine*, *36*(2), 133–149.

Gadenz, C. D., de Campos Moreira, T., Capobianco, D. M., & Cassol, M. (2015). Effects of repetitive transcranial magnetic stimulation in the rehabilitation of communication and deglutition disorders: Systematic review of randomized controlled trials. *Folia Phoniatrica et Logopaedica*, *67*(2), 97–105.

Gallaugher, A. R., Wilson, C. A., & Daniels, S. K. (2012). Cerebro-vascular accidents and dysphagia. In R. Shaker, G. Postma, P. Belafsky, & C. Easterling (Eds.), *Principles of deglutition: A multidisciplinary text for swallowing and its disorders* (pp. 381–394). New York, NY: Springer.

Galovic, M., Leisi, N., Müller, M., Weber, J., Abela, E., Kägi, G., & Weder, B. (2013). Lesion location predicts transient and extended risk of aspiration after supratentorial ischemic stroke. *Stroke*, *44*(10), 2760–2767.

Galovic, M., Leisi, N., Müller, M., Weber, J., Tattenborn, B., Brugger, F., . . . Kägi, G. (2016). Neuroanatomical correlates of tube dependency and impaired oral intake after hemispheric stroke. *European Journal of Neurology*, *23*(5), 926–934.

Garcia, J. M., Chambers, E. T., & Molander, M. (2005). Thickened liquids: Practice patterns of speech-language pathologists. *American Journal of Speech-Language Pathology*, *14*(1), 4–13.

Garcia, J. M., Hakel, M., & Lazarus, C. (2004). Unexpected consequence of effortful swallowing: Case study report. *Journal of Medical Speech-Language Pathology*, *12*(2), 59–67.

Gariballa, S. E., Parker, S. G., Taub, N., & Castleden, M. (1998). Nutritional status of hospitalized acute stroke patients. *British Journal of Nutrition*, *79*(6), 481–487.

Garon, B. R., Engle, M., & Ormiston, C. (1997). A randomized control study to determine the effects of unlimited oral intake of water in patients with identified aspiration. *Journal of Neurologic Rehabilitation*, *11*(3), 139–148.

Gatto, A. R., Cola, P. C., Silva, R. G. D., Spadotto, A. A., Ribeiro, P. W., Schelp, A. O., . . . Henry, M. A. (2013). Sour taste and cold temperature in the oral phase of swallowing in patients after stroke. *CoDAS*, *25*(2), 163–167.

Geng, Z., Hoffman, M. R., Jones, C. A., McCulloch, T. M., & Jiang, J. J. (2013). Three-dimensional analysis of pharyngeal high-resolution manometry data. *Laryngoscope*, *123*(7), 1746–1753.

George, B., Kelly, A., Albert, G., Hwang, D., & Holloway, R. (2017). Timing of percutaneous endoscopic gastrostomy for acute ischemic stroke: An observational study from the US nationwide inpatient sample. *Stroke*, *48*(2), 420–427.

Gilheaney, Ó., Kerr, P., Béchet, S., & Walshe, M. (2016). Effectiveness of endoscopic cricopharyngeal myotomy in adults with neurological disease: Systematic review. *Journal of Laryngology & Otology*, *130*(12), 1077–1085.

Gillman, A., Winkler, R., & Taylor N. F. (2017). Implementing the free water protocol does not result in aspiration pneumonia in carefully selected patients with dysphagia: A systematic review. *Dysphagia*, *32*(3), 345–361.

Glanz, M., Klawansky, S., Stason, W., Berkey, C., & Chalmers, T. C. (1996). Functional electrostimulation in poststroke rehabilitation: A meta-analysis of the randomized controlled trials. *Archives of Physical Medicine and Rehabilitation*, *77*(6), 549–553.

Glickstein, M., & Doron, K. (2008). Cerebellum: Connections and functions. *Cerebellum*, *7*(4), 589–594.

Gomes, C., Andriolo, R., Bennett, C., Lustosa, S., Matos, D., Waisberg, D., & Waisberg, J. (2015). Percutaneous endoscopic gastrostomy versus nasogastric tube feeding for adults with swallowing disturbances. *Cochrane Database Systematic Reviews*, *5*, CD008096.

Gomes, L. M., Silva, R. G., Melo, M., Silva, N. N., Vanderlei, F. M., Garner, D. M., . . . Valenti, V. E. (2016). Effects of effortful swallow on cardiac autonomic regulation. *Dysphagia*, *31*(2), 188–194.

Gomes-Neto, M., Saquetto, M. B., Silva, C. M., Carvalho, V. O., Ribeiro, N., & Conceição, C. S. (2016). Effects of respiratory muscle training on respiratory function, respiratory muscle strength, and exercise tolerance in patients poststroke: A systematic review with meta-analysis. *Archives of Physical Medicine and Rehabilitation*, *97*(11), 1994–2001.

Gonzalez-Fernandez, M., Kleinman, J. T., Ky, P. K., Palmer, J. B., & Hillis, A. E. (2008). Supratentorial regions of acute ischemia associated with clinically important swallowing disorders: A pilot study. *Stroke*, *39*(11), 3022–3028.

Gonzalez-Fernandez, M., Kuhlemeier, K. V., & Palmer, J. B. (2008). Racial disparities in the development of dysphagia after stroke: Analysis of the California (MIRCal) and New York (SPARCS) inpatient databases. *Archives of Physical Medicine and Rehabilitation*, *89*(7), 1358–1365.

Goss, D. A., Hoffman, R. L., & Clark, B. C. (2012). Utilizing transcranial magnetic stimulation to study the human neuromuscular system. *Journal of Visualized Experiments: JoVE*, (59), e3387. https://doi.org/10.3791/3387

Gosselink, R. (2002). Respiratory rehabilitation: Improvement of short and long-term outcome. *European Respiratory Journal*, *20*(1), 4–5.

Gottlieb, D., Kipnis, M., Sister, E., Vardi, Y., & Brill, S. (1996). Validation of the 50 mL drinking test for evaluation of post-stroke dysphagia. *Disability and Rehabilitation*, *18*(10), 529–532.

Goyal, R. K., & Chaudhury, A. (2008). Physiology of normal esophageal motility. *Journal of Clinical Gastroenterology*, *42*(5), 610–619.

Griškova, I., Höppner, J., Rukšėnas, O., & Dapšys, K. (2006). Transcranial magnetic stimulation: The method and application. *Medicina (Kaunas)*, *42*(10), 792–804.

Guertin, P. A., & Steuer, I. (2009). Key central pattern generators of the spinal cord. *Journal of Neuroscience Research, 87*(11), 2399–2405.

Guiu Hernandez, E., Gozdzikowska, K., Apperley, O., & Huckabee, M. L. (2018). Effect of topical nasal anesthetic on swallowing in healthy adults: A double-blind, high-resolution manometry study. *Laryngoscope, 128*(6), 1335–1339.

Gullung, J. L., Hill, E. G., Castell, D. O., & Martin-Harris, B. (2012). Oropharyngeal and esophageal swallowing impairments: Their association and the predictive value of the modified barium swallow impairment profile and combined multichannel intraluminal impedance—esophageal manometry. *Annals of Otology, Rhinology & Laryngology, 121*(11), 738–745.

Haapaniemi, J. J., Laurikainen, E. A., Pulkkinen, J., & Marttila, R. J. (2001). Botulinum toxin in the treatment of cricopharyngeal dysphagia. *Dysphagia, 16*(3), 171–175.

Hadjikoutis, S., Pickersgill, T. P., Dawson, K., & Wiles, C. M. (2000). Abnormal patterns of breathing during swallowing in neurological disorders. *Brain, 123*(Pt. 9), 1863–1873.

Hamanaka-Kondoh, S., Kondoh, J., Tamine, K. I., Hori, K., Fujiwara, S., Maeda, Y., . . . Ono, T. (2014). Tongue pressure during swallowing is decreased in patients with Duchenne muscular dystrophy. *Neuromuscular Disorders, 24*(6), 474–481.

Hamdy, S., Aziz, Q., Rothwell, J. C., Crone, R., Hughes, D., Tallis, R. C., & Thompson, D. G. (1997). Explaining oropharyngeal dysphagia after unilateral hemispheric stroke. *Lancet, 350*(9079), 686–692.

Hamdy, S., Aziz, Q., Rothwell, J. C., Power, M., Singh, K. D., Nicholson, D. A., . . . Thompson, D. G. (1998). Recovery of swallowing after dysphagic stroke relates to functional reorganization in the intact motor cortex. *Gastroenterology, 115*(5), 1104–1112.

Hamdy, S., Aziz, Q., Rothwell, J. C., Singh, K. D., Barlow, J., Hughes, D. G., . . . Thompson, D. G. (1996). The cortical topography of human swallowing musculature in health and disease. *Nature Medicine, 2*(11), 1217–1224.

Hamdy, S., Mikulis, D. J., Crawley, A., Xue, S., Lau, H., Henry, S., & Diamant, N. E. (1999). Cortical activation during human volitional swallowing: An event-related fMRI study. *American Journal of Physiology-Gastrointestinal and Liver Physiology, 277*(1), G219–G225.

Hamdy, S., Rothwell, J. C., Brooks, D. J., Bailey, D., Aziz, Q., & Thompson, D. G. (1999). Identification of the cerebral loci processing human swallowing with H2(15)O PET activation. *Journal of Neurophysiology, 81*(4), 1917–1926.

Hamidon, B. B., Abdullah, S. A., Zawawi, M. F., Sukumar, N., Aminuddin, A., & Raymond, A. A. (2006). A prospective comparison of percutaneous endoscopic gastrostomy and nasogastric tube feeding in patients with acute dysphagic stroke. *Medical Journal of Malaysia, 61*(1), 59–66.

Hamlet, S. L., Nelson, R. J., & Patterson, R. L. (1990). Interpreting the sounds of swallowing: Fluid flow through the cricopharyngeus. *Annals of Otology, Rhinology & Laryngology, 99*(9 Pt. 1), 749–752.

Hammer, M. J., Jones, C. A., Mielens, J. D., Kim, C. H., & McCulloch, T. M. (2014). Evaluating the tongue-hold maneuver using high-resolution manometry and electromyography. *Dysphagia*, *29*(5), 564–570.

Hanna-Pladdy, B., Heilman, K. M., & Foundas, A. L. (2003). Ecological implications of ideomotor apraxia: Evidence from physical activities of daily living. *Neurology*, *60*(3), 487–490.

Harris-Warrick, R. M. (2010). General principles of rhythmogenesis in central pattern generator networks. In *Progress in brain research* (Vol. 187, pp. 213–222). Cambridge, MA: Elsevier.

Hanson, L., Garrett, J., Lewis, C., Phifer, N., Jackman, A., & Carey, T. (2008). Physicians' expectations of benefit from tube feeding. *Journal of Palliative Medicine*, *11*(8), 1130–1134.

Hasan, M., Meara, R. J., Bhowmick, B. K., & Woodhouse, K. (1995). Percutaneous endoscopic gastrostomy in geriatric patients: Attitudes of health care professionals. *Gerontology*, *41*(6), 326–331.

Hegland, K. W., Davenport, P. W., Brandimore, A. E., Singletary, F. F., & Troche, M. S. (2016). Rehabilitation of swallowing and cough functions following stroke: An expiratory muscle strength training trial. *Archives of Physical Medicine and Rehabilitation*, *97*(8), 1345–1351.

Hegland, K. W., Huber, J. E., Pitts, T., Davenport, P. W., & Sapienza, C. M. (2011). Lung volume measured during sequential swallowing in healthy young adults. *Journal of Speech, Language, and Hearing Research*, *54*(3), 777–786.

Hegland, K. W., Okun, M. S., & Troche, M. S. (2014). Sequential voluntary cough and aspiration or aspiration risk in Parkinson's disease. *Lung*, *192*(4), 601–608.

Heilman, K. M., Watson, R. T., & Valenstein, E. (2011). Neglect and related disorders. In K. M. Heilman & E. Valenstein (Eds.), *Clinical neuropsychology* (5th ed., pp. 296–348). New York, NY: Oxford University Press.

Hey, C., Pluschinski, P., Pajunk, R., Almahameed, A., Girth, L., Sader, R., . . . Zaretsky, Y. (2015). Penetration–aspiration: Is their detection in FEES® reliable without video recording? *Dysphagia*, *30*(4), 418–422.

Hiiemae, K. M., & Palmer, J. B. (1999). Food transport and bolus formation during complete feeding sequences on foods of different initial consistency. *Dysphagia*, *14*(1), 31–42.

Hinchey, J. A., Shephard, T., Furie, K., Smith, D., Wang, D., & Tonn, S. (2005). Formal dysphagia screening protocols prevent pneumonia. *Stroke*, *36*(9), 1972–1976.

Hinckley, J. J., & Craig, H. K. (1998). Influence of rate of treatment on the naming ability of adults with chronic aphasia. *Aphasiology*, *12*(11), 989–1006.

Hind, J. A., Nicosia, M. A., Roecker, E. B., Carnes, M. L., & Robbins, J. (2001). Comparison of effortful and non-effortful swallows in healthy middle-aged and older adults. *Archives of Physical Medicine and Rehabilitation*, *82*(12), 1661–1665.

Hirst, L. J., Ford, G. A., Gibson, G. J., & Wilson, J. A. (2002). Swallow-induced alterations in breathing in normal older people. *Dysphagia*, *17*(2), 152–161.

Hiss, S. G., & Huckabee, M. L. (2005). Timing of pharyngeal and upper esophageal sphincter pressures as a function of normal and effortful swallowing in young healthy adults. *Dysphagia, 20*(2), 149–156.

Hiss, S. G., Strauss, M., Treole, K., Stuart, A., & Boutilier, S. (2003). Swallowing apnea as a function of airway closure. *Dysphagia, 18*(4), 293–300.

Hiss, S. G., Strauss, M., Treole, K., Stuart, A., & Boutilier, S. (2004). Effects of age, gender, bolus volume, bolus viscosity, and gustation on swallowing apnea onset relative to lingual bolus propulsion onset in normal adults. *Journal of Speech, Language, and Hearing Research, 47*(3), 572–583.

Hiss, S. G., Treole, K., & Stuart, A. (2001). Effects of age, gender, bolus volume, and trial on swallowing apnea duration and swallow/respiratory phase relationships of normal adults. *Dysphagia, 16*(2), 128–135.

Hockman, C. H., Bieger, D., & Weerasuriya, A. (1979). Supranuclear pathways of swallowing. *Progress in Neurobiology, 12*(1), 15–32.

Hodges, P. W., Pengel, L. H. M., Herbert, R. D., & Gandevia, S. C. (2003). Measurement of muscle contraction with ultrasound imaging. *Muscle & Nerve, 27*(6), 682–692.

Hoffman, M. R., Ciucci, M. R., Mielens, J. D., Jiang, J. J., & McCulloch, T. M. (2010). Pharyngeal swallow adaptations to bolus volume measured with high-resolution manometry. *Laryngoscope, 120*(12), 2367–2373.

Hoffman, M. R., Jones, C. A., Geng, Z., Abelhalim, S. M., Walczak, C. C., Mitchell, A. R., . . . McCulloch, T. M. (2013). Classification of high-resolution manometry data according to videofluoroscopic parameters using pattern recognition. *Otolaryngology–Head and Neck Surgery, 149*(1), 126–133.

Hoffman, M. R., Mielens, J. D., Ciucci, M. R., Jones, C., Jiang, J. J., & McCulloch, T. M. (2012). High-resolution manometry of pharyngeal swallow pressure events associated with effortful swallow and the Mendelsohn maneuver. *Dysphagia, 27*(3), 418–426.

Hogan, N., Krebs, H. I., Rohrer, B., Palazzolo, J. J., Dipietro, L., Fasoli, S. E., . . . Volpe, B. T. (2006). Motions or muscles? Some behavioral factors underlying robotic assistance of motor recovery. *Journal of Rehabilitation Research & Development, 43*(5), 605–618.

Holas, M. A., DePippo, K. L., & Reding, M. J. (1994). Aspiration and relative risk of medical complications following stroke. *Archives of Neurology, 51*(10), 1051–1053.

Hori, K., Ono, T., Iwata, H., Nokubi, T., & Kumakura, I. (2005). Tongue pressure against hard palate during swallowing in post-stroke patients. *Gerodontology, 22*(4), 227–233.

Horner, J., Brazer, S. R., & Massey, E. W. (1993). Aspiration in bilateral stroke patients: A validation study. *Neurology, 43*(2), 430–433.

Horner, J., Buoyer, F. G., Alberts, M. J., & Helms, M. J. (1991). Dysphagia following brainstem stroke. Clinical correlates and outcome. *Archives of Neurology, 48*(11), 1170–1173.

Horner, J., Massey, E. W., & Brazer, S. R. (1990). Aspiration in bilateral stroke patients. *Neurology, 40*(11), 1686–1688.

Horner, J., Massey, E. W., Riski, J. E., Lathrop, D. L., & Chase, K. N. (1988). Aspiration following stroke: Clinical correlates and outcome. *Neurology, 38*(9), 1359–1362.

Hrycyshyn, A. W., & Basmajian, J. V. (1972). Electromyography of the oral stage of swallowing in man. *Developmental Dynamics, 133*(3), 333–340.

Hsiao, M. Y., Chang, Y. C., Chen, W. S., Chang, H. Y., & Wang, T. G. (2012). Application of ultrasonography in assessing oropharyngeal dysphagia in stroke patients. *Ultrasound in Medicine and Biology, 38*(9), 1522–1528.

Hu, S. H., Wang, S. S., Zhang, M. M., Wang, J. W., Hu, J. B., Huang, M. L., . . . Xu, Y. (2011). Repetitive transcranial magnetic stimulation-induced seizure of a patient with adolescent-onset depression: A case report and literature review. *Journal of International Medical Research, 39*(5), 2039–2044.

Huang, Y. L., Hsieh, S. F., Chang, Y. C., Chen, H. C., & Wang, T. G. (2009). Ultrasonographic evaluation of hyoid–larynx approximation in dysphagic stroke patients. *Ultrasound in Medicine and Biology, 35*(7), 1103–1108.

Huckabee, M. L., Butler, S. G., Barclay, M., & Jit, S. (2005). Submental surface electromyographic measurement and pharyngeal pressures during normal and effortful swallowing. *Archives of Physical Medicine and Rehabilitation, 86*(11), 2144–2149.

Huckabee, M. L., & Cannito, M. P. (1999). Outcomes of swallowing rehabilitation in chronic brainstem dysphagia: A retrospective evaluation. *Dysphagia, 14*(2), 93–109.

Huckabee, M. L., Deecke, L., Cannito, M. P., Gould, H. J., & Mayr, W. (2003). Cortical control mechanisms in volitional swallowing: The Bereitschaftspotential. *Brain Topography, 16*(1), 3–17.

Huckabee, M. L., & Doeltgen, S. H. (2007). Emerging modalities in dysphagia rehabilitation: Neuromuscular electrical stimulation. *New Zealand Medical Journal, 120*(1263), 1–9.

Huckabee, M. L., & Lamvik-Gozdzikowska, K. (2018). Reconsidering rehabilitation for neurogenic dysphagia: Strengthening skill in swallowing. *Current Physical Medicine and Rehabilitation Reports 6*(3), 186–191.

Huckabee, M. L., Lamvik, K., & Jones, R. (2014). Pharyngeal mis-sequencing in dysphagia: Characteristics, rehabilitative response, and etiological speculation. *Journal of the Neurological Sciences, 343*(1), 153–158.

Huckabee, M. L., & Macrae, P. (2014). Rethinking rehab: Skill-based training for swallowing impairment. *Perspectives on Swallowing and Swallowing Disorders (Dysphagia), 23*(1), 46–53.

Huckabee, M. L., Macrae, P., & Lamvik, K. (2015). Expanding instrumental options for dysphagia diagnosis and research: Ultrasound and manometry. *Folia Phoniatrica et Logopaedica, 67*(6), 269–284.

Huckabee, M. L., McIntosh, T., Fuller, L., Curry, M., Thomas, P., Walshe, M., . . . Sella-Weiss, O. (2018). The Test of Masticating and Swallowing Solids (TOMASS): Reliability, validity and international normative data. *International Journal of Language & Communication Disorders, 53*(1), 144–156.

Huckabee, M. L., & Pelletier, C. A. (1999). *Management of adult neurogenic dysphagia*. San Diego, CA: Singular.

Huckabee, M. L., & Steele, C. M. (2006). An analysis of lingual contribution to submental surface electromyographic measures and pharyngeal pressure during effortful swallow. *Archives of Physical Medicine and Rehabilitation, 87*(8), 1067–1072.

Hudash, G., Albright, J. P., McAuley, E., Martin, R. K., & Fulton, M. (1985). Cross-sectional thigh components: Computerized tomographic assessment. *Medicine and Science in Sports and Exercise, 17*(4), 417–421

Huggins, P. S., Tuomi, S. K., & Young, C. (1999). Effects of nasogastric tubes on the young, normal swallowing mechanism. *Dysphagia, 14*(3), 157–161.

Hughes, T. A., & Wiles, C. M. (1996). Clinical measurement of swallowing in health and in neurogenic dysphagia. *Quarterly Journal of Medicine, 89*(2), 109–116.

Humbert, I. A., Fitzgerald, M. E., McLaren, D. G., Johnson, S., Porcaro, E., Kosmatka, K., . . . Robbins, J. (2009). Neurophysiology of swallowing: Effects of age and bolus type. *NeuroImage, 44*(3), 982–991.

Humbert, I. A., & German, R. Z. (2013). New directions for understanding neural control in swallowing: The potential and promise of motor learning. *Dysphagia, 28*(1), 1–10.

Humbert, I. A., & Joel, S. (2012). Tactile, gustatory, and visual biofeedback stimuli modulate neural substrates of deglutition. *NeuroImage, 59*(2), 1485–1490.

Humbert, I. A., Poletto, C. J., Saxon, K. G., Kearney, P. R., Crujido, L., Wright-Harp, W., . . . Ludlow, C. (2006). The effect of surface electrical stimulation on hyolaryngeal movement in normal individuals at rest and during swallowing. *Journal of Applied Physiology, 101*(6), 1657–1663.

Hummel, F. C., & Cohen, L. G. (2006). Non-invasive brain stimulation: A new strategy to improve neurorehabilitation after stroke? *Lancet Neurology, 5*(8), 708–712.

Hutcheson, K. A., Hammer, M. J., Rosen, S. P., Jones, C. A., & McCulloch, T. M. (2017). Expiratory muscle strength training evaluated with simultaneous high-resolution manometry and electromyography. *Laryngoscope, 127*(4), 797–804.

Iinuma, T., Arai, Y., Abe, Y., Takayama, M., Fukumoto, M., Fukui, Y., . . . Komiyama, K. (2015). Denture wearing during sleep doubles the risk of pneumonia in the very elderly. *Journal of Dental Research, 94*(3 Suppl.), 28S–36S.

Iizuka, M., & Reding, M. (2005). Use of percutaneous endoscopic gastrostomy feeding tubes and functional recovery in stroke rehabilitation: A case-matched controlled study. *Archives of Physical Medicine and Rehabilitation, 86*(5), 1049–1052.

Inamoto, Y., Fujii, N., Saitoh, E., Baba, M., Okada, S., Katada, K., . . . Palmer, J. B. (2011). Evaluation of swallowing using 320-detector-row multislice CT. Part II: Kinematic analysis of laryngeal closure during normal swallowing. *Dysphagia, 26*(3), 209–217.

Inamoto, Y., Saitoh, E., Ito, Y., Kagaya, H., Aoyagi, Y., Shibata, S., . . . Palmer, J. B. (2018). The Mendelsohn maneuver and its effects on swallowing: Kinematic analysis in three dimensions using dynamic area detector CT. *Dysphagia, 33*(4), 419–430.

Inokuchi, H., González-Fernández, M., Matsuo, K., Brodsky, M. B., Yoda, M., Taniguchi, H., . . . Palmer, J. B. (2014). Electromyography of swallowing with fine wire intramuscular electrodes in healthy human: Activation sequence of selected hyoid muscles. *Dysphagia, 29*(6), 713–721.

Irie, H., & Lu, C. C. (1995). Dynamic evaluation of swallowing in patients with cerebrovascular accident. *Clinical Imaging, 19*(4), 240–243.

Ishikawa, A., Yoneyama, T., Hirota, K., Miyake, Y., & Miyatake, K. (2008). Professional oral health care reduces the number of oropharyngeal bacteria. *Journal of Dental Research, 87*(6), 594–598.

Jaafar, M., Mahadeva, S., Morgan, K., & Tan, M. (2016). Systematic review of qualitative and quantitative studies on the attitudes and barriers to percutaneous endoscopic gastrostomy feeding. *Clinical Nutrition, 35*(6), 1226–1235.

Jacob, P., Kahrilas, P. J., Logemann, J. A., Shah, V., & Ha, T. (1989). Upper esophageal sphincter opening and modulation during swallowing. *Gastroenterology, 97*(6), 1469–1478.

Jacobs, J. R., Logemann, J., Pajak, T. F., Pauloski, B. R., Collins, S., Casiano, R. R., & Schuller, D. E. (1999). Failure of cricopharyngeal myotomy to improve dysphagia following head and neck cancer surgery. *Archives of Otolaryngology–Head and Neck Surgery, 125*(9), 942–946.

James, A., Kapur, K., & Hawthorne, A. B. (1998). Long-term outcome of percutaneous endoscopic gastrostomy feeding in patients with dysphagic stroke. *Age and Ageing, 27*(6), 671–676.

Jankel, W. R. (1978). Bell palsy: Muscle reeducation by electromyograph feedback. *Archives of Physical Medicine and Rehabilitation, 59*(5), 240–242.

Jauch, E. C., Saver, J. L., Adams, H. P., Bruno, A., Demaerschalk, B. M., Khatri, P., . . . Yonas, H. (2013). Guidelines for the early management of patients with acute ischemic stroke: A guideline for healthcare professionals from the American Heart Association/American Stroke Association. *Stroke, 44*(3), 870–947.

Jayasekeran, V., Singh, S., Tyrrell, P., Michou, E., Jefferson, S., Mistry, S., . . . Hamdy, S. (2010). Adjunctive functional pharyngeal electrical stimulation reverses swallowing disability after brain lesions. *Gastroenterology, 138*(5), 1737–1746.

Jayatilake, D., Suzuki, K., Teramoto, Y., Ueno, T., Nakai, K., Hidaka, K., . . . Matsumura, A. (2014, June). Swallowscope: A smartphone based device for the assessment of swallowing ability. In *Biomedical and Health Informatics (BHI), 2014 IEEE-EMBS International Conference* (pp. 697–700).

Jayatilake, D., Ueno, T., Teramoto, Y., Nakai, K., Hidaka, K., Ayuzawa, S., . . . Suzuki, K. (2015). Smartphone-based real-time assessment of swallowing ability from the swallowing sound. *IEEE Journal of Translational Engineering in Health and Medicine*, *3*, 1–10.

Jean, A. (1984a). Brainstem organization of the swallowing network. *Brain, Behavior, and Evolution*, *25*(2–3), 109–116.

Jean, A. (1984b). Control of the central swallowing program by inputs from the peripheral receptors. A review. *Journal of Autonomic Nervous System*, *10*(3–4), 225–233.

Jean, A. (1990). Brainstem control of swallowing: Localization and organization of the central pattern generator for swallowing. In A. Taylor (Ed.), *Neurophysiology of the jaws and teeth* (pp. 294–321). London, UK: Macmillan Press.

Jean, A. (2001). Brainstem control of swallowing: Neuronal network and cellular mechanisms. *Physiological Reviews*, *81*(2), 929–969.

Jean, A., Amri, M., & Calas, A. (1983). Connections between the ventral medullary swallowing area and the trigeminal motor nucleus of the sheep studied by tracing techniques. *Journal of the Autonomic Nervous System*, *7*(2), 87–96.

Jean, A., & Car, A. (1979). Inputs to the swallowing medullary neurons from the peripheral afferent fibers and the swallowing cortical area. *Brain Research*, *178*(2–3), 567–572.

Jefferson, S., Mistry, S., Michou, E., Singh, S., Rothwell, J. C., & Hamdy, S. (2009). Reversal of a virtual lesion in human pharyngeal motor cortex by high-frequency contralesional brain stimulation. *Gastroenterology*, *137*(3), 841–849.

Jefferson, S., Mistry, S., Singh, S., Rothwell, J., & Hamdy, S. (2009). Characterizing the application of transcranial direct current stimulation in human pharyngeal motor cortex. *American Journal of Physiology–Gastrointestinal and Liver Physiology*, *297*(6), G1035–G1040.

Jenkinson, H. F., & Lamont, R. J. (2005). Oral microbial communities in sickness and in health. *Trends in Microbiology*, *13*(12), 589–595.

Jennings, K. S., Siroky, D., & Jackson, C. G. (1992). Swallowing problems after excision of tumors of the skull base: Diagnosis and management in 12 patients. *Dysphagia*, *7*(1), 40–44.

Jensen, J. L., Marstrand, P. C., & Nielsen, J. B. (2005). Motor skill training and strength training are associated with different plastic changes in the central nervous system. *Journal of Applied Physiology*, *99*(4), 1558–1568.

Jeon, W. H., Park, G. W., Lee, J. H., Jeong, H. J., & Sim, Y. J. (2014). Association between location of brain lesion and clinical factors and findings of videofluoroscopic swallowing study in subacute stroke patients. *Brain & Neurorehabilitation*, *7*(1), 54–60.

Johnson, E. R., McKenzie, S. W., & Sievers, A. (1993). Aspiration pneumonia in stroke. *Archives of Physical Medicine and Rehabilitation*, *74*(9), 973–976.

Jones, C. A., Ciucci, M. R., Hammer, M. J., & McCulloch, T. M. (2015). A multisensor approach to improve manometric analysis of the upper esophageal sphincter. *Laryngoscope*, *126*(3), 657–664.

Jones, C. A., Hammer, M. J., Hoffman, M. R., & McCulloch, T. M. (2014). Quantifying contributions of the cricopharyngeus to upper esophageal sphincter pressure changes by means of intramuscular electromyography and high-resolution manometry. *Annals of Otology, Rhinology & Laryngology*, *123*(3), 174–182.

Jones, C. A., Hoffman, M. R., Geng, Z., Abdelhalim, S. M., Jiang, J. J., & McCulloch, T. M. (2014). Reliability of an automated high-resolution manometry analysis program across expert users, novice users, and speech-language pathologists. *Journal of Speech, Language, and Hearing Research*, *57*(3), 831–836.

Jones, C. A., Knigge, M. A., & McCulloch, T. M. (2014). Speech pathologist practice patterns for evaluation and management of suspected cricopharyngeal dysfunction. *Dysphagia*, *29*(3), 332–339.

Jones, D. A., Rutherford, O. M., & Parker, D. F. (1989). Physiological changes in skeletal muscle as a result of strength training. *Experimental Physiology*, *74*(3), 233–256.

Joundi, R. A., Martino, R., Saposnik, G., Giannakeas, V., Fang, J., & Kapral, M. K. (2017). Predictors and outcomes of dysphagia screening after acute ischemic stroke. *Stroke*, *48*(4), 900–906.

Juan, J., Hind, J., Jones, C., McCulloch, T., Gangnon, R., & Robbins, J. (2013). Case study: Application of isometric progressive resistance oropharyngeal therapy using the Madison Oral Strengthening Therapeutic device. *Topics in Stroke Rehabilitation*, *20*(5), 450–470.

Jung, S. H., Lee, K. J., Hong, J. B., & Han, T. R. (2005). Validation of clinical dysphagia scale: Based on videofluoroscopic swallowing study. *Journal of Korean Academy of Rehabilitation Medicine*, *29*(4), 343–350.

Kaatzke-McDonald, M. N., Post, E., & Davis, P. J. (1996). The effects of cold, touch, and chemical stimulation of the anterior faucial pillar on human swallowing. *Dysphagia*, *11*(3), 198–206.

Kahrilas, P. J., Dodds, W. J., Dent, J., Logemann, J. A., & Shaker, R. (1988). Upper esophageal sphincter function during deglutition. *Gastroenterology*, *95*(1), 52–62.

Kahrilas, P. J., Lin, S., Logemann, J. A., Ergun, G. A., & Facchini, F. (1993). Deglutitive tongue action: Volume accommodation and bolus propulsion. *Gastroenterology*, *104*(1), 152–162.

Kahrilas, P. J., Logemann, J. A., Krugler, C., & Flanagan, E. (1991). Volitional augmentation of upper esophageal sphincter opening during swallowing. *American Journal of Physiology–Gastrointestinal and Liver Physiology*, *260*(3 Pt. 1), G450–G456.

Kahrilas, P. J., Logemann, J. A., Lin, S., & Ergun, G. A. (1992). Pharyngeal clearance during swallowing: A combined manometric and videofluoroscopic study. *Gastroenterology*, *103*(1), 128–136.

Kahrilas, P. J., & Shi, G. (1998). First measurement standards, then catheter standards, for manofluorography. *Dysphagia*, *13*(2), 111–112.

Kahrilas, P. J., & Sifrim, D. (2008). High-resolution manometry and impedance-pH/manometry: Valuable tools in clinical and investigational esophagology. *Gastroenterology*, *135*(3), 756–769.

Kajisa, E., Tohara, H., Nakane, A., Wakasugi, Y., Hara, K., Yamaguchi, K., . . . Minakuchi, S. (2018). The relationship between jaw-opening force and the cross-sectional area of the suprahyoid muscles in healthy elderly. *Journal of Oral Rehabilitation, 45*(3), 222–227.

Kanehisa, H., Nagareda, H., Kawakami, Y., Akima, H., Masani, K., Kouzaki, M., & Fukunaga, T. (2002). Effects of equivolume isometric training programs comprising medium or high resistance on muscle size and strength. *European Journal of Applied Physiology, 87*(2), 112–119.

Kaneoka, A. S., Langmore, S. E., Krisciunas, G. P., Field, K., Scheel, R., McNally, E., . . . Cabral, H. (2013). The Boston Residue and Clearance Scale: Preliminary reliability and validity testing. *Folia Phoniatrica et Logopaëdica, 65*(6), 312–317.

Kaneoka, A., Pisegna, J. M., Saito, H., Lo, M., Felling, K., Haga, N., . . . Langmore, S. E. (2017). A systematic review and meta-analysis of pneumonia associated with thin liquid vs. thickened liquid intake in patients who aspirate. *Clinical Rehabilitation, 31*(8), 1116–1125.

Karagiannis, M. J. P., Chivers, L., & Karagiannis, T. C. (2011). Effects of oral intake of water in patients with oropharyngeal dysphagia. *BMC Geriatrics, 11*(9). https://doi.org/10.1186/1471-2318-11-9

Karagiannis, M., & Karagiannis, T. C. (2014). Oropharyngeal dysphagia, free water protocol, and quality of life: An update from a prospective clinical trial. *Hellenic Journal of Nuclear Medicine, 17*(Suppl. 1), 26–29.

Kasman, G. (1996). Motor learning with EMG biofeedback: An information processing perspective for rehabilitation. *Biofeedback, 24*, 4–7.

Kastelik, J. A., Thompson, R. H., Aziz, I., Ojoo, J. C., Redington, A. E., & Morice, A. H. (2002). Sex-related differences in cough reflex sensitivity in patients with chronic cough. *American Journal of Respiration and Critical Care Medicine, 166*(7), 961–964.

Kawai, T., Watanabe, Y., Tonogi, M., Yamane, G. Y., Abe, S., Yamada, Y., & Callan, A. (2009). Visual and auditory stimuli associated with swallowing: An FMRI study. *The Bulletin of Tokyo Dental College, 50*(4), 169–181.

Kayser-Jones, J., & Schell, E. S. (1997). Staffing and the mealtime experience of nursing home residents on a special care unit. *American Journal of Alzheimer's Disease, 12*(2), 67–72.

Kelly, A. M., Drinnan, M. J., & Leslie, P. (2007). Assessing penetration and aspiration: How do videofluoroscopy and fiberoptic endoscopic evaluation of swallowing compare? *Laryngoscope, 117*(10), 1723–1727.

Kelly, A. M., Leslie, P., Beale, T., Payten, C., & Drinnan, M. J. (2006). Fibreoptic endoscopic evaluation of swallowing and videofluoroscopy: Does examination type influence perception of pharyngeal residue severity? *Clinical Otolaryngology, 31*(5), 425–432.

Kelly, B. N., Huckabee, M. L., Jones, R. D., & Carroll, G. J. (2007). The influence of volition on breathing-swallowing coordination in healthy adults. *Behavioral Neuroscience, 121*(6), 1174–1179.

Kent, R. D. (2004). The uniqueness of speech among motor systems. *Clinical Linguistics & Phonetics, 18*(6-8), 495–505.

Kern, M., Bardan, E., Arndorfer, R., Hofmann, C., Ren, J., & Shaker, R. (1999). Comparison of upper esophageal sphincter opening in healthy asymptomatic young and elderly volunteers. *Annals of Otology, Rhinology & Laryngology, 108*(10), 982–989.

Kern, M. K., Jaradeh, S., Arndorfer, R. C., & Shaker, R. (2001). Cerebral cortical representation of reflexive and volitional swallowing in humans. *American Journal of Physiology–Gastrointestinal and Liver Physiology, 280*(3), G354–G360.

Kertscher, B., Speyer, R., Plamieri, M., & Plant, C. (2014). Bedside screening to detect oropharyngeal dysphagia in patients with neurological disorders: An updated systematic review. *Dysphagia, 29*(2), 204–212.

Kessler, J. P., & Jean, A. (1985). Identification of the medullary swallowing regions in the rat. *Experimental Brain Research, 57*(2), 256–263.

Khedr, E. M., & Abo-Elfetoh, N. (2010). Therapeutic role of rTMS on recovery of dysphagia in patients with lateral medullary syndrome and brainstem infarction. *Journal of Neurology, Neurosurgery, & Psychiatry, 81*(5), 495–499.

Khedr, E. M., Abo-Elfetoh, N., & Rothwell, J. C. (2009). Treatment of post-stroke dysphagia with repetitive magnetic stimulation. *Acta Neurologica Scandinavica, 119*(3), 155–161.

Kidd, D., Lawson, J., Nesbitt, R., & MacMahon, J. (1993). Aspiration in acute stroke: A clinical study with videofluoroscopy. *Quarterly Journal of Medicine, 86*(12), 825–829.

Kiger, M., Brown, C. S., & Watkins, L. (2006). Dysphagia management: An analysis of patient outcomes using VitalStim therapy compared to traditional swallow therapy. *Dysphagia, 21*(4), 243–253.

Kim, H., Chung, C. S., Lee, K. H., & Robbins, J. (2000). Aspiration subsequent to a pure medullary infarction: Lesion sites, clinical variables, and outcome. *Archives of Neurology, 57*(4), 478–483.

Kim, H., Park, J. W., & Nam, K. (2017). Effortful swallow with resistive electrical stimulation training improves pharyngeal constriction in patients post-stroke with dysphagia. *Journal of Oral Rehabilitation, 44*(10), 763–769.

Kim, J., Davenport, P., & Sapienza, C. (2009). Effect of expiratory muscle strength training on elderly cough function. *Archives of Gerontology and Geriatrics, 48*(3), 361–366.

Kim, J., Oh, B. M., Kim, J. Y., Lee, G. J., Lee, S. A., & Han, T. R. (2014). Validation of the videofluoroscopic dysphagia scale in various etiologies. *Dysphagia, 29*(4), 438–443.

Kim, J. H., & Kim, M. S. (2012). Lateral pharyngeal wall motion analysis using ultrasonography in stroke patients with dysphagia. *Ultrasound in Medicine and Biology, 38*(12), 2058–2064.

Kim, Y., McCullough, G. H., & Asp, C. W. (2005). Temporal measurements of pharyngeal swallowing in normal populations. *Dysphagia, 20*(4), 290–296.

Kim, J., & Sapienza, C. M. (2005). Implications of expiratory muscle strength training for rehabilitation of the elderly: Tutorial. *Journal of Rehabilitation Research and Development*, *42*(2), 211–224.

Kirchner, J. A., Scatliff, J. H., Dey, F. L., & Shedd, D. P. (1963). The pharynx after laryngectomy. Changes in its structure and function. *Laryngoscope*, *73*(1), 18–33.

Kirton, A., Chen, R., Friefeld, S., Gunraj, C., Pontigon, A. M., & deVeber, G. (2008). Contralesional repetitive transcranial magnetic stimulation for chronic hemiparesis in subcortical paediatric stroke: A randomised trial. *Lancet Neurology*, *7*(6), 507–513.

Kirton, A., Gunraj, C., & Chen, R. (2010). Cortical excitability and interhemispheric inhibition after subcortical pediatric stroke: Plastic organization and effects of rTMS. *Clinical Neurophysiology*, *121*(11), 1922–1929.

Kitago, T., & Krakauer, J. W. (2013). Motor learning principles for neurorehabilitation. In M. P. Barnes & D. C. Good (Eds.), *Handbook of clinical neurology* (Vol. 110, pp. 93–103). Cambridge, MA: Elsevier.

Klahn, M. S., & Perlman, A. L. (1999). Temporal and durational patterns associating respiration and swallowing. *Dysphagia*, *14*(3), 131–138.

Kleim, J. A., & Jones, T. A. (2008). Principles of experience-dependent neural plasticity: Implications for rehabilitation after brain damage. *Journal of Speech, Language, and Hearing Research*, *51*(1), S225–S239.

Klomjai, W., Katz, R., & Lackmy-Vallée, A. (2015). Basic principles of transcranial magnetic stimulation (TMS) and repetitive TMS (rTMS). *Annals of Physical and Rehabilitation Medicine*, *58*(4), 208–213.

Klor, B. M., & Milianti, F. J. (1999). Rehabilitation of neurogenic dysphagia with percutaneous endoscopic gastrostomy. *Dysphagia*, *14*(3), 162–164.

Knigge, M. A., & Thibeault, S. (2016). Relationship between tongue base region pressures and vallecular clearance. *Dysphagia*, *31*(3), 391–397.

Knigge, M. A., Thibeault, S., & McCulloch, T. M. (2014). Implementation of high-resolution manometry in the clinical practice of speech-language pathology. *Dysphagia*, *29*(1), 2–16.

Kobayashi, H., Hoshino, M., Okayama, K., Sekizawa, K., & Sasaki, H. (1994). Swallowing and cough reflexes after onset of stroke. *Chest*, *105*(5), 1623.

Kobayashi, M., & Pascual-Leone, A. (2003). Transcranial magnetic stimulation in neurology. *Lancet Neurology*, *2*(3), 145–156.

Kober, S. E., & Wood, G. (2014). Changes in hemodynamic signals accompanying motor imagery and motor execution of swallowing: A near-infrared spectroscopy study. *NeuroImage*, *93*, 1–10.

Kocdor, P., Siegel, E. R., & Tulunay-Ugur, O. E. (2016). Cricopharyngeal dysfunction: A systematic review comparing outcomes of dilatation, botulinum toxin injection, and myotomy. *Laryngoscope*, *126*(1), 135–141.

Kokura, Y., Maeda, K., Wakabayashi, H., Nishioka, S., & Higashi, S. (2016). High nutritional-related risk on admission predicts less improvement of functional independence measure in geriatric stroke patients: A retrospective cohort study. *Journal of Stroke and Cerebrovascular Diseases, 25*(6), 1335–1341

Kos, M. P., David, E. F., Klinkenberg-Knol, E. C., & Mahieu, H. F. (2010). Long-term results of external upper esophageal sphincter myotomy for oropharyngeal dysphagia. *Dysphagia, 25*(3), 169–176.

Koshi, N., Matsumoto, H., Hiramatsu, T., Shimizu, Y., & Hagino, H. (2018). Influence of backrest angle on swallowing musculature activity and physical strain during the head lift exercise in elderly women compared with young women. *Journal of Oral Rehabilitation, 45*(7), 532–538.

Kostadima, E., Kaditis, A., Alexopoulos, E., Zakynthinos, E., & Sfyras, D. (2005). Early gastrostomy reduces the rate of ventilator-associated pneumonia in stroke or head injury patients. *European Respiratory Journal, 26*(1), 106–111.

Krakauer, J. W. (2006). Motor learning: Its relevance to stroke recovery and neurorehabilitation. *Current Opinion in Neurology, 19*(1), 84–90.

Krespi, Y. P., Quatela, V. C., Sisson, G. A., & Som, M. L. (1984). Modified tracheoesophageal diversion for chronic aspiration. *Laryngoscope, 94*(10), 1298–1301.

Krishnamurthi, R. V., Feigin, V. L., Forouzanfar, M. H., Mensah, G. A., Connor, M., Bennett, D. A., . . . Murray, C. (2013). Global and regional burden of first-ever ischaemic and haemorrhagic stroke during 1990–2010: Findings from the Global Burden Disease Study 2010. *Lancet Global Health, 1*(5), e259–e281.

Krishnan, C., Santos, L., Peterson, M. D., & Ehinger, M. (2015). Safety of noninvasive brain stimulation in children and adolescents. *Brain Stimulation, 8*(1), 76–87.

Krival, K., & Bates, C. (2012). Effects of club soda and ginger brew on linguapalatal pressures in healthy adults. *Dysphagia, 27*(2), 228–239.

Kuhlemeier, K. V., Palmer, J. B., & Rosenberg, D. (2001). Effect of liquid bolus consistency and delivery method on aspiration and pharyngeal retention in dysphagia patients. *Dysphagia, 16*(2), 119–122.

Kuhlemeier, K. V., Yates, P., & Palmer, J. B. (1998). Intra and inter-rater variation in the evaluation of videofluorographic swallowing studies. *Dysphagia, 13*(3), 142–147.

Kumar, S., Wagner, C. W., Frayne, C., Zhu, L., Selim, M., Feng, W., & Schlaug, G. (2011). Noninvasive brain stimulation may improve stroke-related dysphagia: A pilot study. *Stroke, 42*(4), 1035–1040.

Kuo, P., Holloway, R. H., & Nguyen, N. Q. (2012). Current and future techniques in the evaluation of dysphagia. *Journal of Gastroenterology and Hepatology, 27*(5), 873–881.

Kuramoto, N., Jayatilake, D., Hidaka, K., & Suzuki, K. (2016, August). Smartphone-based swallowing monitoring and feedback device for mealtime assistance in nursing homes. In *Engineering in Medicine and Biology Society (EMBC), 2016 IEEE 38th Annual International Conference* (pp. 5781–5784).

Kuypers, H. G. (1958a). Corticobular connexions to the pons and lower brainstem in man: An anatomical study. *Brain, 81*(3), 364–388.

Kuypers, H. G. (1958b). Some projections from the peri-central cortex to the pons and lower brainstem in monkey and chimpanzee. *Journal of Comparative Neurology, 110*(2), 221–255.

Lagarde, M. L. J., Kamalski, D. M. A., & van den Engel-Hoek, L. (2016). The reliability and validity of cervical auscultation in the diagnosis of dysphagia: A systematic review. *Clinical Rehabilitation, 30*(2), 199–207.

Lakshminarayan, K., Tsai, A. W., Tong, X., Vazquez, G., Peacock, J. M., George, M. G., . . . Anderson, D. C. (2010). Utility of dysphagia screening results in predicting poststroke pneumonia. *Stroke, 41*(12), 2849–2854.

Lamvik, K., Guiu Hernandez, E., Jones, R., & Huckabee, M. L. (2016). Characterization and correction of pressure drift in the ManoScan™ high-resolution manometry system: In vitro and in vivo. *Neurogastroenterology & Motility, 28*(5), 732–742.

Lamvik, K., Jones, R., Sauer, S., Erfmann, K., & Huckabee, M.L. (2015). The capacity for volitional control of pharyngeal swallowing in healthy adults. *Physiology & Behavior, 152*, 257–263.

Lamvik, K., Macrae, P., Doeltgen, S., Collings, A., & Huckabee, M. L. (2014). Normative data for pharyngeal pressure generation during saliva, bolus, and effortful saliva swallowing across age and gender. *Speech, Language, and Hearing, 17*(4), 210–215.

Lan, Y., Ohkubo, M., Berretin-Felix, G., Carnaby-Mann, G. D., & Crary, M. A. (2012). Normalization of temporal aspects of swallowing physiology after the McNeill Dysphagia Therapy Program. *Annals of Otology, Rhinology & Laryngology, 121*(8), 525–532.

Lan, Y., Xu, G., Dou, Z., Wan, G., Yu, F., & Lin, T. (2013). Biomechanical changes in the pharynx and upper esophageal sphincter after modified balloon dilatation in brainstem stroke patients with dysphagia. *Neurogastroenterology & Motility, 25*(12), e821–e829.

Lan, Y., Xu, G., Dou, Z., Lin, T., Yu, F., & Jiang, L. (2015). The correlation between manometric and videofluoroscopic measurements of the swallowing function in brainstem stroke patients with dysphagia. *Journal of Clinical Gastroenterology, 49*(1), 24–30.

Lang, I. M. (2009). Brainstem control of the phases of swallowing. *Dysphagia, 24*(3), 333–348.

Langdon, P. C., Lee, A. H., & Binns, C. W. (2009). High incidence of respiratory infections in 'nil by mouth' tube-fed acute ischemic stroke patients. *Neuroepidemiology, 32*(2), 107–113.

Langhorne, P., & Duncan, P. (2001). Does the organization of postacute stroke care really matter? *Stroke, 32*(1), 268–274.

Langmore, S. E., Terpenning, M. S., Schork, A., Chen, Y., Murray, J. T., Lopatin, D., & Loesche, W. J. (1998). Predictors of aspiration pneumonia: How important is dysphagia? *Dysphagia, 13*(2), 69–81.

Larsen, G. L. (1972). Rehabilitation for dysphagia paralytica. *Journal of Speech and Hearing Disorders*, *37*(2), 187–194.

Lasserson, D., Mills, K., Arunachalam, R., Polkey, M., Moxham, J., & Kalra, L. (2006). Differences in motor activation of voluntary and reflex cough in humans. *Thorax*, *61*(8), 699–705.

Lawless, H. T., Bender, S., Oman, C., & Pelletier, C. (2003). Gender, age, vessel size, cup vs. straw sipping, and sequence effects on sip volume. *Dysphagia*, *18*(3), 196–202.

Lazarus, C., Logemann, J. A., Huang, C. F., & Rademaker, A. W. (2003). Effects of two types of tongue strengthening exercises in young normals. *Folia Phoniatrica et Logopaedica*, *55*(4), 199–205.

Lazarus, C., Logemann, J. A., Song, C. W., Rademaker, A. W., & Kahrilas, P. J. (2002). Effects of voluntary maneuvers on tongue base function for swallowing. *Folia Phoniatrica et Logopaedica*, *54*(4), 171–176.

Lazarus, C. L., Logemann, J. A., Pauloski, B. R., Rademaker, A. W., Larson, C. R., Mittal, B. B., & Pierce, M. (2000). Swallowing and tongue function following treatment for oral and oropharyngeal cancer. *Journal of Speech, Language, and Hearing Research*, *43*(4), 1011–1023.

Lazarus, C. L., Logemann, J. A., Rademaker, A. W., Kahrilas, P. J., Pajak, T., Lazar, R., & Halper, A. (1993). Effects of bolus volume, viscosity, and repeated swallows in nonstroke subjects and stroke patients. *Archives of Physical Medicine and Rehabilitation*, *74*(10), 1066–1070.

Lazzara, G., Lazarus, C., & Logemann, J. A. (1986). Impact of thermal stimulation on the triggering of the swallowing reflex. *Dysphagia*, *1*(2), 73–77.

Leder, S. B. (1996). Gag reflex and dysphagia. *Head and Neck*, *18*(2), 138–141.

Leder, S. B. (1997). Videofluoroscopic evaluation of aspiration with visual examination of the gag reflex and velar movement. *Dysphagia*, *12*(1), 21–23.

Leder, S. B. (2000). Use of arterial oxygen saturation, heart rate, and blood pressure as indirect objective physiologic markers to predict aspiration. *Dysphagia*, *15*(4), 201–205.

Leder, S. B., Acton, L. M., Lisitano, H. L., & Murray, J. T. (2005). Fiberoptic endoscopic evaluation of swallowing (FEES) with and without blue-dyed food. *Dysphagia*, *20*(2), 157–162.

Leder, S. B., & Espinosa, J. F. (2002). Aspiration risk after acute stroke: Comparison of clinical examination and fiberoptic endoscopic evaluation of swallowing. *Dysphagia*, *17*(3), 214–218.

Leder, S. B., Ross, D. A., Briskin, K. B., & Sasaki, C. T. (1997). A prospective, double-blind, randomized study on the use of a topical anesthetic, vasoconstrictor, and placebo during transnasal flexible fiberoptic endoscopy. *Journal of Speech, Language, and Hearing Research*, *40*(6), 1352–1357.

Leder, S. B., & Suiter, D. M. (2008). Effect of nasogastric tubes on incidence of aspiration. *Archives of Physical Medicine & Rehabilitation*, *89*(4), 648–651.

Leder, S. B., & Suiter, D. M. (2014). *The Yale Swallow Protocol: An evidence-based approach to decision making*. Switzerland: Springer.

Lederle, A., Hoit, J. D., & Barkmeier-Kraemer, J. (2012). Effects of sequential swallowing on drive to breathe in young, healthy adults. *Dysphagia*, *27*(2), 221–227.

Lee, J. H., Kim, S. B., Lee, K. W., Lee, S. J., & Lee, J. U. (2015). Effect of repetitive transcranial magnetic stimulation according to the stimulation site in stroke patients with dysphagia. *Annals of Rehabilitation Medicine*, *39*(3), 432–439.

Lee, T. H., Lee, J. S., Hong, S. J., Lee, J. S., Jeon, S. R., Kim, W. J., . . . Park, W. Y. (2014). High-resolution manometry: Reliability of automated analysis of upper esophageal sphincter relaxation parameters. *Turkish Journal of Gastroenterology*, *25*(5), 473–480.

Lee, T. H., Lee, J. S., & Kim, W. J. (2012). High resolution impedance manometric findings in dysphagia of Huntington's disease. *World Journal of Gastroenterology*, *18*(14), 1695–1699.

Lee, Y. S., Lee, K. E., Kang, Y., Yi, T. I., & Kim, J. S. (2016). Usefulness of submental ultrasonographic evaluation for dysphagia patients. *Annals of Rehabilitation Medicine*, *40*(2), 197–205.

Leelamanit, V., Limsakul, C., & Geater, A. (2002). Synchronized electrical stimulation in treating pharyngeal dysphagia. *Laryngoscope*, *112*(12), 2204–2210.

Lefebvre, S., Dricot, L., Laloux, P., Gradkowski, W., Desfontaines, P., Evrard, F., . . . Vandermeeren, Y. (2014). Neural substrates underlying stimulation-enhanced motor skill learning after stroke. *Brain*, *138*(1), 149–163.

Leibovitz, A., Plotnikov, G., Habot, B., Rosenberg, M., Wolf, A., Nagler, R., . . . Segal, R. (2003). Saliva secretion and oral flora in prolonged nasogastric tube-fed elderly patients. *Israel Medical Association Journal*, *5*(5), 329–332.

Leigh, J., Lim, J. Y., Han, M. K., Bae, H. J., Kim, W. S., & Paik, N. J. (2016). A prospective comparison between bedside swallowing screening test and videofluoroscopic swallowing study in post-stroke dysphagia. *Brain & Neurorehabilitation*, *9*(2), e7. https://doi.org/10.12786/bn.2016.9.e7

Leigh, J. H., Oh, B. M., Seo, H. G., Lee, G. J., Min, Y., Kim, K., . . . Han, T. R. (2015). Influence of the chin-down and chin-tuck maneuver on swallowing kinematics of healthy adults. *Dysphagia*, *30*(1), 89–98.

Leonard, R., & Kendall, K. A. (2014). *Dysphagia assessment and treatment planning* (3rd ed.). San Diego, CA: Plural.

Leonard, R., Rees, C. J., Belafsky, P., & Allen, J. (2011). Fluoroscopic surrogate for pharyngeal strength: The pharyngeal constriction ratio (PCR). *Dysphagia*, *26*(1), 13–17.

Leonard, R. J., Kendall, K. A., McKenzie, S., Gonçalves, M. I., & Walker, A. (2000). Structural displacements in normal swallowing: A videofluoroscopic study. *Dysphagia*, *15*(3), 146–152.

Leonard, R. J., White, C., McKenzie, S., & Belafsky, P. C. (2016). Effects of bolus rheology on aspiration in patients with dysphagia. *Journal of the Academy of Nutrition and Dietetics*, *114*(4), 590–594.

Leopold, N. A., & Daniels, S. K. (2010). Supranuclear control of swallowing. *Dysphagia, 25*(3), 250–257.

Leopold, N. A., & Kagel, M. C. (1997). Dysphagia—ingestion or deglutition? A proposed paradigm. *Dysphagia, 12*(4), 202–206.

Leow, L. P., Huckabee, M. L., Sharma, S., & Tooley, T. P. (2007). The influence of taste on swallowing apnea, oral preparation time, and duration and amplitude of submental muscle contraction. *Chemical Senses, 32*(2), 119–128.

Leslie, P., Drinnan, M. J., Finn, P., Ford, G. A., & Wilson, J. A. (2004). Reliability and validity of cervical auscultation: A controlled comparison using videofluoroscopy. *Dysphagia, 19*(4), 231–240.

Leslie, P., Drinnan, M. J., Ford, G. A., & Wilson, J. A. (2002). Swallow respiration patterns in dysphagic patients following acute stroke. *Dysphagia, 17*(3), 202–207.

Li, S., Ma, Z., Tu, S., Zhou, M., Chen, S., Guo, Z., . . . Lui, S. (2014). Altered resting-state functional and white matter tract connectivity in stroke patients with dysphagia. *Neurorehabilitation and Neural Repair, 28*(3), 260–272.

Liew, S. L., Santarnecchi, E., Buch, E. R., & Cohen, L. G. (2014). Non-invasive brain stimulation in neurorehabilitation: Local and distant effects for motor recovery. *Frontiers in Human Neuroscience, 8*, 378. https://doi.org/10.3389/fnhum.2014.00378

Lim, S. H., Lieu, P. K., Phua, S. Y., Seshadri, R., Venketasubramanian, N., Lee, S. H., & Choo, P. W. (2001). Accuracy of bedside clinical methods compared with fiberoptic endoscopic examination of swallowing (FEES) in determining the risk of aspiration in acute stroke patients. *Dysphagia, 16*(1), 1–6.

Lin, T., Xu, G., Dou, Z., Lan, Y., Yu, F., & Jiang, L. (2014). Effect of bolus volume on pharyngeal swallowing assessed by high-resolution manometry. *Physiology & Behavior, 128*, 46–51.

Lin, Y. N., Chen, S. Y., Wang, T. G., Chang, Y. C., Chie, W. C., & Lien, I. N. (2005). Findings of videofluoroscopic swallowing studies are associated with tube feeding dependency at discharge in stroke patients with dysphagia. *Dysphagia, 20*(1), 23–31.

Linden, P., & Siebens, A. A. (1983). Dysphagia: Predicting laryngeal penetration. *Archives of Physical Medicine and Rehabilitation, 64*(6), 281–284.

Liu-Ambrose, T., Taunton, J. E., MacIntyre, D., McConkey, P., & Khan, K. M. (2003). The effects of proprioceptive or strength training on the neuromuscular function of the ACL reconstructed knee: A randomized clinical trial. *Scandinavian Journal of Medicine & Science in Sports, 13*(2), 115–123.

Lof, G. L., & Robbins, J. (1990). Test-retest variability in normal swallowing. *Dysphagia, 4*(4), 236–242.

Logemann, J. A. (1983). *Evaluation and treatment of swallowing disorders* (1st ed.). San Diego, CA: College-Hill.

Logemann, J. A. (1998). *Evaluation and treatment of swallowing disorders* (2nd ed.). Austin, TX: Pro-Ed.

Logemann, J. A., Gensler, G., Robbins, J., Lindblad, A., Brandt, D., Hind, J. A., . . . Miller Gardner, P. J. (2008). A randomized study of three interventions for aspiration of thin liquids in patients with dementia and Parkinson's disease. *Journal of Speech, Language, and Hearing Research*, *51*(1), 173–183.

Logemann, J. A., & Kahrilas, P. J. (1990). Relearning to swallow after stroke—application of maneuvers and indirect biofeedback: A case study. *Neurology*, *40*(7), 1136–1138.

Logemann, J. A., Kahrilas, P. J., Cheng, J. O., Pauloski, B. R., Gibbons, P. J., Rademaker, A. W., & Lin, S. H. (1992). Closure mechanisms of laryngeal vestibule during swallow. *American Journal of Physiology–Gastrointestinal and Liver Physiology*, *262*(2), G338–G344.

Logemann, J. A., Kahrilas, P. J., Kobara, M., & Vakil, N. B. (1989). The benefit of head rotation on pharyngoesophageal dysphagia. *Archives of Physical Medicine and Rehabilitation*, *70*(10), 767–771.

Logemann, J. A., Pauloski, B. R., Colangelo, L., Lazarus, C., Fujiu, M., & Kahrilas, P. J. (1995). Effects of a sour bolus on oropharyngeal swallowing measures in patients with neurogenic dysphagia. *Journal of Speech and Hearing Research*, *38*(3), 556–563.

Logemann, J. A., Pauloski, B. R., Rademaker, A. W., Colangelo, L. A., Kahrilas, P. J., & Smith, C. H. (2000). Temporal and biomechanical characteristics of oropharyngeal swallow in younger and older men. *Journal of Speech, Language, and Hearing Research*, *43*(5), 1264–1274.

Logemann, J. A., Shanahan, T., Rademaker, A. W., Kahrilas, P. J., Lazar, R., & Halper, A. (1993). Oropharyngeal swallowing after stroke in the left basal ganglion/internal capsule. *Dysphagia*, *8*(3), 230–234.

Logemann, J. A., Veis, S., & Colangelo, L. (1999). A screening procedure for oropharyngeal dysphagia. *Dysphagia*, *14*(1), 44–51.

Lowell, S. Y., Poletto, C. J., Knorr-Chung, B. R., Reynolds, R. C., Simonyan, K., & Ludlow, C. L. (2008). Sensory stimulation activates both motor and sensory components of the swallowing system. *NeuroImage*, *42*(1), 285–295.

Lucas, C. E., Yu, P., Vlahos, A., & Ledgerwood, A. M. (1999). Lower esophageal sphincter dysfunction often precludes safe gastric feeding in stroke patients. *Archives of Surgery*, *134*(1), 55–58.

Ludlow, C. L. (2010). Electrical neuromuscular stimulation in dysphagia: Current status. *Current Opinion in Otolaryngology & Head and Neck Surgery*, *18*(3), 159–164.

Ludlow, C. L., Humbert, I., Poletto, C. J., Saxon, K. G., Kearney, P. R., Crujido, L., & Sonies, B. (2005). *The use of coordination training for the onset of intramuscular stimulation in dysphagia*. Paper presented at the 10th annual conference of the International FES Society, Montreal, Quebec, Canada.

Ludlow, C. L., Humbert, I., Saxon, K., Poletto, C., Sonies, B., & Crujido, L. (2007). Effects of surface electrical stimulation both at rest and during swallowing in chronic pharyngeal dysphagia. *Dysphagia*, *22*(1), 1–10.

Luft, A. R., & Buitrago, M. M. (2005). Stages of motor skill learning. *Molecular Neurobiology*, *32*(3), 205–216.

Lund, J. P., & Kolta, A. (2006a). Brainstem circuits that control mastication: Do they have anything to say during speech? *Journal of Communication Disorders*, *39*(5), 381–390.

Lund, J. P., & Kolta, A. (2006b). Generation of the central masticatory pattern and its modification by sensory feedback. *Dysphagia*, *21*(3), 167–174.

Macrae, P., Anderson, C., & Humbert, I. (2014). Mechanisms of airway protection during chin-down swallowing. *Journal of Speech, Language, and Hearing Research*, *57*(4), 1251–1258.

Macrae, P., Anderson, C., Taylor-Kamara, I., & Humbert, I. (2014). The effects of feedback on volitional manipulation of airway protection during swallowing. *Journal of Motor Behavior*, *46*(2), 133–139.

Macrae, P. R., Doeltgen, S. H., Jones, R. D., & Huckabee, M. L. (2012). Intra- and inter-rater reliability for analysis of hyoid displacement measured with sonography. *Journal of Clinical Ultrasound*, *40*(2), 74–78.

Macrae, P. R., Jones, R. D., Myall, D. J., Melzer, T. R., & Huckabee, M. L. (2013). Cross-sectional area of the anterior belly of the digastric muscle: Comparison of MRI and ultrasound measures. *Dysphagia*, *28*(3), 375–380.

Macrae, P. R., Myall, D. J., Jones, R. D., & Huckabee, M. L. (2011). Pharyngeal pressures during swallowing within and across three sessions: Within-subject variance and order effects. *Dysphagia*, *26*(4), 385–391.

Maeda, K., Ono, T., Otsuka, R., Ishiwata, Y., Kuroda, T., & Ohyama, K. (2004). Modulation of voluntary swallowing by visual inputs in humans. *Dysphagia*, *19*(1), 1–6.

Maganaris, C. N., Baltzopoulos, V., & Sargeant, A. J. (2002). Repeated contractions alter the geometry of human skeletal muscle. *Journal of Applied Physiology*, *93*(6), 2089–2094.

Mahoney, C., & Veitch, L. (2018). Interventions for maintaining nasogastric feeding after stroke: An integrative review of effectiveness and acceptability. *Journal of Clinical Nursing*, *27*(3-4), e427–e436.

Malandraki, G. A., Hind, J. A., Gangnon, R., Logemann, J. A., & Robbins, J. (2011). The utility of pitch elevation in the evaluation of oropharyngeal dysphagia: Preliminary findings. *American Journal of Speech-Language Pathology*, *20*(4), 262–268.

Malandraki, G. A., Johnson, S., & Robbins, J. (2011). Functional MRI of swallowing: From neurophysiology to neuroplasticity. *Head & Neck*, *33*(S1), S14–S20.

Malandraki, G. A., Perlman, A. L., Karampinos, D. C., & Sutton, B. P. (2011). Reduced somatosensory activations in swallowing with age. *Human Brain Mapping*, *32*(5), 730–743.

Malandraki, G. A., Sutton, B. P., Perlman, A. L., Karampinos, D. C., & Conway, C. (2009). Neural activation of swallowing and swallowing-related tasks in healthy young adults: An attempt to separate the components of deglutition. *Human Brain Mapping*, *30*(10), 3209–3226.

Mamun, K., & Lim, J. (2005). Role of nasogastric tube in preventing aspiration pneumonia in patients with dysphagia. *Singapore Medical Journal, 46*(11), 627–631.

Mann, G. (2002). *MASA: The Mann Assessment of Swallowing Ability*. Clifton Park, NY: Thomson Delmar Learning.

Mann, G., & Hankey, G. J. (2001). Initial clinical and demographic predictors of swallowing impairment following acute stroke. *Dysphagia, 16*(3), 208–215.

Mann, G., Hankey, G. J., & Cameron, D. (1999). Swallowing function after stroke: Prognosis and prognostic factors at 6 months. *Stroke, 30*(4), 744–748.

Mann, G., Hankey, G. J., & Cameron, D. (2000). Swallowing disorders following acute stroke: Prevalence and diagnostic accuracy. *Cerebrovascular Disorders, 10*(5), 380–386.

Marian, T., Schröder, J., Muhle, P., Claus, I., Oelenberg, S., Hamacher, C., . . . Dziewas, R. (2017). Measurement of oxygen desaturation is not useful for the detection of aspiration in dysphagic stroke patients. *Cerebrovascular Diseases Extra, 7*(1), 44–50.

Martin, B. J., Logemann, J. A., Shaker, R., & Dodds, W. J. (1993). Normal laryngeal valving patterns during three breath-hold maneuvers: A pilot investigation. *Dysphagia, 8*(1), 11–20.

Martin, B. J., Logemann, J. A., Shaker, R., & Dodds, W. J. (1994). Coordination between respiration and swallowing: Respiratory phase relationships and temporal integration. *Journal of Applied Physiology, 76*(2), 714–723.

Martin, R. E. (2009). Neuroplasticity and swallowing. *Dysphagia, 24*(2), 218–229.

Martin, R. E., Goodyear, B. G., Gati, J. S., & Menon, R. S. (2001). Cerebral cortical representation of automatic and volitional swallowing in humans. *Journal of Neurophysiology, 85*(2), 938–950.

Martin-Harris, B., Brodsky, M. B., Michel, Y., Castell, D. O., Schleicher, M., Sandidge, J., . . . Blair, J. (2008). MBS measurement tool for swallow impairment—MBSImp: Establishing a standard. *Dysphagia, 23*(4), 392–405.

Martin-Harris, B., Brodsky, M. B., Michel, Y., Ford, C. L., Walters, B., & Heffner, J. (2005). Breathing and swallowing dynamics across the adult lifespan. *Archives of Otolaryngology–Head and Neck Surgery, 131*(9), 762–770.

Martin-Harris, B., Brodsky, M. B., Michel, Y., Lee, F. S., & Walters, B. (2007). Delayed initiation of the pharyngeal swallow: Normal variability in adult swallows. *Journal of Speech, Language, and Hearing Research, 50*(3), 585–594.

Martin-Harris, B., & Easterling, C. S. (2006). *Esophageal swallowing physiology and disorders* [Electronic presentation]. Rockville, MD: American Speech-Language-Hearing Association.

Martin-Harris, B., McFarland, D., Hill, E. G., Strange, C. B., Focht, K. L., Wan, Z., . . . McGrattan, K. (2015). Respiratory-swallow training in patients with head and neck cancer. *Archives of Physical Medicine and Rehabilitation, 96*(5), 885–893.

Martino, R., Maki, E., & Diamant, N. (2014). Identification of dysphagia using the Toronto Bedside Swallowing Screening Test (TOR-BSST©): Are 10 teaspoons of water necessary? *International Journal of Speech-Language Pathology, 16*(3), 193–198.

Martino, R., & McCulloch, T. (2016). Therapeutic intervention in oropharyngeal dysphagia. *Nature Reviews Gastroenterology and Hepatology, 13*(11), 665–669.

Martino, R., Pron, G., & Diamant, N. (2000). Screening for oropharyngeal dysphagia in stroke: Insufficient evidence for guidelines. *Dysphagia, 15*(1), 19–30.

Martino, R., Silver, F., Teasell, R., Bayley, M., Nicholson, G., Streiner, D. L., & Diamant, N. E. (2009). The Toronto Bedside Swallowing Screening Test (TOR-BSST). Development and validation of a dysphagia screening tool for patients with stroke. *Stroke, 40*(2), 555–561.

Martino, R., Terrault, N., Ezerzer, F., Mikulis, D., & Diamant, N. E. (2001). Dysphagia in a patient with lateral medullary syndrome: Insight into the central control of swallowing. *Gastroenterology, 121*(2), 420–426.

Martner, J. (1975). Cerebellar influences on autonomic mechanisms. An experimental study in the cat with special reference to the fastigial nucleus. *Acta Physiologica Scandinavica Supplementum, 425*, 1–42.

Marvin, S., Gustafson, S., & Thibeault, S. (2016). Detecting aspiration and penetration using FEES with and without food dye. *Dysphagia, 31*(4), 498–504.

Masrur, S., Smith, E. E., Saver, J. L., Reeves, M. J., Bhatt, D. L., Zhao, X., . . . Schwamm, L. H. (2013). Dysphagia screening and hospital-acquired pneumonia in patients with acute ischemic stroke: Findings from Get with the Guidelines–Stroke. *Journal of Stroke and Cerebrovascular Diseases, 22*(8), e301–e309.

Matsuo, K., Hiiemae, K. M., Gonzalez-Fernandez, M., & Palmer, J. B. (2008). Respiration during feeding on solid food: Alterations in breathing during mastication, pharyngeal bolus aggregation, and swallowing. *Journal of Applied Physiology, 104*(3), 674–681.

Matsuo, K., & Palmer, J. B. (2015). Coordination of oro-pharyngeal food transport during chewing and respiratory phase. *Physiology & Behavior, 142*, 52–56.

Mattay, V. S., Fera, F., Tessitore, A., Hariri, A. R., Das, S., Callicott, J. H., & Weinberger, D. R. (2002). Neurophysiological correlates of age-related changes in human motor function. *Neurology, 58*(4), 630–635.

Matthews, P. M., Johansen-Berg, H., & Reddy, H. (2004). Non-invasive mapping of brain functions and brain recovery: Applying lessons from cognitive neuroscience to neurorehabilitation. *Restorative Neurology and Neuroscience, 22*(3-5), 245–260.

McConnel, F. M. (1988). Analysis of pressure generation and bolus transit during pharyngeal swallowing. *Laryngoscope, 98*(1), 71–78.

McCulloch, T. M., Hoffman, M. R., & Ciucci, M. R. (2010). High resolution manometry of pharyngeal swallow pressure events associated with head turn and chin tuck. *Annals of Otology, Rhinology & Laryngology, 119*(6), 369–376.

McCullough, G. H., Kamarunas, E., Mann, G. C., Schmidley, J. W., Robbins, J. A., & Crary, M. A. (2012). Effects of Mendelsohn maneuver on measures of swallowing duration post stroke. *Topics in Stroke Rehabilitation, 19*(3), 234–243.

McCullough, G. H., & Kim, Y. (2013). Effects of the Mendelsohn maneuver on extent of hyoid movement and UES opening post-stroke. *Dysphagia*, *28*(4), 511–519.

McCullough, G. H., Rosenbek, J. C., Wertz, R. T., McCoy, S., Mann, G., & McCullough, K. (2005). Utility of clinical swallowing examination measures for detecting aspiration post-stroke. *Journal of Speech, Language, and Hearing Research*, *48*(6), 1280–1293.

McCullough, G. H., Rosenbek, J. C., Wertz, R. T., Suiter, D., & McCoy, S. C. (2007). Defining swallowing function by age: Promises and pitfalls of pigeonholing. *Topics in Geriatric Rehabilitation*, *23*(4), 290–307.

McCullough, G. H., Wertz, R. T., & Rosenbek, J. C. (2001). Sensitivity and specificity of clinical/bedside examination signs for detecting aspiration in adults subsequent to stroke. *Journal of Communication Disorders*, *34*(1–2), 55–72.

McCullough, G. H., Wertz, R. T., Rosenbek, J. C., Mills, R. H., Ross, K. B., & Ashford, J. R. (2000). Inter and intrajudge reliability of a clinical examination of swallowing in adults. *Dysphagia*, *15*(2), 58–67.

McCullough, G. H., Wertz, R. T., Rosenbek, J. C., Mills, R. H., Webb, W. G., & Ross, K. B. (2001). Inter and intrajudge reliability for videofluoroscopic swallowing evaluation measures. *Dysphagia*, *16*(2), 110–118.

McDonnell, M. N., Hillier, S. L., Miles, T., Thompson, P. D., & Ridding, M. C. (2007). Influence of combined afferent stimulation and task-specific training following stroke: A pilot randomized controlled trial. *Neurorehabilitation and Neural Repair*, *21*(5), 435–443.

McFarland, A. (2017). A cost utility analysis of the clinical algorithm for nasogastric tube placement confirmation in adult hospital patients. *Journal of Advanced Nursing*, *73*(1), 201–216.

McFarland, D. H., Martin-Harris, B., Fortin, A. J., Humphries, K., Hill, E., & Armeson, K. (2016). Respiratory-swallowing coordination in normal subjects: Lung volume at swallowing initiation. *Respiratory Physiology & Neurobiology*, *234*, 89–96.

McHorney, C. A., Martin-Harris, B., Robbins, J., & Rosenbek, J. (2006). Clinical validity of the SWAL-QOL and SWAL-CARE outcome tools with respect to bolus flow measures. *Dysphagia*, *21*(3), 141–148.

McHorney, C. A., Robbins, J., Lomax, K., Rosenbek, J. C., Chignell, K., Kramer, A. E., & Bricker, D. E. (2002). The SWAL-QOL and SWAL-CARE outcomes tool for oropharyngeal dysphagia in adults: III. Documentation of reliability and validity. *Dysphagia*, *17*(2), 97–114.

Meier-Ewert, H. K., van Herwaarden, M. A., Gideon, R. M., Castell, J. A., Achem, S., & Castell, D. O. (2001). Effect of age on differences in upper esophageal sphincter and pharynx pressures between patients with dysphagia and control subjects. *American Journal of Gastroenterology*, *96*(1), 35–40.

Mendelsohn, M. S., & Martin, R. E. (1993). Airway protection during breath-holding. *Annals of Otology, Rhinology & Laryngology*, *102*(12), 941–944.

Menezes, K. K., Nascimento, L. R., Ada, L., Polese, J. C., Avelino, P. R., & Teixeira-Salmela, L. F. (2016). Respiratory muscle training increases respiratory muscle strength and reduces respiratory complications after stroke: A systematic review. *Journal of Physiotherapy*, *62*(3), 138–144.

Meng, N. H., Wang, T. G., & Lien, I. N. (2000). Dysphagia in patients with brainstem stroke: Incidence and outcome. *American Journal of Physical Medicine and Rehabilitation*, *79*(2), 170–175.

Mepani, R., Antonik, S., Massey, B., Kern, M., Logemann, J., Pauloski, B., . . . Shaker, R. (2009) Augmentation of deglutitive thyrohyoid muscle shortening by the Shaker exercise. *Dysphagia*, *24*(1), 26–31.

Mesulam, M. M., & Mufson, E. J. (1985). The insula of Reil in man and monkey: Architectonics, connectivity, and function. In A. Peters & E. G. Jones (Eds.), *Cerebral cortex, Volume 4, Association and auditory cortices* (pp. 179–226). New York, NY: Plenum.

Metzger, B. L., & Therrien, B. (1990). Effect of position on cardiovascular response during the Valsalva maneuver. *Nursing Research*, *39*(4), 198–202.

Michou, E., & Hamdy, S. (2009). Cortical input in control of swallowing. *Current Opinion in Otolaryngology & Head and Neck Surgery*, *17*(3), 166–171.

Michou, E., Mastan, A., Ahmed, S., Mistry, S., & Hamdy, S. (2012). Examining the role of carbonation and temperature on water swallowing performance: A swallow reaction-time study. *Chemical Senses*, *37*(9), 799–907.

Michou, E., Raginis-Zborowska, A., Watanabe, M., Lodhi, T., & Hamdy, S. (2016). Repetitive transcranial magnetic stimulation: A novel approach for treating oropharyngeal dysphagia. *Current Gastroenterology Reports*, *18*(2), 10. https://doi.org/10.1007/s11894-015-0483-8

Midgren, B., Hansson, L., Karlsson, J. A., Simonsson, B. G., & Persson, C. G. (1992). Capsaicin-induced cough in humans. *American Review of Respiratory Disease*, *146*(2), 347–351.

Mielens, J. D., Hoffman, M. R., Ciucci, M. R., McCulloch, T. M., & Jiang, J. J. (2012). Application of classification models to pharyngeal high-resolution manometry. *Journal of Speech, Language, and Hearing Research*, *55*(3), 892–902.

Mihai, P. G., Otto, M., Platz, T., Eickhoff, S. B., & Lotze, A. M. (2014). Sequential evolution of cortical activity and effective connectivity of swallowing using fMRI. *Human Brain Mapping*, *35*(12), 5962–5973.

Miles, A., McFarlane, M., Scott, S., & Hunting, A. (2018). Cough response to aspiration in thin and thick fluids during FEES in hospitalized inpatients. *International Journal of Language & Communication Disorders*, *53*(5), 909–918.

Miles, A., Moore, S., McFarlane, M., Lee, F., Allen, J., & Huckabee, M. L. (2013). Comparison of cough reflex test against instrumental assessment of aspiration. *Physiology & Behavior*, *118*(1), 25–31.

Miles, A., Zeng, I. S., McLauchlan, H., & Huckabee, M. L. (2013). Cough reflex testing in dysphagia following stroke: A randomized controlled trial. *Journal of Clinical Medicine Research*, *5*(3), 222–233.

Miller, A. J. (1972). Characteristics of the swallowing reflex induced by peripheral nerve and brainstem stimulation. *Experimental Neurology*, *34*(2), 210–222.

Miller, A. J. (1999). *The neuroscientific principles of swallowing and dysphagia*. San Diego, CA: Singular.

Miller, A. J. (2002). Oral and pharyngeal reflexes in the mammalian nervous system: Their diverse range in complexity and the pivotal role of the tongue. *Critical Reviews in Oral Biology & Medicine*, *13*(5), 409–425.

Miller, A. J. (2008). The neurobiology of swallowing and dysphagia. *Developmental Disabilities Research Reviews*, *14*(2), 77–86.

Miller, A. J., Bieger, D., & Conklin, J. L. (1997). Functional controls of deglutition. In A. L. Perlman & K. Schulze-Delreiu (Eds.), *Deglutition and its disorders* (pp. 43–98). San Diego, CA: Singular.

Miller, A. J., & Bowman, J. P. (1977). Precentral cortical modulation of mastication and swallowing. *Journal of Dental Research*, *56*(10), 1154.

Miller, F. R., & Sherrington, C. S. (1915). Some observations on the buccopharyngeal stage of reflex deglutition in the cat. *Quarterly Journal of Experimental Physiology*, *9*(2), 147–186.

Miller, J. L., & Watkin, K. L. (1996). The influence of bolus volume and viscosity on anterior lingual force during the oral stage of swallowing. *Dysphagia*, *11*(2), 117–124.

Miller, J. L., & Watkin, K. L. (1997). Lateral pharyngeal wall motion during swallowing using real-time ultrasound. *Dysphagia*, *12*(3), 125–132.

Millns, B., Gosney, M., Jack, C. I. A., Martin, M. V., & Wright, A. E. (2003). Acute stroke predisposes to oral gram-negative bacilli—a cause of aspiration pneumonia? *Gerontology*, *49*(3), 173–176.

Mills, C., Jones, R., & Huckabee, M. L. (2017). Measuring voluntary and reflexive cough strength in healthy individuals. *Respiratory Medicine*, *132*, 95–101.

Minnerup, J., Wersching, H., Brokinkel, B., Dziewas, R., Heuschmann, P. U., Nabavi, D. G., . . . Ritter, M. A. (2010). The impact of lesion location and lesion size on poststroke infection frequency. *Journal of Neurology, Neurosurgery, and Psychiatry*, *81*(2), 198–202.

Mishra, A., Rajappa, A., Tipton, E., & Malandraki, G. A. (2015). The recline exercise: Comparisons with the head lift exercise in healthy adults. *Dysphagia*, *30*(6), 730–737.

Mistry, S., Michou, E., Rothwell, J., & Hamdy, S. (2012). Remote effects of intermittent theta burst stimulation of the human pharyngeal motor system. *European Journal of Neuroscience*, *36*(4), 2493–2499.

Mistry, S., Verin, E., Singh, S., Jefferson, S., Rothwell, J. C., Thompson, D. G., & Hamdy, S. (2007). Unilateral suppression of pharyngeal motor cortex to repetitive transcranial magnetic stimulation reveals functional asymmetry in the hemispheric projections to human swallowing. *Journal of Physiology*, *585*(2), 525–538.

Miura, Y., Nakagami, G., Yabunaka, K., Tohara, H., Murayama, R., Noguchi, H., . . . Sanada, H. (2014). Method for detection of aspiration based on B-mode video ultrasonography. *Radiological Physics and Technology*, *7*(2), 290–295.

Miyaoka, Y., Haishima, K., Takagi, M., Haishima, H., Asari, J., & Yamada, Y. (2006). Influences of thermal and gustatory characteristics on sensory and motor aspects of swallowing. *Dysphagia*, *21*(1), 38–48.

Mojon, P., Budtz-Jørgensen, E., Miche, J. P., & Limeback, H. (1997). Oral health and history of respiratory tract infection in frail institutionalised elders. *Gerodontology*, *14*(1), 9–16.

Molfenter, S. M., Amin, M. R., Branski, R. C., Brumm, J. D., Hagiwara, M., Roof, S. A., & Lazarus, C. L. (2015). Age-related changes in pharyngeal lumen size: A retrospective MRI analysis. *Dysphagia*, *30*(3), 321–327.

Molfenter, S. M., Hsu, C. Y., Lu, Y., & Lazarus, C. L. (2018). Alterations to swallowing physiology as the result of effortful swallowing in healthy seniors. *Dysphagia*, *33*(3), 380–388.

Molfenter, S. M., & Steele, C. M. (2011). Physiological variability in the deglutition literature: Hyoid and laryngeal kinematics. *Dysphagia*, *26*(1), 67–74.

Molfenter, S. M., & Steele, C. M. (2013). Variation in temporal measures of swallowing: Sex and volume effects. *Dysphagia*, *28*(2), 226–233.

Molkov, Y. I., Bacak, B. J., Dick, T. E., & Rybak, I. A. (2013). Control of breathing by interacting pontine and pulmonary feedback loops. *Frontiers in Neural Circuits*, *7*, 16. https://doi.org/10.3389/fncir.2013.00016

Moon, J. H., Jung, J. H., Won, Y. S., Cho, H. Y., & Cho, K. (2017). Effects of expiratory muscle strength training on swallowing function in acute stroke patients with dysphagia. *Journal of Physical Therapy Science*, *29*(4), 609–612.

Morice, A. H., Kastelik, J. A., & Thompson, R. (2001). Cough challenge in the assessment of cough reflex. *British Journal of Clinical Pharmacology*, *52*(4), 365–375.

Morinière, S., Hammoudi, K., Marmouset, F., Bakhos, D., Beutter, P., & Patat, F. (2013). Ultrasound analysis of the upper esophageal sphincter during swallowing in the healthy subject. *European Annals of Otorhinolaryngology, Head and Neck Diseases*, *130*(6), 321–325.

Morquette, P., Lavoie, R., Fhima, M. D., Lamoureux, X., Verdier, D., & Kolta, A. (2012). Generation of the masticatory central pattern and its modulation by sensory feedback. *Progress in Neurobiology*, *96*(3), 340–355.

Morrell, K., Hyers, M., Stuchiner, T., Lucas, L., Schwartz, K., Mako, J., . . . Yanase, L. (2017). Telehealth stroke dysphagia evaluation is safe and effective. *Cerebrovascular Diseases*, *44*(3–4), 225–231.

Mosier, K., & Bereznaya, I. (2001). Parallel cortical networks for volitional control of swallowing in humans. *Experimental Brain Research*, *140*(3), 280–289.

Mosier, K., Patel, R., Liu, W. C., Kalnin, A., Maldjian, J., & Baredes, S. (1999). Cortical representation of swallowing in normal adults: Functional implications. *Laryngoscope*, *109*(9), 1417–1423.

Movahedi, F., Kurosu, A., Coyle, J. L., Perera, S., & Sejdić, E. (2017). A comparison between swallowing sounds and vibrations in patients with dysphagia. *Computer Methods and Programs in Biomedicine, 144*, 179–187.

Mozaffarian, D., Benjamin, E. J., Go, A. S., Arnett, D., K., Blaha, M. J., Cushman, M., . . . Turner, M. B. (2016). Heart disease and stroke statistics—2016 update: A report from the American Heart Association. *Circulation, 131*(4), e38–e360.

Mufson, E. J., & Mesulam, M. M. (1984). Thalamic connections of the insula in the rhesus monkey and comments on the paralimbic connectivity of the medial pulvinar nucleus. *Journal of Comparative Neurology, 227*(1), 109–120.

Muhle, P., Suntrup-Krueger, S., Bittner, S., Ruck, T., Claus, I., Marian, T., . . . Dziewas, R. (2017). Increase of Substance P concentration in saliva after pharyngeal electrical stimulation in severely dysphagic stroke patients—an indicator of decannulation success? *Neurosignals, 25*(1), 74–87.

Mullan, H., Roubenoff, R. A., & Roubenoff, R. (1992). Risk of pulmonary aspiration among patients receiving enteral nutrition support. *JPEN Journal of Parenteral and Enteral Nutrition, 16*(2), 160–164.

Murray, J. (1999). *Manual of dysphagia assessment in adults.* San Diego, CA: Singular.

Murray, J., Ashworth, R., Forster, A., & Young, J. (2003). Developing a primary care-based stroke service: A review of the qualitative literature. *British Journal of General Practice, 53*(487), 137–142.

Murray, J., Doeltgen, S., Miller, M., & Scholten, I. (2016). Does a water protocol improve the hydration and health status of individuals with thin liquid aspiration following stroke? A randomized controlled trial. *Dysphagia, 31*(3), 424–433.

Murray, J., Langmore, S. E., Ginsberg, S., & Dostie, A. (1996). The significance of accumulated oropharyngeal secretions and swallowing frequency in predicting aspiration. *Dysphagia, 11*(2), 99–103.

Murray, J., Miller, M., Doeltgen, S., & Scholten, I. (2014). Intake of thickened liquids by hospitalized adults with dysphagia after stroke. *International Journal of Speech-Language Pathology, 16*(5), 486–494.

Mussen, A. T. (1927). Symposium on the cerebellum: (4) Experimental investigations on the cerebellum. *Brain, 50*(3-4), 313–349.

Naghavi, M., Wang, H., Lozano, R., Davis, A, Liang, X., & Zhou, M. (2015). Global, regional, and national age-sex specific all-cause and cause-specific mortality for 240 causes of death, 1990-2013: A systematic analysis for the Global Burden of Disease Study 2013. *Lancet, 385*(9963), 117–171.

Nagy, A., Leigh, C., Hori, S. F., Molfenter, S. M., Shariff, T., & Steele, C. M. (2013). Timing differences between cued and noncued swallows in healthy young adults. *Dysphagia, 28*(3), 428–434.

Nagy, A., Molfenter, S. M., Péladeau-Pigeon, M., Stokely, S., & Steele, C. M. (2014). The effect of bolus volume on hyoid kinematics in healthy swallowing. *BioMed Research International*, article ID 738971. https://doi.org/10.1155/2014/738971

Nagy, A., Molfenter, S. M., Péladeau-Pigeon, M., Stokely, S., & Steele, C. M. (2015). The effect of bolus consistency on hyoid velocity in healthy swallowing. *Dysphagia, 30*(4), 445–451.

Nagy, A., Steele, C. M., & Pelletier, C. A. (2014). Differences in swallowing between high and low concentration taste stimuli. *BioMed Research International*, article ID 813084. https://doi.org/10.1155/2014/813084

Nakadate, A., Otaka, Y., Kondo, K., Yamamoto, R., Matsuura, D., Honaga, K., . . . Liu, M. (2016). Age, body mass index, and white blood cell count predict the resumption of oral intake in subacute stroke patients. *Journal of Stroke and Cerebrovascular Disorders, 25*(12), 2801–2808.

Nakajoh, K., Nakagawa, T., Sekizawa, K., Matsui, T., Arai, H., & Sasaki, H. (2000). Relation between incidence of pneumonia and protective reflexes in post-stroke patients with oral or tube feeding. *Journal of Internal Medicine, 247*(1), 39–42.

Nam, H. S., Beom, J., Oh, B. M., & Han, T. R. (2013). Kinematic effects of hyolaryngeal electrical stimulation therapy on hyoid excursion and laryngeal elevation. *Dysphagia, 28*(4), 548–556.

Nam, H. S., Oh, B. M., & Han, T. R. (2015). Temporal characteristics of hyolaryngeal structural movements in normal swallowing. *Laryngoscope, 125*(9), 2129–2133.

Nathadwarawala, K. M., Nicklin, J., & Wiles, C. M. (1992). A timed test of swallowing capacity for neurological patients. *Journal of Neurology, Neurosurgery, and Psychiatry, 55*(9), 822–825.

Nativ-Zeltzer, N., Kahrilas, P. J., & Logemann, J. (2012). Manofluorography in the evaluation of oropharyngeal dysphagia. *Dysphagia, 27*(2), 151–161.

Nativ-Zeltzer, N., Kuhn, M. A., Imai, D. M., Traslavina, R. P., Domer, A. S., Litts, J. K., . . . Belafsky, P. C. (2018). The effects of aspirated thickened water on survival and pulmonary injury in a rabbit model. *Laryngoscope, 128*(2), 327–331.

McNaughton, H., McRae, A., Green, G., Abernethy, G., & Gommans, J. (2014). Stroke rehabilitation services in New Zealand: A survey of service configuration, capacity and guideline adherence. *New Zealand Medical Journal (Online), 127*(1402), 10–19.

Nelles, G., Jentzen, W., Jueptner, M., Müller, S., & Diener, H. C. (2001). Arm training induced brain plasticity in stroke studied with serial positron emission tomography. *NeuroImage, 13*(6), 1146–1154.

Netsell, R., & Cleeland, C. S. (1973). Modification of lip hypertonia in dysarthria using EMG feedback. *Journal of Speech and Hearing Disorders, 38*(1), 131–140.

Neubauer, P. D., Hersey, D. P., & Leder, S. B. (2016). Pharyngeal residue severity rating scales based on fiberoptic endoscopic evaluation of swallowing: A systematic review. *Dysphagia, 31*(3), 352–359.

Neubauer, P. D., Rademaker, A. W., & Leder, S. B. (2015). The Yale Pharyngeal Residue Severity Rating Scale: An anatomically defined and image-based tool. *Dysphagia, 30*(5), 521–528.

Neumann, S. (1993). Swallowing therapy with neurologic patients: Results of direct and indirect therapy methods in 66 patients suffering from neurological disorders. *Dysphagia*, *8*(2), 150–153.

Neumann, S., Bartolome, G., Buchholz, D., & Prosiegel, M. (1995). Swallowing therapy of neurologic patients: Correlation of outcome with pretreatment variables and therapeutic methods. *Dysphagia*, *10*(1), 1–5.

Newman, R., Vilardell, N., Clavé, P., & Speyer, R. (2016). Effect of bolus viscosity on safety and efficacy of swallowing and the kinematics of the swallowing response in patients with oropharyngeal dysphagia: White paper by the European Society for Swallowing Disorders (ESSD). *Dysphagia*, *31*(2), 232–249.

NICE Guidelines. (2008, updated 2017). *Stroke and transient ischemic attack in over 16s: Diagnosis and initial management*. Retrieved from https://www.nice.org.uk/guidance/cg68/chapter/1-Guidance#nutrition-and-hydration

Nicosia, M. A., Hind, J. A., Roecker, E. B., Carnes, M., Doyle, J., Dengel, G. A., & Robbins, J. (2000). Age effects on the temporal evolution of isometric and swallowing pressure. *Journals of Gerontology Series A: Biological Sciences and Medical Sciences*, *55*(11), M634–M640.

Nilsson, H., Ekberg, O., Bülow, M., & Hindfelt, B. (1997). Assessment of respiration during video fluoroscopy of dysphagic patients. *Academic Radiology*, *4*(7), 503–507.

Nishino, T., & Hiraga, K. (1991). Coordination of swallowing and respiration in unconscious subjects. *Journal of Applied Physiology*, *70*(3), 988–993.

Nishiwaki, K., Tsuji, T., Liu, M., Hase, K., Tanaka, N., & Fujiwara, T. (2005). Identification of a simple screening tool for dysphagia in patients with stroke using factor analysis of multiple dysphagia variables. *Journal of Rehabilitation Medicine*, *37*(4), 247–251.

Nitsche, M. A., & Paulus, W. (2001). Sustained excitability elevations induced by transcranial DC motor cortex stimulation in humans. *Neurology*, *57*(10), 1899–1901.

Norton, B., Homer-Ward, M., Donnelly, M. T., Long, R. G., & Holmes, G. K. (1996). A randomised prospective comparison of percutaneous endoscopic gastrostomy and nasogastric tube feeding after acute dysphagic stroke. *British Medical Journal*, *312*(7022), 13–16.

O'Dea, M. B., Langmore, S. E., Krisciunas, G. P., Walsh, M., Zanchetti, L. L., Scheel, R., . . . Butler, S. G. (2015). Effect of lidocaine on swallowing during FEES in patients with dysphagia. *Annals of Otology, Rhinology & Laryngology*, *124*(7), 537–544.

Odderson, I. R., Keaton, J. C., & McKenna, B. S. (1995). Swallow management in patients on an acute stroke pathway: Quality is cost effective. *Archives of Physical Medicine and Rehabilitation*, *76*(12), 1130–1133.

Odderson, I. R., & McKenna, B. S. (1993). A model for management of patients with stroke during the acute phase. Outcome and economic implications. *Stroke*, *24*(12), 1823–1827.

Ogawa, N., Mori, T., Fujishima, I., Wakabayashi, H., Itoda, M., Kunieda, K., . . . Ogawa, S. (2017). Ultrasonography to measure swallowing muscle mass and quality in older patients with sarcopenic dysphagia. *Journal of the American Medical Directors Association*, *19*(6), 516–522.

Oh, J. C., Park, J. W., Cha, T. H., Woo, H. S., & Kim, D. K. (2012). Exercise using tongue-holding swallow does not improve swallowing function in normal subjects. *Journal of Oral Rehabilitation*, *39*(5), 364–369.

Ohmae, Y., Logemann, J. A., Kaiser, P., Hanson, D. G., & Kahrilas, P. J. (1995). Timing of glottic closure during normal swallow. *Head and Neck*, *17*(5), 394–402.

Ohmae, Y., Logemann, J. A., Kaiser, P., Hanson, D. G., & Kahrilas, P. J. (1996). Effects of two breath-holding maneuvers on oropharyngeal swallow. *Annals of Otology, Rhinology & Laryngology*, *105*(2), 123–131.

O'Horo, J. C., Rogus-Pulia, N., Garcia-Arguello, L., Robbins, J., & Safdar, N. (2015). Bedside diagnosis of dysphagia: A systematic review. *Journal of Hospital Medicine*, *10*(4), 256–265.

Olsson, R., Kjellin, O., & Ekberg, O. (1996). Videomanometric aspects of pharyngeal constrictor activity. *Dysphagia*, *11*(2), 83–86.

Omari, T. I., Dejaeger, E., Tack, J., Vanbeckevoort, D., & Rommel, N. (2012). An impedance-manometry based method for non-radiological detection of pharyngeal postswallow residue. *Neurogastroenterology & Motility*, *24*(7), 277–284.

Omari, T. I., Dejaeger, E., Tack, J., Van Beckevoort, D., & Rommel, N. (2013). Effect of bolus volume and viscosity on pharyngeal automated impedance manometry variables derived for broad dysphagia patients. *Dysphagia*, *28*(2), 146–152.

Omari, T. I., Dejaeger, E., Van Beckevoort, D., Goeleven, A., De Cock, P., Hoffman, I., . . . Rommel, N. (2011). A novel method for the nonradiological assessment of ineffective swallowing. *American Journal of Gastroenterology*, *106*(10), 1796–1802.

Omari, T. I., Papathanasopoulos, A., Dejaeger, E., Wauters, L., Scarpellini, E., Vos, R., . . . Rommel, N. (2011). Reproducibility and agreement of pharyngeal automated impedance manometry with videofluoroscopy. *Clinical Gastroenterology and Hepatology*, *9*(10), 862–867.

Omari, T., Rommel, N., Szczesniak, M., Fuentealba, S., Dinning, P., Davidson, G., & Cook, I. J. (2006). Assessment of intraluminal impedance for the detection of pharyngeal bolus flow during swallowing in healthy adults. *American Journal of Physiology–Gastrointestinal and Liver Physiology*, *290*(1), G183–G188.

Omari, T. I., Savilampi, J., Kokkinn, K., Schar, M., Lamvik, K., Doeltgen, S., & Cock, C. (2016). The reliability of pharyngeal high resolution manometry with impedance for derivation of measures of swallowing function in healthy volunteers. *International Journal of Otolaryngology*, article ID 2718482. https://doi.org/10.1155/2016/2718482

Omari, T. I., Wiklendt, L., Dinning, P., Costa, M., Rommel, N., & Cock, C. (2015). Upper esophageal sphincter mechanical states analysis: A novel methodology to describe UES relaxation and opening. *Frontiers in Systems Neuroscience, 8*, 241. https://doi.org/10.3389/fnsys.2014.00241

O'Neil, K. H., Purdy, M., Falk, J., & Gallo, L. (1999). The Dysphagia Outcome and Severity Scale. *Dysphagia, 14*(3), 139–145.

Ono, H., Azuma, T., Miyaji, H., Ito, S., Ohtaki, H., Ohtani, M., . . . Kuriyama, M. (2003). Effects of percutaneous endoscopic gastrostomy tube placement on gastric antral motility and gastric emptying. *Journal of Gastroenterology, 38*(10), 930–936.

O'Rourke, A., & Humphries, K. (2017). The use of high-resolution pharyngeal manometry as biofeedback in dysphagia therapy. *Ear, Nose & Throat Journal, 96*(2), 56–58.

O'Rourke, A., Morgan, L. B., Coss-Adame, E., Morrison, M., Weinberger, P., & Postma, G. (2014). The effect of voluntary pharyngeal swallowing maneuvers on esophageal swallowing physiology. *Dysphagia, 29*(2), 262–268.

Paik, N. J., Kim, I. S., Kim, J. H., Oh, B. M., & Han, T. R. (2005). Clinical validity of the functional dysphagia scale based on videofluoroscopic swallowing study. *Journal of Korean Academy of Rehabilitation Medicine, 29*(1), 43–49.

Palmer, J. B., & Hiiemae, K. M. (2003). Eating and breathing: Interactions between respiration and feeding on solid food. *Dysphagia, 18*(3), 169–178.

Palmer, J. B., Rudin, N. J., Lara, G., & Crompton, A. W. (1992). Coordination of mastication and swallowing. *Dysphagia, 7*(4), 187–200.

Palmer, P. M., McCulloch, T. M., Jaffe, D., & Neel, A. T. (2005). Effects of a sour bolus on the intramuscular electromyographic (EMG) activity of muscles in the submental region. *Dysphagia, 20*(3), 210–217.

Pandolfino, J. E., Fox, M. R., Bredenoord, A. J., & Kahrilas, P. J. (2009). High-resolution manometry in clinical practice: Utilizing pressure topography to classify oesophageal motility abnormalities. *Neurogastroenterology & Motility, 21*(8), 796–806.

Panther, K. (2005). The Frazier free water protocol. *Perspectives on Swallowing and Swallowing Disorders, 14*(1), 4–9.

Parameswaran, M. S., & Soliman, A. M. (2002). Endoscopic botulinum toxin injection for cricopharyngeal dysphagia. *Annals of Otology, Rhinology & Laryngology, 111*(10), 871–874.

Park, C. L., O'Neill, P. A., & Martin, D. F. (1997). A pilot exploratory study of oral electrical stimulation on swallow function following stroke: An innovative technique. *Dysphagia, 12*(3), 161–166.

Park, E., Kim, M. S., Chang, W. H., Oh, S. M., Kim, Y. K., Lee, A., & Kim, Y. H. (2017). Effects of bilateral repetitive transcranial magnetic stimulation on post-stroke dysphagia. *Brain Stimulation, 10*(1), 75–82.

Park, J. S., Hwang, N. K., Oh, D. H., & Chang, M. Y. (2017). Effect of head lift exercise on kinematic motion of the hyolaryngeal complex and aspiration in patients with dysphagic stroke. *Journal of Oral Rehabilitation, 44*(5), 385–391.

Park, J. S., Oh, D. H., Chang, M. Y., & Kim, K. M. (2016). Effects of expiratory muscle strength training on oropharyngeal dysphagia in subacute stroke patients: A randomised controlled trial. *Journal of Oral Rehabilitation*, *43*(5), 364–372.

Park, J. W., Oh, J. C., Lee, J. W., Yeo, J. S., & Ryu, K. H. (2013). The effect of 5Hz high-frequency rTMS over contralesional pharyngeal motor cortex in post-stroke oropharyngeal dysphagia: A randomized controlled study. *Neurogastroenterology & Motility*, *25*(4), 324–e250.

Park, R. H., Allison, M. C., Lang, J., Spence, E., Morris, A. J., Danesh, B. J., . . . Mills, P. R. (1992). Randomised comparison of percutaneous endoscopic gastrostomy and nasogastric tube feeding in patients with persisting neurological dysphagia. *British Medical Journal*, *304*(6839), 1406–1409.

Park, Y. H., Bang, H. L., Han, H. R., & Chang, H. K. (2015). Dysphagia screening measures for use in nursing homes: A systematic review. *Journal of Korean Academy of Nursing*, *45*(1), 1–13.

Parker, C., Power, M., Hamdy, S., Bowen, A., Tyrrell, P., & Thompson, D. G. (2004). Awareness of dysphagia by patients following stroke predicts swallowing performance. *Dysphagia*, *19*(1), 28–35.

Pauloski, B. R., Rademaker, A. W., Lazarus, C., Boeckxstaens, G., Kahrilas, P. J., & Logemann, J. A. (2009). Relationship between manometric and videofluoroscopic measures of swallow function in healthy adults and patients treated for head and neck cancer with various modalities. *Dysphagia*, *24*(2), 196–203.

Passingham, R. (1993). *The frontal lobes and voluntary action*. Oxford, UK: Oxford University Press.

Pearson, W. G., Molfenter, S. M., Smith, Z. M., & Steele, C. M. (2013). Image-based measurement of post-swallow residue: The normalized residue ratio scale. *Dysphagia*, *28*(2), 167–177.

Peladeau-Pigeon, M., & Steele, C. M. (2013). Technical aspects of the videofluoroscopic swallowing study. *Canadian Journal of Speech-Language Pathology and Audiology*, *37*(3), 216–226.

Peladeau-Pigeon, M., & Steele, C. M. (2017). Age-related variability in tongue pressure patterns for maximum isometric and saliva swallowing tasks. *Journal of Speech, Language, and Hearing Research*, *60*(11), 3177–3184.

Pelletier, C. A., & Dhanaraj, G. E. (2006). The effect of taste and palatability on lingual swallowing pressure. *Dysphagia*, *21*(2), 121–128.

Pelletier, C. A., & Lawless, H. T. (2003). Effect of citric acid and citric acid-sucrose mixtures on swallowing in neurogenic oropharyngeal dysphagia. *Dysphagia*, *18*(4), 231–241.

Pelletier, C. A., & Steele, C. M. (2014). Influence of the perceived taste intensity of chemesthetic stimuli on swallowing parameters given age and genetic taste differences in healthy adult women. *Journal of Speech, Language, and Hearing Research*, *57*(1), 46–56.

Perlman, A. L., Booth, B. M., & Grayhack, J. P. (1994). Videofluoroscopic predictors of aspiration in patients with oropharyngeal dysphagia. *Dysphagia*, *9*(2), 90–95.

Perlman, A. L., He, X., Barkmeier, J., & Van Leer, E. (2005). Bolus location associated with videofluoroscopic and respirodeglutometric events. *Journal of Speech, Language, and Hearing Research*, *48*(1), 21–33.

Perlman, A. L., Schultz, J. G., & VanDaele, D. J. (1993). Effects of age, gender, bolus volume, and bolus viscosity on oropharyngeal pressure during swallowing. *Journal of Applied Physiology*, *75*(1), 33–37.

Perrini, P., Tiezzi, G., Castagna, M., & Vannozzi, R. (2013). Three-dimensional microsurgical anatomy of cerebellar peduncles. *Neurosurgical Review*, *36*(2), 215–225.

Perry, L., & Love, C. P. (2001). Screening for dysphagia and aspiration in acute stroke: A systematic review. *Dysphagia*, *16*(1), 7–18.

Perry, S. E., Miles, A., Fink, J. N., & Huckabee, M. L. (2018). The dysphagia in stroke protocol reduces aspiration pneumonia in patients with dysphagia following acute stroke: A clinical audit. *Translational Stroke Research*. https://doi.org/10.1007/s12975-018-0625-z

Perry, S. E., Winkelman, C. J., & Huckabee, M. L. (2016). Variability in ultrasound Measurement of hyoid bone displacement and submental muscle size using 2 methods of data acquisition. *Folia Phoniatrica et Logopaedica*, *68*(5), 205–210.

Pilz, W., Vanbelle, S., Kremer, B., van Hooren, M. R., van Becelaere, T., Roodenburg, N., & Baijens, L. W. (2016). Observers' agreement on measurements in fiberoptic endoscopic evaluation of swallowing. *Dysphagia*, *31*(2), 180–187.

Pisegna, J. M., Kaneoka, A., Pearson, W. G., Kumar, S., & Langmore, S. E. (2016). Effects of non-invasive brain stimulation on post-stroke dysphagia: A systematic review and meta-analysis of randomized controlled trials. *Clinical Neurophysiology*, *127*(1), 956–968.

Pitts, T., Bolser, D., Rosenbek, J., Troche, M., Okun, M. S., & Sapienza, C. (2009). Impact of expiratory muscle strength training on voluntary cough and swallow function in Parkinson disease. *Chest*, *135*(5), 1301–1308.

Plautz, E. J., Milliken, G. W., & Nudo, R. J. (2000). Effects of repetitive motor training on movement representations in adult squirrel monkeys: Role of use versus learning. *Neurobiology of Learning and Memory*, *74*(1), 27–55.

Pluschinski, P., Zaretsky, E., Stöver, T., Murray, J., Sader, R., & Hey, C. (2016). Validation of the secretion severity rating scale. *European Archives of Oto-Rhino-Laryngology*, *273*(10), 3215–3218.

Poirier, N. C., Bonavina, L., Taillefer, R., Nosadini, A., Peracchia, A., & Duranceau, A. (1997). Cricopharyngeal myotomy for neurogenic oropharyngeal dysphagia. *Journal of Thoracic and Cardiovascular Surgery*, *113*(2), 233–240.

Poorjavad, M., & Jalaie, S. (2014). Systematic review on highly qualified screening tests for swallowing disorders following stroke: Validity and reliability issues. *Journal of Research in Medical Sciences*, *19*(8), 776–785.

Pooyania, S., Vandurme, L., Daun, R., & Buchel, C. (2015). Effects of a free water protocol on inpatients in a neuro-rehabilitation setting. *Open Journal of Therapy and Rehabilitation, 3*, 132–138.

Popa Nita, S., Murith, M., Chisholm, H., & Engmann, J. (2012). Matching the rheological properties of videofluoroscopic contrast agents and thickened liquid prescriptions. *Dysphagia, 28*(2), 245–252.

Popovtzer, A., Cao, Y., Feng, F. Y., & Eisbruch, A. (2009). Anatomical changes in the pharyngeal constrictors after chemo-irradiation of head and neck cancer and their dose–effect relationships: MRI-based study. *Radiotherapy and Oncology, 93*(3), 510–515.

Pouderoux, P., & Kahrilas, P. J. (1995). Deglutitive tongue force modulation by volition, volume, and viscosity in humans. *Gastroenterology, 108*(5), 1418–1426.

Pouderoux, P., Logemann, J. A., & Kahrilas, P. J. (1996). Pharyngeal swallowing elicited by fluid infusion: Role of volition and vallecular containment. *American Journal of Physiology–Gastrointestinal and Liver Physiology, 270*(2), G347–G354.

Pounsford, J. C., & Saunders, K. B. (1985). Diurnal variation and adaptation of the cough response to citric acid in normal subjects. *Thorax, 40*(9), 657–661.

Power, M. L., Cross, S. P., Roberts, S., & Tyrrell, P. J. (2007). Evaluation of service development to implement the top three process indicators for quality stroke care. *Journal of Evaluation in Clinical Practice, 13*(1), 90–94.

Power, M., Fraser, C., Hobson, A., Rothwell, J. C., Mistry, S., Nicholson, D. A., . . . Hamdy, S. (2004). Changes in pharyngeal corticobulbar excitability and swallowing behavior after oral stimulation. *American Journal of Physiology–Gastrointestinal and Liver Physiology, 286*(1), G45–G50.

Power, M., Fraser, C. H., Hobson, A., Singh, S., Tyrrell, P., Nicholson, D. A., . . . Hamdy, S. (2006). Evaluating oral stimulation as a treatment for dysphagia after stroke. *Dysphagia, 21*(1), 49–55.

Powers, W. J., Rabinstein, A. A., Ackerson, T., Adeoye, O. M., Bambakidis, N. C., Becker, K., . . . Tirschwell, D. L. (2018). 2018 guidelines for the early management of patients with acute ischemic stroke: A guideline for healthcare professionals from the American Heart Association/American Stroke Association. *Stroke, 49*(3), e46–e110.

Preiksaitis, H. G., & Mills, C. A. (1996). Coordination of breathing and swallowing: Effects of bolus consistency and presentation in normal adults. *Journal of Applied Physiology, 81*(4), 1707–1714.

Pryor, L. N., Ward, E. C., Cornwell, P. L., O'Connor, S. N., Finnis, M. E., & Chapman, M. J. (2015). Impact of nasogastric tubes on swallowing physiology in older healthy subjects: A randomized controlled crossover trial. *Clinical Nutrition, 34*, 572–578.

Quinn, B., Baker D. L., Cohen, S., Stewart, J. L., Lima, C. A., & Parise C. (2014). Basic nursing care to prevent nonventilator hospital-acquired pneumonia. *Journal of Nursing Scholarship, 46*(1), 11–19.

Quintero, A., Ichesco, E., Schutt, R., Myers, C., Peltier, S., & Gerstner, G. E. (2013). Functional connectivity of human chewing: An fMRI study. *Journal of Dental Research, 92*(3), 272–278.

Rademaker, A. W., Pauloski, B. R., Colangelo, L. A., & Logemann, J. A. (1998). Age and volume effects on liquid swallowing function in normal women. *Journal of Speech, Language, and Hearing Research, 41*(2), 275–284.

Ragnarsson, K. T. (1994). The physiologic aspects and clinical application of functional electrical stimulation in rehabilitation. In J. A. Downey, S. J. Myers, E. G. Gonzalez, & J. S. Lieberman (Eds.), *The physiological basis of rehabilitation medicine* (2nd ed., pp. 573–597). Boston, MA: Butterworth-Heinemann.

Rajappa, A. T., Soriano, K. R., Ziemer, C., Troche, M. S., Malandraki, J. B., & Malandraki, G. A. (2017). Reduced maximum pitch elevation predicts silent aspiration of small liquid volumes in stroke patients. *Frontiers in Neurology, 8*, 436. https://doi.org/10.3389/fneur.2017.00436

Ramsey, D., Smithard, D., Donaldson, N., & Kalra, L. (2005). Is the gag reflex useful in the management of swallowing problems in acute stroke? *Dysphagia, 20*(2), 105–107.

Ramsey, D., Smithard, D. G., & Kalra, L. (2003). Early assessment of dysphagia and aspiration risk in acute stroke patients. *Stroke, 34*(5), 1252–1257.

Rangarathnam, B., Kamarunas, E., & McCullough, G. H. (2014). Role of cerebellum in deglutition and deglutition disorders. *The Cerebellum, 13*(6), 767–776.

Rasley, A., Logemann, J. A., Kahrilas, P. J., Rademaker, A. W., Pauloski, B. R., & Dodds, W. J. (1993). Prevention of barium aspiration during videofluoroscopic swallowing studies: Value of change in posture. *AJR American Journal of Roentgenology, 160*(5), 1005–1009.

Ravich, W. J. (1995). The unrealized potential of pharyngeal manometry. *Dysphagia, 10*(1), 42–43.

Ravich, W. J. (2001). Botulinum toxin for UES dysfunction: Therapy or poison? *Dysphagia, 16*(3), 168–170.

Regan, J., Murphy, A., Chiang, M., McMahon, B., Coughlan, T., & Walshe, M. (2014). Botulinum toxin for upper oesophageal sphincter dysfunction in neurological swallowing disorders. *Cochrane Database of Systematic Reviews, 5*, CD009968.

Reimers, C. D., Harder, T., & Saxe, H. (1998). Age-related muscle atrophy does not affect all muscles and can partly be compensated by physical activity: An ultrasound study. *Journal of the Neurological Sciences, 159*(1), 60–66.

Reimers-Neils, L., Logemann, J., & Larson, C. (1994). Viscosity effects on EMG activity in normal swallow. *Dysphagia, 9*(2), 101–106.

Reitsma, J. B., Rutjes, A. W. S., Whiting, P., Vlassov, V., Leeflang, M. M. G., & Deeks, J. J. (2009). Assessing methodological quality: Version 1.0.0. *Cochrane Handbook for Systematic Reviews of Diagnostic Test Accuracy*.

Remple, M. S., Bruneau, R. M., VandenBerg, P. M., Goertzen, C., & Kleim, J. A. (2001). Sensitivity of cortical movement representations to motor experience:

evidence that skill learning but not strength training induces cortical reorganization. *Behavioural Brain Research, 123*(2), 133–141.

Ren, J., Shaker, R., Zamir, Z., Dodds, W. J., Hogan, W. J., & Hoffmann, R. G. (1993). Effect of age and bolus variables on the coordination of the glottis and upper esophageal sphincter during swallowing. *American Journal of Gastroenterology, 88*(5), 665–669.

Rensink, M., Schuurmans, M., Lindeman, E., & Hafsteinsdottir, T. (2009). Task-oriented training in rehabilitation after stroke: Systematic review. *Journal of Advanced Nursing, 65*(4), 737–754.

Restivo, D., & Hamdy, S. (2018). Pharyngeal electrical stimulation device for the treatment of neurogenic dysphagia: Technology update. *Medical Devices: Evidence and Research, 11*, 21–26.

Rice, T. W., & Shay, S. S. (2011). A primer of high-resolution esophageal manometry. *Seminars in Thoracic and Cardiovascular Surgery, 23*(3), 181–190.

Richter, J. E., & Castell, J. A. (1989). Esophageal manometry. In D. W. Gelfand & J. E. Richter (Eds.), *Dysphagia: Diagnosis and treatment* (pp. 83–114). New York, NY: IgatsuShoin.

Ridding, M. C., & Rothwell, J. C. (2007). Is there a future for therapeutic use of transcranial magnetic stimulation? *Nature Reviews Neuroscience, 8*(7), 559–567.

Risberg, M. A., Holm, I., Myklebust, G., & Engebretsen, L. (2007). Neuromuscular training versus strength training during first 6 months after anterior cruciate ligament reconstruction: A randomized clinical trial. *Physical Therapy, 87*(6), 737–750.

Robbins, J., Butler, S. G., Daniels, S. K., Diez Gross, R., Langmore, S., Lazarus, C. L., . . . Rosenbek, J. (2008). Swallowing and dysphagia rehabilitation: Translating principles of neural plasticity into clinically oriented evidence. *Journal of Speech, Language, and Hearing Research, 51*(1), S276–S300.

Robbins, J., Coyle, J., Rosenbek, J., Roecker, E., & Wood, J. (1999). Differentiation of normal and abnormal airway protection during swallowing using the penetration-aspiration scale. *Dysphagia, 14*(4), 228–232.

Robbins, J., Gangnon, R. E., Theis, S. M., Kays, S. A., Hewitt, A. L., & Hind, J. A. (2005). The effects of lingual exercise on swallowing in older adults. *Journal of the American Geriatrics Society, 53*(9), 1483–1489.

Robbins, J., Gensler, G., Hind, J., Logemann, J. A., Lindblad, A. S., & Brandt, D. (2008). Comparison of 2 interventions for liquid aspiration on pneumonia incidence: A randomized trial. *Annals of Internal Medicine, 148*(7), 509–518.

Robbins, J., Hamilton, J. W., Lof, G. L., & Kempster, G. B. (1992). Oropharyngeal swallowing in normal adults of different ages. *Gastroenterology, 103*(3), 823–829.

Robbins, J., Kays, S. A., Gangnon, R. E., Hind, J. A., Hewitt, A. L., Gentry, L. R., & Taylor, A. J. (2007). The effects of lingual exercise in stroke patients with dysphagia. *Archives of Physical Medicine and Rehabilitation, 88*(2), 150–158.

Robbins, J., & Levine, R. (1993). Swallowing after lateral medullary syndrome plus. *Clinics in Communication Disorders, 3*(4), 45–55.

Robbins, J., Levine, R., Wood, J., Roecker, E. B., & Luschei, E. (1995). Age effects on lingual pressure generation as a risk factor for dysphagia. *Journals of Gerontology Series: A Biological Sciences and Medical Sciences, 50*(5), M257–M262.

Robbins, J., & Levine, R. L. (1988). Swallowing after unilateral stroke of the cerebral cortex: Preliminary experience. *Dysphagia, 3*(1), 11–17.

Robbins, J., Levine, R. L., Maser, A., Rosenbek, J. C., & Kempster, G. B. (1993). Swallowing after unilateral stroke of the cerebral cortex. *Archives of Physical Medicine and Rehabilitation, 74*(12), 1295–1300.

Robertson, E. V., Lee, Y. Y., Derakhshan, M. H., Wirz, A. A., Whiting, J. R. H., Seenan, J. P., . . . McColl, K. E. L. (2012). High-resolution esophageal manometry: Addressing thermal drift of the manoscan system. *Neurogastroenterology & Motility, 24*(1), 61–65.

Robin, D. G., Somodi, L. B., & Luschei, E. S. (1991) Measurement of tongue strength and endurance in normal and articulation disordered subjects. In C. A. Moore, K. M. Yorkston, & D. R. Beukelman (Eds.), *Dysarthria and apraxia of speech: Perspectives on management* (pp. 173–184). Baltimore, MD: Brookes.

Roe, G., Harris, K., Lambie, H., & Tolan, D. (2017). Radiographer workforce role expansion to improve patient safety related to nasogastric tube placement for feeding in adults. *Clinical Radiology, 72*(6), 518.e1. https://doi.org/10.1016/j.crad.2016.12.018

Rofes, L., Arreola, V., Martin, A., & Clavé, P. (2013). Natural capsaicinoids improve swallow response in older patients with oropharyngeal dysphagia. *Gut, 62*(9), 1280–1287.

Rofes, L., Arreola, V., Martin, A., & Clavé, P. (2014). Effect of oral piperine on the swallow response of patients with oropharyngeal dysphagia. *Journal of Gastroenterology, 49*(12), 1517–1523.

Rogus-Pulia, N., Rusche, N., Hind, J. A., Zielinski, J., Gangnon, R., Safdar, N., & Robbins, J. (2016). Effects of device-facilitated isometric progressive resistance oropharyngeal therapy on swallowing and health-related outcomes in older adults with dysphagia. *Journal of the American Geriatrics Society, 64*(2), 417–424.

Roland, P. E., Larsen, B., Lassen, N. A., & Skinhoj, E. (1980). Supplementary motor area and other cortical areas in organization of voluntary movements in man. *Journal of Neurophysiology, 43*(1), 118–136.

Roman, C. (1986). Neural control of deglutition and esophageal motility in mammals [in French]. *Journal of Physiology (Paris), 81*(2), 118–131.

Rose, D. J., & Christina, R. W. (2006). *Multilevel approach to the study of motor control and learning* (2nd ed.). San Francisco, CA: Pearson.

Rosenbek, J. C., McCullough, G. H., & Wertz, R. T. (2004). Is the information about a test important? Applying the methods of evidence-based medicine to the clinical examination of swallowing. *Journal of Communication Disorders, 37*(5), 437–450.

Rosenbek, J. C., Robbins, J., Fishback, B., & Levine, R. L. (1991). Effects of thermal application on dysphagia after stroke. *Journal of Speech and Hearing Research, 34*(6), 1257–1268.

Rosenbek, J. C., Robbins, J., Willford, W. O., Kirk, G., Schiltz, A., Sowell, T. W., . . . Hansen, J. E. (1998). Comparing treatment intensities of tactile-thermal application. *Dysphagia, 13*(1), 1–9.

Rosenbek, J. C., Robbins, J. A., Roecker, E. B., Coyle, J. L., & Wood, J. L. (1996). A Penetration-Aspiration Scale. *Dysphagia, 11*(2), 93–98.

Rosenbek, J. C., Roecker, E. B., Wood, J. L., & Robbins, J. (1996). Thermal application reduces the duration of stage transition in dysphagia after stroke. *Dysphagia, 11*(4), 225–233.

Rossi, S., Hallett, M., Rossini, P. M., & Pascual-Leone, A. (2009). Safety, ethical considerations, and application guidelines for the use of transcranial magnetic stimulation in clinical practice and research. *Clinical Neurophysiology, 120*(12), 2008–2039.

Rossignol, S., & Dubuc, R. (1994). Spinal pattern generation. *Current Opinions in Neurobiology, 4*(6), 894–902.

Rossini, P. M., & Rossi, S. (2007). Transcranial magnetic stimulation: Diagnostic, therapeutic, and research potential. *Neurology, 68*(7), 484–488.

Rubow, R. (1984). Reinforcement and compliance on training and transfer in biofeedback-based rehabilitation of motor speech disorders. In M. R. McNeil, J. C. Rosenbek, & A. E. Aronson (Eds.), *The dysarthrias: Physiology, acoustics, perception, and managment* (pp. 207–229). San Diego, CA: College-Hill Press.

Rugiu, M. G. (2007). Role of videofluoroscopy in evaluation of neurologic dysphagia. *ACTA Otorhinolaryngologica Italica, 27*(6), 306–316.

Rybak, I. A., Shevtsova, N. A., Paton, J. F. R., Dick, T. E., John, W. S., Mörschel, M., & Dutschmann, M. (2004). Modeling the ponto-medullary respiratory network. *Respiratory Physiology & Neurobiology, 143*(2-3), 307–319.

Ryu, J. S., Park, D., & Kang, J. Y. (2015). Application and interpretation of high-resolution manometry for pharyngeal dysphagia. *Journal of Neurogastroenterology and Motility, 21*(2), 283–287.

Sackett, D. L., Haynes, R. B., Guyatt, G. H., & Tugwell, P. (1991). *Clinical epidemiology: A basic science for clinical medicine.* Boston, MA: Little Brown.

Sackett, D. L., Strauss, S. E., Richardson, W. S., Rosenberg, W., & Haynes, R. B. (2000). *Evidence-based medicine* (2nd ed.). New York, NY: Churchill Livingstone.

Sakakura, K., Tazawa, M., Otani, N., Takagi, M., Morita, M., Kurosaki, M., . . . Chikamatsu, K. (2017). Impact of a multidisciplinary round visit for the management of dysphagia utilizing a Wi-Fi–based wireless flexible endoscopic evaluation of swallowing. *Annals of Otology, Rhinology & Laryngology, 126*(1), 47–53.

Saito, Y., Ezure, K., Tanaka, I., & Osawa, M. (2003). Activity of neurons in ventrolateral respiratory groups during swallowing in decerebrate rats. *Brain Development, 25*(5), 338–345.

Salassa, J. R., DeVault, K. R., & McConnel, F. M. (1998). Proposed catheter standards for pharyngeal manofluorography (videomanometry). *Dysphagia*, *13*(2), 105–110.

Saleem, A. F., Sapienza, C. M., & Okun, M. S. (2005). Respiratory muscle strength training: treatment and response duration in a patient with early idiopathic Parkinson's disease. *NeuroRehabilitation*, *20*(4), 323–333.

Salmoni, A. W., Schmidt, R. A., & Walter, C. B. (1984). Knowledge of results and motor learning: A review and critical reappraisal. *Psychological Bulletin*, *95*(3), 355–386.

Samson, N., Praud, J. P., Quenet, B., Similowski, T., & Straus, C. (2017). New insights into sucking, swallowing and breathing central generators: A complexity analysis of rhythmic motor behaviors. *Neuroscience Letters*, *638*, 90–95.

Sanders, H. N., Hoffman, S. B., & Lund, C. A. (1992). Feeding strategy for dependent eaters. *Journal of the American Dietetic Association*, *92*(11), 1389–1390.

Sandrini, M., & Cohen, L. G. (2013). Noninvasive brain stimulation in neurorehabilitation. In A. M. Lozano & M. Hallett (Eds.), *Handbook of clinical neurology* (Vol. 116, pp. 499–524). Cambridge, MA: Elsevier.

Sapienza, C. M., Davenport, P. W., & Martin, A. D. (2002). Expiratory muscle training increases pressure support in high school band students. *Journal of Voice*, *16*(4), 495–501.

Sapienza, C. M., & Wheeler, K. (2006). Respiratory muscle strength training: Functional outcomes versus plasticity. *Seminars in Speech and Language*, *27*(4), 236–244.

Scannapieco, F. A. (2006). Pneumonia in nonambulatory patients: The role of oral bacteria and oral hygiene. *Journal of the American Dental Association*, *137*(Suppl. 2), S21–S25.

Scharitzer, M., Pokieser, P., Schober, E., Schima, W., Eisenhuber, E., Stadler, A., . . . Ekberg, O. (2002). Morphological findings in dynamic swallowing studies of symptomatic patients. *European Radiology*, *12*(5), 1139–1144.

Schaser, A. J., Ciucci, M. R., & Connor, N. P. (2016). Cross-activation and detraining effects of tongue exercise in aged rats. *Behavioural Brain Research*, *297*, 285–296.

Schepp, S. K., Tirschwell, D. L., Miller, R. M., & Longstreth, W. T. (2012). Swallowing screens after acute stroke: A systematic review. *Stroke*, *43*(3), 869–871.

Schiffman, S. S. (1993). Perception of taste and smell in elderly persons. *Critical Reviews in Food Science and Nutrition*, *33*(1), 17–26.

Schlaug, G., Renga, V., & Nair, D. (2008). Transcranial direct current stimulation in stroke recovery. *Archives of Neurology*, *65*(12), 1571–1576.

Schmidt, R. A., & Lee, T. D. (1999). *Motor control and learning: A behavioral emphasis* (3rd ed.). Champaign, IL: Human Kinetics.

Schroeder, M. F., Daniels, S. K., McClain, M., Corey, D. M., & Foundas, A. L. (2006). Clinical and cognitive predictors of swallowing recovery in stroke. *Journal of Rehabilitation, Research, and Development*, *43*(3), 301–310.

Schulz, M. L. (1994). *The somatotopic arrangement of motor fibers in the periventricular white matter and internal capsule in the Rhesus monkey* (Dissertation). Boston University, Boston, MA.

Schulze-Delrieu, K., & Miller, R. (1997). Clinical assessment of dysphagia. In A. L. Perlman & K. Schulze-Delreiu (Eds.), *Deglutition and its disorders* (pp. 125–152). San Diego, CA: Singular.

Scott, A., Perry, A., & Bench, J. (1998). A study of inter-rater reliability when using videofluoroscopy as an assessment of swallowing. *Dysphagia, 13*(4), 223–227.

Scutt, P., Lee, H. S., Hamdy, S., & Bath, P. M. (2015). Pharyngeal electrical stimulation for treatment of poststroke dysphagia: Individual patient data meta-analysis of randomised controlled trials. *Stroke Research and Treatment*, article ID 429053. https://doi.org/10.1155/2015/429053

Sdravou, K., Walshe, M., & Dagdilelis, L. (2012). Effects of carbonated liquids on oropharyngeal swallowing measures in people with neurogenic dysphagia, *Dysphagia, 27*(2), 240–250.

Selinger, M., Prescott, T. E., & Hoffman, I. (1994). Temperature acceleration in cold oral stimulation. *Dysphagia, 9*(2), 83–87.

Selley, W. G., Flack, F. C., Ellis, R. E., & Brooks, W. A. (1989a). Respiratory patterns associated with swallowing: Part 1. The normal adult pattern and changes with age. *Age and Ageing, 18*(3), 168–172.

Selley, W. G., Flack, F. C., Ellis, R. E., & Brooks, W. A. (1989b). Respiratory patterns associated with swallowing: Part 2. Neurologically impaired dysphagic patients. *Age and Ageing, 18*(3), 173–176.

Sessle, B. J., Adachi, K., Avivi-Arber, L., Lee, J., Nishiura, H., Yao, D., & Yoshino, K. (2007). Neuroplasticity of face primary motor cortex control of orofacial movements. *Archives of Oral Biology, 52*(4), 334–337.

Sessle, B. J., Yao, D., Nishiura, H., Yoshino, K., Lee, J. C., Martin, R. E., & Murray, G. M. (2005). Properties and plasticity of the primate somatosensory and motor cortex related to orofacial sensorimotor function. *Clinical and Experimental Pharmacology and Physiology, 32*(1-2), 109–114.

Shaker, R., Cook, I. J., Dodds, W. J., & Hogan, W. J. (1988). Pressure-flow dynamics of the oral phase of swallowing. *Dysphagia, 3*(2), 79–84.

Shaker, R., Dodds, W. J., Dantas, R. O., Hogan, W. J., & Arndorfer, R. C. (1990) Coordination of deglutitive glottic closure with oropharyngeal swallowing. *Gastroenterology, 98*(6), 1478–1484.

Shaker, R., Easterling, C., Kern, M., Nitschke, T., Massey, B., Daniels, S., . . . Dikeman, K. (2002). Rehabilitation of swallowing by exercise in tube-fed patients with pharyngeal dysphagia secondary to abnormal UES opening. *Gastroenterology, 122*(5), 1314–1321.

Shaker, R., Kern, M., Bardan, E., Taylor, A., Stewart, E. T., Hoffmann, R. G., . . . Bonnevier, J. (1997). Augmentation of deglutitive upper esophageal sphincter opening in the elderly by exercise. *American Journal of Physiology–Gastrointestinal and Liver Physiology, 272*(6 Pt. 1), G1518–G1522.

Shaker, R., Ren, J., Bardan, E., Easterling, C., Dua, K., Xie, P., & Kern, M. (2003). Pharyngoglottal closure reflex: Characterization in healthy young, elderly and dysphagic patients with predeglutitive aspiration. *Gerontology*, *49*(1), 12–20.

Shaker, R., Ren, J., Podvrsan, B., Dodds, W. J., Hogan, W. J., Kern, M., . . . Hintz, J. (1993). Effect of aging and bolus variables on pharyngeal and upper esophageal sphincter motor function. *American Journal of Physiology–Gastrointestinal and Liver Physiology*, *264*(3), G427–G432.

Shaker, R., Ren, J., Zamir, Z., Sarna, A., Liu, J., & Sui, Z. (1994). Effect of aging, position, and temperature on the threshold volume triggering pharyngeal swallows. *Gastroenterology*, *107*(2), 396–402.

Shanahan, T. K., Logemann, J. A., Rademaker, A. W., Pauloski, B. R., & Kahrilas, P. J. (1993). Chin-down posture effect on aspiration in dysphagic patients. *Archives of Physical Medicine and Rehabilitation*, *74*(7), 736–739.

Shaw, D. W., Cook, I. J., Gabb, M., Holloway, R. H., Simula, M. E., Panagopoulos, V., & Dent, J. (1995). Influence of normal aging on oral-pharyngeal and upper esophageal sphincter function during swallowing. *American Journal of Physiology–Gastrointestinal and Liver Physiology*, *268*(3), G389–G396.

Shaw, G. Y., & Searl, J. P. (2001). Botulinum toxin treatment for cricopharyngeal dysfunction. *Dysphagia*, *16*(3), 161–167.

Shiba, K., Satoh, I., Kobayashi, N., & Hayashi, F. (1999). Multifunctional laryngeal motoneurons: An intracellular study in the cat. *Journal of Neuroscience*, *19*(7), 2717–2727.

Shigematsu, T., Fujishima, I., & Ohno, K. (2013). Transcranial direct current stimulation improves swallowing function in stroke patients. *Neurorehabilitation and Neural Repair*, *27*(4), 363–369.

Sia, I., Carvajal, P., Carnaby-Mann, G. D., & Crary, M. A. (2012). Measurement of hyoid and laryngeal displacement in video fluoroscopic swallowing studies: Variability, reliability, and measurement error. *Dysphagia*, *27*(2), 192–197.

Sia, I., Carvajal, P., Lacy, A. A., Carnaby, G. D., & Crary, M. A. (2015). Hyoid and laryngeal excursion kinematics—magnitude, duration and velocity—changes following successful exercise-based dysphagia rehabilitation: MDTP. *Journal of Oral Rehabilitation*, *42*(5), 331–339.

Silverman, E. P., Sapienza, C. M., Saleem, A., Carmichael, C., Davenport, P. W., Hoffman-Ruddy, B., & Okun, M. S. (2006). Tutorial on maximum inspiratory and expiratory mouth pressures in individuals with idiopathic Parkinson disease (IPD) and the preliminary results of an expiratory muscle strength training program. *NeuroRehabilitation*, *21*(1), 71–79.

Simons, A., & Hamdy, S. (2017). The use of brain stimulation in dysphagia management. *Dysphagia*, *32*(2), 209–215.

Sinha, U. K., James, A., & Hasan, M. (2001). Audit of percutaneous endoscopic gastrostomy (PEG): A questionnaire survey of hospital consultants. *Archives of Gerontology and Geriatrics*, *32*(2), 113–118.

Sjögren, P., Nilsson, E., Forsell, M., Johansson, O., & Hoogstraate, J. (2008). A systematic review of the preventative effect of oral hygiene on pneumonia and respiratory tract infection in elderly people in hospitals and nursing homes: Effect estimates and methodological quality of randomized control trials. *Journal of the American Geriatrics Society, 56*(11), 2124–2130.

Skolnick, M. L., Zagzebski, J. A., & Watkin, K. L. (1975). Two dimensional ultrasonic demonstration of lateral pharyngeal wall movement in real time—a preliminary report. *The Cleft Palate Journal, 12*, 299–303.

Slack, J. P. (2016). Molecular pharmacology of chemesthesis. In F. Zufall & S. D. Munger (Eds.), *Chemosensory transduction* (pp. 375–391). London, UK: Elsevier.

Smeltzer, S. C., Lavietes, M. H., & Cook, S. D. (1996). Expiratory training in multiple sclerosis. *Archives of Physical Medicine and Rehabilitation*, 77(9), 909–912.

Smith, D. F., Ott, D. J., Gelfand, D. W., & Chen, M. Y. (1998). Lower esophageal mucosal ring: Correlation of referred symptoms with radiographic findings using a marshmallow bolus. *AJR American Journal of Roentgenology, 171*(5), 1361–1365.

Smith, E. E., Kent, D. M., Bulsara, K. R., Leung, L. Y., Lichtman, J. H., Reeves, M. J., . . . Zahuranec, D. B. (2018). Effect of dysphagia screening strategies on clinical outcomes after stroke: A systematic review for the 2018 guidelines for the early management of patients with acute ischemic stroke. *Stroke, 49*(3), e123–e128.

Smithard, D. G., O'Neill, P. A., England, R. E., Park, C. L., Wyatt, R., Martin, D. F., & Morris, J. (1997). The natural history of dysphagia following a stroke. *Dysphagia, 12*(4), 188–193.

Smithard, D. G., O'Neill, P. A., Park, C., England, R., Renwick, D. S., Wyatt, R., . . . Martin, D. F. (1998). Can bedside assessment reliably exclude aspiration following acute stroke? *Age and Ageing, 27*(2), 99–106.

Smith Hammond, C. A., Goldstein, L. B., Horner, R. D., Ying, J., Gray, L., Gonzalez-Rothi, L., & Bolser, D. C. (2009). Predicting aspiration in patients with ischemic stroke. *Chest, 135*(3), 769–777.

Smith Hammond, C. A., Goldstein, L. B., Zajac, D. J., Gray, L., Davenport, P. W., & Bolser, D. C. (2001). Assessment of aspiration risk in stroke patients with quantification of voluntary cough. *Neurology, 56*(4), 502–506.

Solomon, N. P., Clark, H. M., Makashay, M. J., & Newman, L. A. (2008). Assessment of orofacial strength in patients with dysarthria. *Journal of Medical Speech-Language Pathology, 16*(4), 251–258.

Sörös, P., Lalone, E., Smith, R., Stevens, B., Theurer, J., Menon, R. S., & Martin, R. E. (2008). Functional MRI of oropharyngeal air-pulse stimulation. *Neuroscience, 153*(4), 1300–1308.

Steele, C. M. (2002). Emergency room assessment and intervention for dysphagia: A pilot project. *Journal of Speech-Language Pathology and Audiology, 26*(2), 100–110.

Steele, C. M. (2017). *Mapping Bracco's Varibar® barium products to the IDDSI framework.* Retrieved from http://iddsi.org/wp-content/uploads/2017/07/Mapping-Varibar_Short-version-1.pdf

Steele, C. M., Bailey, G. L., Polacco, R. E. C., Hori, S. F., Molfenter, S. M., Oshalla, M., & Yeates, E. M. (2013). Outcomes of tongue-pressure strength and accuracy training for dysphagia following acquired brain injury. *International Journal of Speech-Language Pathology, 15*(5), 492–502.

Steele, C. M., Bayley, M. T., Peladeau-Pigeon, M., Nagy, A., Namasivayam, A. M., Stokely, S. L., & Wolkin, T. (2016). A randomized trial comparing two tongue-pressure resistance training protocols for post-stroke dysphagia. *Dysphagia, 31*(3), 452–461.

Steele, C. M., & Huckabee, M. L. (2007). The influence of orolingual pressure on the timing of pharyngeal pressure events. *Dysphagia, 22*(1), 30–36.

Steele, C. M., & Miller, A. J. (2010). Sensory input pathways and mechanisms in swallowing: A review. *Dysphagia, 25*(4), 323–333.

Steele, C. M., Molfenter, S. M., Péladeau-Pigeon, M., & Stokely, S. (2013). Challenges in preparing contrast media for videofluoroscopy. *Dysphagia, 28*(3), 464–467.

Steele, C. M., Namasivayam-MacDonald, A. M., Guida, B. T., Cichero, J. A. Y., Duivestein, J., Hanson, B., . . . Riquelme, L. F. (2018). Creation and initial validation of the International Dysphagia Diet Standardisation Initiative Functional Diet Scale. *Archives of Physical Medicine and Rehabilitation, 99*(5), 934–944.

Steele, C. M., Thrasher, A. T., & Popovic, M. R. (2007). Electric stimulation approaches to the restoration and rehabilitation of swallowing: A review. *Neurological Research, 29*(1), 9–15.

Steele, C. M., van Lieshout, P. H. H. M., & Pelletier, C. A. (2012). The influence of stimulus taste and chemesthesis on tongue movement timing in swallowing. *Journal of Speech, Language, and Hearing Research, 55*(1), 262–275.

Steinhagen, V., Grossmann, A., Benecke, R., & Walter, U. (2009). Swallowing disturbance pattern relates to brain lesion location in acute stroke patients. *Stroke, 40*(5), 1903–1906.

Stephen, J. R., Taves, D. H., Smith, R. C., & Martin, R. E. (2005). Bolus location at the initiation of the pharyngeal stage of swallowing in healthy older adults. *Dysphagia, 20*(4), 266–272.

Stepp, C. E., Britton, D., Chang, C., Merati, A. L., & Matsuoka, Y. (2011, April). Feasibility of game-based electromyographic biofeedback for dysphagia rehabilitation. In *Neural Engineering (NER), 5th International IEEE/EMBS Conference* (pp. 233–236).

Sterr, A., Elbert, T., Berthold, I., Kolbel, S., Rockstroh, B., & Taub, E. (2002). Longer versus shorter daily constraint-induced movement therapy of chronic hemiparesis: An exploratory study. *Archives of Physical Medicine and Rehabilitation, 83*(10), 1374–1377.

Stevens, D. (1978). Ultrasound swallow. *British Medical Journal, 2*(6154), 1789–1790.

Stevenson, R. D., & Allaire, J. H. (1991). The development of normal feeding and swallowing. *Pediatric Clinics of North America, 38*(6), 1439–1453.

Stierwalt, J. A. G., & Youmans, S. R. (2007). Tongue measures in individuals with normal and impaired swallowing. *American Journal of Speech-Language Pathology, 16*(2), 148–156.

St.-John, W. M., & Paton, J. F. R. (2004). Role of pontile mechanisms in the neurogenesis of eupnea. *Respiratory Physiology & Neurobiology, 143*(2–3), 321–332.

Stoeckli, S. J., Huisman, T. A., Seifert, B., & Martin-Harris, B. J. (2003). Inter-rater reliability of videofluoroscopic swallow evaluation. *Dysphagia, 18*(1), 53–57.

Stone, M. (2005). A guide to analysing tongue motion from ultrasound images. *Clinical Linguistics & Phonetics, 19*(6-7), 455–501.

Streckfus, C. F. (1995). Salivary function and hypertension: A review of the literature and a case report. *Journal of the American Dental Association, 126*(7), 1012–1017.

Streiner, D. L. (2003). Diagnosing tests: Using and misusing diagnostic and screening tests. *Journal of Personality Assessment, 81*(3), 209–219.

Strub, R. L., & Black, F. W. (2000). *The mental status examination in neurology* (4th ed.). Philadelphia, PA: F. A. Davis.

Suiter, D. M., Sloggy, J., & Leder, S. B. (2014). Validation of the Yale Swallow Protocol: A prospective double-blind videofluoroscopic study. *Dysphagia, 29*(2), 199–203.

Suiter, D. M., & Leder, S. B. (2008). Clinical utility of the 3-ounce water swallow test. *Dysphagia, 23*(3), 244–250.

Suiter, D. M., Leder, S. B., & Ruark, J. L. (2006). Effects of neuromuscular electrical stimulation on submental muscle activity. *Dysphagia, 21*(1), 56–60.

Sumi, T. (1969). Some properties of cortically-evoked swallowing and chewing in rabbits. *Brain Research, 15*(1), 107–120.

Sumi, T. (1972). Reticular ascending activation of frontal cortical neurons in rabbits, with special reference to the regulation of deglutition. *Brain Research, 46*, 43–54.

Sumi, Y., Miura, H., Sunakawa, M., Michiwaki, Y., & Sakagami, N. (2002). Colonization of denture plaque by respiratory pathogens in dependent elderly. *Gerodontology, 19*(1), 25–29.

Suntrup, S., Kemling, A., Warnecke, T., Hamacher, C., Oelenberg, S., Niederstadt, T., . . . Dziewas, R. (2015). The impact of lesion location on dysphagia incidence, pattern and complications in acute stroke. Part 1: Dysphagia incidence, severity and aspiration. *European Journal of Neurology, 22*(5), 832–838.

Suntrup, S., Marian, T., Schröder, J., Suttrup, I., Muhle, P., Oelenberg, S., . . . Dziewas, R. (2015). Electrical pharyngeal stimulation for dysphagia treatment in tracheotomized stroke patients: A randomized controlled trial. *Intensive Care Medicine, 41*(9), 1629–1637.

Suntrup, S., Teismann, I., Wollbrink, A., Winkels, M., Warnecke, T., Flöel, A., . . . Dziewas, R. (2013). Magnetoencephalographic evidence for the modulation of cortical swallowing processing by transcranial direct current stimulation. *NeuroImage, 83*, 346–354.

Suntrup-Krueger, S., Kemling, A., Warnecke, T., Hamacher, C., Oelenberg, S., Niederstadt, T., . . . Dziewas, R. (2017). The impact of lesion location on dysphagia incidence, pattern and complications in acute stroke. Part 2: Oropharyngeal residue, swallow and cough response, and pneumonia. *European Journal of Neurology, 24*(6), 867–874.

Svensson, P., Romaniello, A., Arendt-Nielsen, L., & Sessle, B. J. (2003). Plasticity in corticomotor control of the human tongue musculature induced by tongue-task training. *Experimental Brain Research, 152*(1), 42–51.

Svensson, P., Romaniello, A., Wang, K., Arendt-Nielsen, L., & Sessle, B. J. (2006). One hour of tongue-task training is associated with plasticity in corticomotor control of the human tongue musculature. *Experimental Brain Research, 173*(1), 165–173.

Swan, K., Speyer, R., Heijnen, B. J., Wagg, B., & Cordier, R. (2015). Living with oropharyngeal dysphagia: Effects of bolus modification on health-related quality of life—a systematic review. *Quality of Life Research, 24*(10), 2447–2456.

Szczesniak, M., Rommel, N., Dinning, P., Fuentealba, S., Cook, I., & Omari, T. (2008). Optimal criteria for detecting bolus passage across the pharyngo-oesophageal segment during the normal swallow using intraluminal impedance recording. *Neurogastroenterology and Motility, 20*(5), 440–447.

Szczesniak, M., Rommel, N., Dinning, P., Fuentealba, S., Cook, I., & Omari, T. (2009) Intraluminal impedance detects failure of pharyngeal bolus clearance during swallowing: A validation study in adults with dysphagia. *Neurogastroenterology and Motility, 21*(3), 244–252.

Sze, W. P., Yoon, W. L., Escoffier, N., & Liow, S. J. R. (2016). Evaluating the training effects of two swallowing rehabilitation therapies using surface electromyography—chin tuck against resistance (CTAR) exercise and the Shaker exercise. *Dysphagia, 31*(2), 195–205.

Takahashi, K., Groher, M. E., & Michi, K. (1994). Methodology for detecting swallowing sounds. *Dysphagia, 9*(1), 54–62.

Takasaki, K., Umeki, H., Enatsu, K., Tanaka, F., Sakihama, N., Kumagami, H., & Takahashi, H. (2008). Investigation of pharyngeal swallowing function using high-resolution manometry. *Laryngoscope, 118*(10), 1729–1732.

Takasaki, K., Umeki, H., Hara, M., Kumagami, H., & Takahashi, H. (2011). Influence of effortful swallow on pharyngeal pressure: Evaluation using a high-resolution manometry. *Otolaryngology–Head and Neck Surgery, 144*(1), 16–20.

Takeuchi, N., & Izumi, S. I. (2012). Maladaptive plasticity for motor recovery after stroke: Mechanisms and approaches. *Neural Plasticity*, article ID 359728. http://doi.org/10.1155/2012/359728

Tan, C., Liu, Y., Li, W., Liu, J., & Chen, L. (2013). Transcutaneous neuromuscular electrical stimulation can improve swallowing function in patients with dysphagia caused by non-stroke diseases: A meta-analysis. *Journal of Oral Rehabilitation*, *40*(6), 472–480.

Taniguchi, H., Matsuo, K., Okazaki, H., Yoda, M., Inokuchi, H., Gonzalez-Fernandez, M., . . . Palmer, J. B. (2013). Fluoroscopic evaluation of tongue and jaw movements during mastication in healthy humans. *Dysphagia*, *28*(3), 419–427.

Teasell, R., Foley, N., Fisher, J., & Finestone, H. (2002). The incidence, management, and complications of dysphagia in patients with medullary strokes admitted to a rehabilitation unit. *Dysphagia*, *17*(2), 115–120.

Teismann, I. K., Steinstraeter, O., Stoeckigt, K., Suntrup, S., Wollbrink, A., Pantev, C., & Dziewas, R. (2007). Functional oropharyngeal sensory disruption interferes with the cortical control of swallowing. *BMC Neuroscience*, *8*, 62. http://doi.org/10.1186/1471-2202-8-62

Terpenning, M., Taylor, G. W., Lopatin, D., Kerr, C., Dominguez, B., & Loesche, W. (2001). Aspiration pneumonia: Dental and oral risk factors in an older veteran population. *Journal of the American Geriatrics Society*, *49*(5), 557–563.

Theurer, J. A., Bihari, F., Barr, A. M., & Martin, R. E. (2005). Oropharyngeal stimulation with air-pulse trains increases swallowing frequency in healthy adults. *Dysphagia*, *20*(4), 254–260.

Theurer, J. A., Czachorowski, K. A., Martin, L. P., & Martin, R. E. (2009). Effects of oropharyngeal air-pulse stimulation on swallowing in healthy older adults. *Dysphagia*, *24*, 302–313.

Theurer, J. A., Johnston, J. L., Taves, D. H., Bach, D., Hachinski, V., & Martin, R. E. (2008). Swallowing after right hemisphere stroke: Oral versus pharyngeal deficits. *Canadian Journal of Speech-Language Pathology and Audiology*, *32*(3), 114–122.

Toogood, J. A., Barr, A. M., Stevens, T. K., Gati, J. S., Menon, R. S., & Martin, R. E. (2005). Discrete functional contributions of cerebral cortical foci in voluntary swallowing: A functional magnetic resonance imaging (fMRI) "Go, No-Go" study. *Experimental Brain Research*, *161*(1), 81–90.

Tracy, J. F., Logemann, J. A., Kahrilas, P. J., Jacob, P., Kobara, M., & Krugler, C. (1989). Preliminary observations on the effects of age on oropharyngeal deglutition. *Dysphagia*, *4*(2), 90–94.

Trapl, M., Enderle, P., Nowotny, M., Teuschel, Y., Matz, K., Dachenhausen, A., & Brainin, M. (2007). Dysphagia bedside screening for acute-stroke patients. The Gugging Swallowing Screen. *Stroke*, *38*(11), 2948–2952.

Troche, M. S., Okun, M. S., Rosenbek, J. C., Musson, N., Fernandez, H. H., Rodriguez, R., . . . Sapienza, C. M. (2010). Aspiration and swallowing in Parkinson disease and rehabilitation with EMST: A randomized trial. *Neurology*, *75*(21), 1912–1919.

Troche, M. S., Schumann, B., Brandimore, A. E., Okun, M. S. & Hegland, K. W. (2016). Reflex cough and disease duration as predictors of swallowing dysfunction in Parkinson's disease. *Dysphagia*, *31*(6), 757–764.

Tsuga, K., Maruyama, M., Yoshikawa, M., Yoshida, M., & Akagawa, Y. (2011). Manometric evaluation of oral function with a hand-held balloon probe. *Journal of Oral Rehabilitation, 38*(9), 680–685.

Tsukamoto, Y. (2000). CT study of closure of the hemipharynx with head rotation in a case of lateral medullary syndrome. *Dysphagia, 15*(1), 17–18.

Turkington, L., Nund, R. L., Ward, E. C., & Farrell, A. (2017). Exploring current sensory enhancement practices with videofluoroscopic swallow study (VFSS) clinics. *Dysphagia, 32*(2), 225–235.

Turkington, L. G., Ward, E. C., & Farrell, A. M. (2017). Carbonation as a sensory enhancement strategy: A narrative synthesis of existing evidence. *Disability and Rehabilitation, 39*(19), 1958–1967.

Ushioda, T., Watanabe, Y., Sanjo, Y., Yamane, G., Abe, S., Tsuji, Y., & Ishiyama, A. (2012). Visual and auditory stimuli associated with swallowing activate mirror neurons: A magnetoencephalography study. *Dysphagia, 27*(4), 504–513.

van der Maarel-Wierink, C. D., Vanobbergen, J. N., Bronkhorst, E. M., Schols, J. M., & de Baat, C. (2013). Oral health care and aspiration pneumonia in frail older people: A systematic literature review. *Gerodontology, 30*(1), 3–9.

Vanderwegen, J., Guns, C., Van Nuffelen, G., Elen, R., & De Bodt, M. (2013). The influence of age, sex, bulb position, visual feedback, and the order of testing on maximum anterior and posterior tongue strength and endurance in healthy Belgian adults. *Dysphagia, 28*(2), 159–166.

van Herwaarden, M. A., Katz, P. O., Gideon, R. M., Barrett, J., Castell, J. A., Achem, S., & Castell, D. O. (2003). Are manometric parameters of the upper esophageal sphincter and pharynx affected by age and gender? *Dysphagia, 18*(3), 211–217.

Van Riper, C. (1954). *Speech correction: Principles and methods* (3rd ed.). Englewood Cliffs, NJ: Prentice-Hall.

van Wijk, M. P., Sifrim, D., Rommel, N., Benninga, M. A., Davidson, G. P., & Omari, T. I. (2009). Characterization of intraluminal impedance patterns associated with gas reflux in healthy volunteers. *Neurogastroenterology & Motility, 21*(8), e25–e55.

Vasant, D. H., Michou, E., O'Leary, N., Vail, A., Mistry, S., Hamdy, S., & Greater Manchester Stroke Research Network. (2016). Pharyngeal electrical stimulation in dysphagia poststroke: A prospective, randomized single-blinded interventional study. *Neurorehabilitation and Neural Repair, 30*(9), 866–875.

Vasant, D. H., Mistry, S., Michou, E., Jefferson, S., Rothwell, J. C., & Hamdy, S. (2014). Transcranial direct current stimulation reverses neurophysiological and behavioural effects of focal inhibition of human pharyngeal motor cortex on swallowing. *Journal of Physiology, 592*(4), 695–709.

Veis, S. L., & Logemann, J. A. (1985). Swallowing disorders in persons with cerebrovascular accident. *Archives of Physical Medicine and Rehabilitation, 66*(6), 372–375.

Vilardell, N., Rofes, L., Arreola, V., Speyer, R., & Clavé, P. (2016). A comparative study between modified starch and xanthan gum thickeners in post-stroke oropharyngeal dysphagia. *Dysphagia, 31*(2), 169–179.

Wakasugi, Y., Tohara, H., Hattori, F., Motohashi, Y., Nakane, A., Goto, S., . . . Uematsu, H. (2008). Screening test for silent aspiration at the bedside. *Dysphagia, 23*(4), 364–370.

Walczak, C. C., Jones, C. A., & McCulloch, T. M. (2017). Pharyngeal pressure and timing during bolus transit. *Dysphagia, 32*(1), 104–114.

Wallace, K. G., Middleton, S., & Cook, I. J. (2000). Development and validation of a self-report symptom inventory to assess the severity of oral-pharyngeal dysphagia. *Gastroenterology, 118*(4), 678–687.

Walters, D. N., Battle, J. W., Portera, C. A., Blizzard, J. D., & Browder, I. W. (1998). Zenker's diverticulum in the elderly: A neurologic etiology? *The American Surgeon, 64*(9), 909–911.

Wang, T. G., Wu, M. C., Chang, Y. C., Hsiao, T. Y., & Lien, I. N. (2006). The effect of nasogastric tubes on swallowing function in persons with dysphagia following stroke. *Archives of Physical Medicine and Rehabilitation, 87*(9), 1270–1273.

Warnecke, T., Ritter, M. A., Kröger, B., Oelenberg, S., Teismann, I., Heuschmann, P. U., . . . Dziewas, R. (2009). Fiberoptic endoscopic dysphagia severity scale predicts outcome after acute stroke. *Cerebrovascular Diseases, 28*(3), 283–289.

Warnecke, T., Teismann, I., Oelenberg, S., Hamacher, C., Ringelstein, E. B., Schäbitz, W. R., & Dziewas, R. (2009a). The safety of fiberoptic endoscopic evaluation of swallowing in acute stroke patients. *Stroke, 40*(2), 482–486.

Warnecke, T., Teismann, I., Oelenberg, S., Hamacher, C., Ringelstein, E. B., Schäbitz, W. R., & Dziewas, R. (2009b). Towards a basic endoscopic evaluation of swallowing in acute stroke–Identification of salient findings by the inexperienced examiner. *BMC Medical Education, 9*(1), 13. https://doi.org/10.1186/1472-6920-9–13

Warner, H. L., Suiter, D. M., Nystrom, K. V., Poskus, K., & Leder, S. B. (2014). Comparing accuracy of the Yale Swallow Protocol when administered by registered nurses and speech-language pathologists. *Journal of Clinical Nursing, 23*(13–14), 1908–1914.

Wassermann, E. M. (1998). Risk and safety of repetitive transcranial magnetic stimulation: Report and suggested guidelines from the International Workshop on the Safety of Repetitive Transcranial Magnetic Stimulation. *Electroencephalography and Clinical Neurophysiology, 108*(1), 1–16.

Watando, A., Ebihara, S., Ebihara, T., Okazaki, T., Takahashi, H., Asada, M., & Sasaki, H. (2004). Daily oral care and cough reflex sensitivity in elderly nursing home patients. *Chest, 126*(4), 1066–1070.

Watkin, K. L., Diouf, I., Gallagher, T. M., Logemann, J. A., Rademaker, A. W., & Ettema, S. L. (2001). Ultrasonic quantification of geniohyoid cross-sectional area and tissue composition: A preliminary study of age and radiation effects. *Head & Neck, 23*(6), 467–474.

Wei, X., Yu, F., Dai, M., Xie, C., Wan, G., Wang, Y., & Dou, Z. (2017). Change in excitability of cortical projection after modified catheter balloon dilatation therapy in brainstem stroke patients with dysphagia: A prospective controlled study. *Dysphagia, 32*(5), 645–656.

Welch, M. V., Logemann, J. A., Rademaker, A. W., & Kahrilas, P. J. (1993). Changes in pharyngeal dimensions effected by chin tuck. *Archives of Physical Medicine and Rehabilitation*, *74*(2), 178–181.

Wheeler, K. M., Chiara, T., & Sapienza, C. M. (2007). Surface electromyographic activity of the submental muscles during swallow and expiratory pressure threshold training tasks. *Dysphagia*, *22*(2), 108–116.

Wheeler-Hegland, K. M., Rosenbek, J. C., & Sapienza, C. M. (2008). Submental sEMG and hyoid movement during Mendelsohn maneuver, effortful swallow, and expiratory muscle strength training. *Journal of Speech, Language, and Hearing Research*, *51*(5), 1072–1087.

Whiting, P., Rutjes, A. W. S., Reitsma, J. B., Bossuyt, P. M., & Kleijnen, J. (2003). The development of QUADAS: A tool for the quality assessment of studies of diagnostic accuracy included in systematic reviews. *BMC Medical Research Methodology*, *3*(25). https://doi.org/10.1186/1471-2288-3-25

Whiting, P. F., Rutjes, A. W. S., Westwood, M. E., Mallett, S., Deeks, J. J. Reitsma, J. B., . . . Bossuyt, P. M. M. (2011). QUADAS-2: A revised tool for the quality assessment of diagnostic accuracy studies. *Annals of Internal Medicine*, *155*(8), 529–536.

Widdicombe, J. G. (1986). *Reflexes from the upper respiratory tract (Volume 2: Control of breathing, part 1)*. Bethesda, MD: American Physiological Association.

Widdicombe, J. G., Addington, W. R., Fontana, G. A., & Stephens, R. E. (2011). Voluntary and reflex cough and the expiration reflex; implications for aspiration after stroke. *Pulmonary Pharmacology & Therapeutics*, *24*(3), 312–317.

Wilcox, F., Liss, J. M., & Siegel, G. M. (1996). Interjudge agreement in videofluoroscopic studies of swallowing. *Journal of Speech and Hearing Research*, *39*(1), 144–152.

Williams, R. B., Pal, A., Brasseur, J. G., & Cook, I. J. (2001). Space-time pressure structure of pharyngo-esophageal segment during swallowing. *American Journal of Physiology-Gastrointestinal and Liver Physiology*, *281*(5), G1290–G1300.

Wilmskoetter, J., Martin-Harris, B., Pearson, W. G., Bonilha, L., Elm, J. J., Horn, J., & Bonilha, H. S. (2018). Differences in swallow physiology in patients with left and right hemispheric strokes. *Physiology & Behavior*, *194*, 144–152.

Wilmskoetter, J., Simpson, A., Logan, S., Simpson, K., & Bonilha, H. (2018). Impact of gastrostomy feeding tube placement on the 1-year trajectory of care in patients after stroke. *Nutrition in Clinical Practice*, *33*(4), 553–566.

Wilmskoetter, J., Simpson, A., Simpson, K., & Bonilha, H. (2016). Practice patterns of percutaneous endoscopic gastrostomy tube placement in acute stroke: Are the guidelines achievable? *Journal of Stroke and Cerebrovascular Diseases*, *25*(11), 2694–2700.

Wilmskoetter, J., Simpson, K., & Bonilha, H. (2016). Hospital readmissions of stroke patients with percutaneous endoscopic gastrostomy feeding tubes. *Journal of Stroke and Cerebrovascular Diseases*, *25*(10), 2535–2542.

Wilson, M. (2005). *Microbial inhabitants of humans.* Cambridge, UK: Cambridge University Press.

Wilson, R. D. (2012). Mortality and cost of pneumonia after stroke for different risk groups. *Journal of Stroke and Cerebrovascular Diseases, 21*(1), 61–67.

Wilson, R. D., & Howe, E. C. (2012). A cost-effectiveness analysis of screening methods for dysphagia after stroke. *Physical Medicine & Rehabilitation, 4*(4), 273–782.

Wise, S. P., & Strick, R. L. (1984). Anatomical and physiological organization of the non-primary motor cortex. *Trends in Neuroscience, 7*(11), 442–446.

Witte, U., Huckabee, M. L., Doeltgen, S. H., Gumbley, F., & Robb, M. (2008). The effect of effortful swallow on pharyngeal manometric measurements during saliva and water swallowing in healthy participants. *Archives of Physical Medicine and Rehabilitation, 89*(5), 822–828.

Wojner, A. W., & Alexandrov, A. V. (2000). Predictors of tube feeding in acute stroke patients with dysphagia. *AACN Clinical Issues, 11*(4), 531–540.

Wolf, S. L. (1994). Biofeedback. In J. A. Downey, S. J. Myers, E. G. Gonzales, & J. S. Lieberman (Eds.), *The physiological basis of rehabilitation medicine* (2nd ed., pp. 563–572). Stoneham, MA: Butterworth-Heinemann.

Wu, M. C., Chang, Y. C., Wang, T. G., & Lin, L. C. (2004). Evaluating swallowing dysfunction using a 100-ml water swallowing test. *Dysphagia, 19*(1), 43–47.

Yang, E. J., Baek, S. R., Shin, J., Lim, J. Y., Jang, H. J., Kim, Y. K., & Paik, N. J. (2012). Effects of transcranial direct current stimulation (tDCS) on post-stroke dysphagia. *Restorative Neurology and Neuroscience, 30*(4), 303–311.

Yang, S. N., Pyun, S. B., Kim, H. J., Ahn, H. S., & Rhyu, B. J. (2015). Effectiveness of non-invasive brain stimulation in dysphagia subsequent to stroke: A systemic review and meta-analysis. *Dysphagia, 30*(4), 383–391.

Yilmaz, E. Y., Gupta, S. R., Mlcoch, A. G., & Moritz, T. (1998). Aspiration following stroke. *Neurorehabilitation and Neural Repair, 12*(2), 61–64.

Yim, H. B., Kaushik, S. P., Lau, T. C., & Tan, C. C. (2000). An audit of percutaneous endoscopic gastrostomy in a general hospital in Singapore. *European Journal of Gastroenterology and Hepatology, 12*(2), 183–186.

Yoneyama, T., Yoshida, M., Ohrui, T., Mukaiyama, H., Okamoto, H., Hoshiba, K., . . . Sasaki, H. (2002). Oral care reduces pneumonia in older patients in nursing homes. *Journal of the American Geriatrics Society, 50*(3), 430–433.

Yoon, W. L., Khoo, J. K. P., & Liow, S. J. R. (2014). Chin tuck against resistance (CTAR): New method for enhancing suprahyoid muscle activity using a Shaker-type exercise. *Dysphagia, 29*(2), 243–248.

Yoshino, A., Ebihara, T., Ebihara, S., Fuji, H., & Sasaki, H. (2001). Daily oral care and risk factors for pneumonia among elderly nursing home patients. *Journal of the American Medical Association, 286*(18), 2233–2236.

Youmans, S. R., & Stierwalt, J. A. G. (2006). Measures of tongue function related to normal swallowing. *Dysphagia, 21*(2), 102–111.

Yuan, Y, Zhao, Y, Xie, T, & Hu, Y. (2016). Percutaneous endoscopic gastrostomy versus percutaneous radiological gastrostomy for swallowing disturbances. *Cochrane Database Systematic Review, 2*, CD009198.

Zaidi, N. H., Smith, H. A., King, S. C., Park, C., O'Neill, P. A., & Connolly, M. J. (1995). Oxygen desaturation on swallowing as a potential marker of aspiration in acute stroke. *Age and Ageing, 24*(4), 267–270.

Zald, D. H., & Pardo, J. V. (1999). The functional neuroanatomy of voluntary swallowing. *Annals of Neurology, 46*(3), 281–286.

Zenner, P. M., Losinski, D. S., & Mills, R. H. (1995). Using cervical auscultation in the clinical dysphagia examination in long-term care. *Dysphagia, 10*(1), 27–31.

Index

Note: Page numbers in **bold** reference non-text material.

B

C

E

I

K

L

M

P

Q

R

S

U

V

W

X

Y

Z